Memory, Aging and the Brain

Memory, Aging and the Brain brings together some of the best known experts in their fields to offer a cross-disciplinary summary of current research on human memory. More than this however, the book pays tribute to the work of Lars-Göran Nilsson and his many contributions to the psychology of human memory.

The book is divided into three subsections, which deal with general issues in human memory; memory and aging; and memory and the brain. These sections represent the three cornerstones in Lars-Göran's scientific career and comprise contributions from senior collaborators, colleagues and former students.

Areas of discussion include:

- long-term and working memory: how do they interact?
- an epidemiological approach to cognitive health in aging
- the cognitive neuroscience of signed language.

Covering a broad range of topics, this book will be of great interest to all those involved in the study and research of human memory.

Lars Bäckman is Professor at the Aging Research Center, Karolinska Institute, Stockholm, Sweden, as well as a member of the Royal Swedish Academy of Sciences and the European Academy of Sciences. His primary research area is cognition in normal and pathological aging, with special focus on memory. He was recently a recipient of the Humboldt Research Award.

Lars Nyberg is Professor of Neuroscience at Umeå University, Sweden, as well as a member of the Royal Swedish Academy of Sciences. His main area of research is cognitive neuroscience, with special focus on memory functions and he received the Göran Gustafsson Prize in Medicine in 2007 for his studies on brain functions.

Memory, Aging and the Brain

A Festschrift in Honour of Lars-Göran Nilsson

Edited by Lars Bäckman and Lars Nyberg

Psychology Press
Taylor & Francis Group
HOVE AND NEW YORK

First published 2010
by Psychology Press
27 Church Road, Hove, East Sussex BN3 2FA

Simultaneously published in the USA and Canada
by Psychology Press
711 Third Avenue, New York NY 10017

Psychology Press is an imprint of the Taylor & Francis Group, an Informa business

First issued in paperback 2012

Typeset in Times by RefineCatch Limited, Bungay, Suffolk

Cover design by Jim Wilkie

This publication has been produced with paper manufactured to strict environmental standards and with pulp derived from sustainable forests.

British Library Cataloguing in Publication Data
A catalogue record for this book is available from the British Library

Library of Congress Cataloging-in-Publication Data
Memory, aging and the brain : a festschrift in honor of Lars-Göran Nilsson / edited by Lars Bäckman & Lars Nyberg.
p. cm.
Includes index.
1. Memory. 2. Aging. 3. Brain. 4. Nilsson, Lars-Göran, 1944– I. Bäckman, Lars. II. Nyberg, Lars, 1966–
BF378.A33M46 2009
153.1′2–dc22

2009002259

ISBN: 978–1–84169–692–8 (hbk)

ISBN: 978–0–415–65008–3 (pbk)

Contents

Contributors

Lars Bäckman Karolinska Institutet, Aging Research Center, Gävlegatan 16, SE-113 30 Stockholm, Sweden

Alan Baddeley University of York, Department of Psychology, YO10 5DD, York, UK

Oliver Baumann The University of Queensland, Queensland Brain Institute, St Lucia, 4072 Queensland, Australia

Ellen Bialystok York University, Cognitive Development Laboratory, Behavioral Sciences Building, 234, 4700 Keele Street, Toronto, Ontario M3J 1P3

Matthias Brand University of Bielefeld, Department of Psychology, PO Box 1001 31, D-33501 Bielefeld, Germany

Fergus I. M. Craik Rotman Research Institute, Baycrest, 3560 Bathurst Street, 944, Toronto, Ontario, Canada M6A 2E1

Roger A. Dixon University of Alberta, Department of Psychology, P-217 Biological Sciences Building, Edmonton, Alberta, Canada T6G 2E9

Tor Endestad University of Oslo, Department of Psychology, Postboks 1094 Blindern, 0317 Oslo, Norway

Catharina Foo Linköping University, Department of Behavioral Sciences and Learning, 581 83 Linköping, Sweden

Mark W. Greenlee Universität Regensburg, Institut für Experimentelle Psychologie, 93040 Regensburg, Germany

Agneta Herlitz Karolinska Institutet, Aging Research Center, Gävlegatan 16, SE-113 30 Stockholm, Sweden

Kairi Kreegipuu University of Tartu, Institute for Psychology, EE 504 10, Tartu, Estonia

Johanna Lind University of Oslo, Department of Psychology, Postboks 1094 Blindern, 0317 Oslo, Norway

Martin Lövdén Lund University, Department of Psychology, Box 213, 221 00 Lund, Sweden

Johanna Lovén Karolinska Institutet, Aging Research Center, Gävlegatan 16, SE-113 30 Stockholm, Sweden

Svein Magnussen University of Oslo, Department of Psychology, Postboks 1094 Blindern, 0317 Oslo, Norway

Timo Mäntylä University of Umeå, Department of Psychology, 901 87 Umeå, Sweden

Hans J. Markowitsch University of Bielefeld, Department of Psychology, PO Box 1001 31, D-33501 Bielefeld, Germany

Risto Näätänen University of Tartu, Institute for Psychology, EE 504 10, Tartu, Estonia

Lars Nyberg University of Umeå, IMB/Physiology, 901 87 Umeå, Sweden

Arne Öhman Karolinska Institutet, Department of Clinical Neuroscience, Psychology Section, 171 76 Stockholm, Sweden

Jenny Rehnman Karolinska Institutet, Aging Research Center, Gävlegatan 16, SE-113 30 Stockholm, Sweden

Henry L. Roediger, III Washington University in St. Louis, Department of Psychology, One Brookings Drive, Campus Box 1125, St. Louis, MO 63130, USA

Jerker Rönnberg Linköping University, Linnaeus Centre HEAD (HEaring And Deafness), Swedish Institute for Disability Research, Department of Behavioral Sciences and Learning, 581 83 Linköping, Sweden

Mary Rudner Linköping University, Linnaeus Centre HEAD (HEaring And Deafness), Swedish Institute for Disability Research, Department of Behavioral Sciences and Learning, 581 83 Linköping, Sweden

Petra Thilers Karolinska Institutet, Aging Research Center, Gävlegatan 16, SE-113 30 Stockholm, Sweden

Endel Tulving Rotman Research Institute, Baycrest, 3560 Bathurst Street, 932, Toronto, Ontario, Canada M6A 2E1

Franklin M. Zaromb Washington University in St. Louis, Department of Psychology, One Brookings Drive, Campus Box 1125, St. Louis, MO 63130, USA

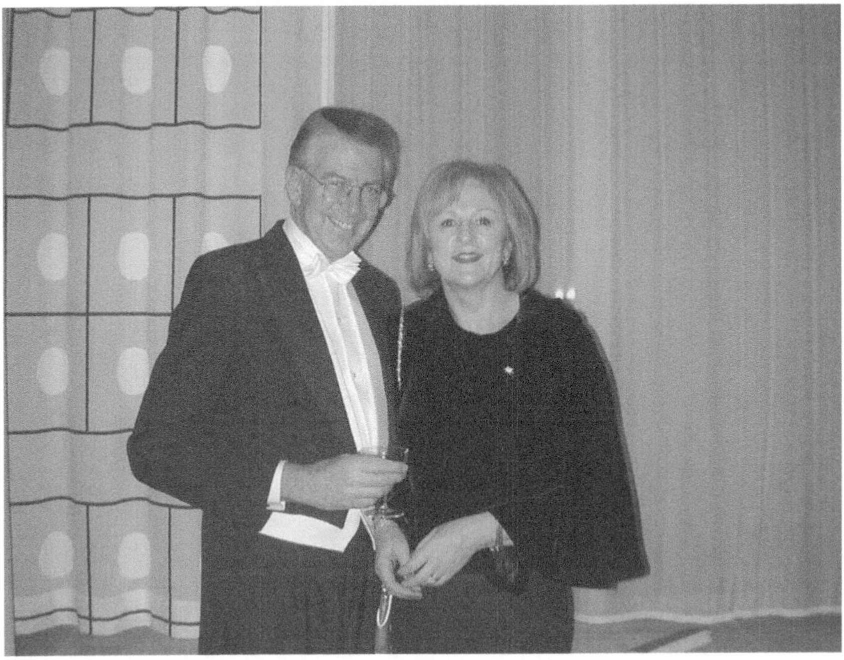

Lars-Göran Nilsson and Gun Nilsson at Umeå University's annual autumn ceremony, October 1999 (courtesy of Bo Molander).

1 Introduction

Lars Bäckman and Lars Nyberg

This volume is based on the proceedings from a conference arranged at Näsby Castle outside Stockholm in the fall of 2006. The purpose of the meeting was to honour the many contributions by Lars-Göran Nilsson to the psychology of human memory. The chapter authors constitute a mixture of senior collaborators and colleagues as well as former students of Lars-Göran from Sweden and abroad.

A son of a farmer, Lars-Göran was born in 1944 in the small village of Trönö in Hälsingland County in Northern Sweden. Although his family background was all but academic, the parents were highly supportive of their oldest son pursuing university studies (an attitude that was rather rare for that birth cohort in that part of Sweden!). Besides, the farm represented a basic security for Lars-Göran, something to fall back on if the academic ambitions were to fail.

A key influence in Lars-Göran's early professional development was the late Ronald Cohen. Not only did Ronald serve as supervisor for Lars-Göran's PhD thesis on motivation and memory at Uppsala University (Nilsson, 1973); he was also instrumental in establishing the long-standing relationship between Swedish and Canadian memory research. Ronald, then a professor at Glendon College in Toronto, invited Lars-Göran over from Sweden shortly after the defence of the dissertation. This invitation paved the way for regular contacts with members of the famous Ebbinghaus Empire in the psychology department at the University of Toronto, featuring persons such as Fergus Craik, Endel Tulving, Bennett Murdock, Norman Slamecka, Paul Kolers, and Robert Lockhart. The transatlantic interactions have been immense during the past 30 years, opening up possibilities for many Swedish students of memory.

Lars-Göran's international perspective on research also involves the European scene. He has had major functions in the European Society for Cognitive Psychology, including serving as Editor-in-Chief of its journal, as well as in the European Academy of Sciences. He has also collaborated actively over the years with a variety of top European memory scholars such as John Gardiner, Svein Magnussen, Hans Markowitsch, Cesare Cornoldi, and Ulman Lindenberger. Lars-Göran's international outlook is further evidenced by the fact that he served as President for the 27th International Congress of Psychology held in Stockholm in 2000.

As his former students, we would like to highlight an important aspect of Lars-Göran's legacy in addition to his scientific merits: His role as a mentor, a role model for new generations of memory researchers. A key feature in this regard is the setting of standards. This includes always being present at the office on Saturdays, as well as pushing beginning graduate students hard to submit their papers to the best possible peer-reviewed journals and attend international conferences. The latter demands deviated from traditional norms and have contributed greatly, we believe, to the professionalism of Swedish memory research. Finding the optimal balance between demand and support in interacting with students and junior colleagues is a unique talent that Lars-Göran possesses.

The theme of this book – memory, aging, and brain – represents three cornerstones in Lars-Göran's scientific activities over the past 35 years. His research in the 1970s primarily dealt with then-hot-topics in basic memory research, such as modality effects in free recall, organization in short-term memory, processing and storage operations, and output interference (e.g., Nilsson, 1974, 1976; Nilsson, Wright, & Murdock, 1975). However, there was an early interest in cognitive aging, as exemplified in Lars-Göran's work on the relative importance of encoding and retrieval factors in age-related memory deficits (Shaps & Nilsson, 1980). Although Lars-Göran's interest in basic memory research (e.g., action memory, cue utilization, the recall–recognition relationship) has remained over the years (e.g., Bäckman, Nilsson, & Chalom, 1986; Mäntylä & Nilsson, 1988; Nilsson, Law, & Tulving, 1988), the focus on aging was intensified in the late 1980s when he launched the highly influential Betula project, a large-scale longitudinal study on memory, health, and aging, the fifth wave of data collection for which is ongoing at this time (Nilsson, Adolfsson, Bäckman, Molander, & Nyberg, 2004; Nilsson et al., 1997).

Interest in the neural underpinnings of memory processes also commenced in the 1980s, notably in work on epilepsy (Nilsson et al., 1984), sensory handicaps (Rönnberg, Öhngren, & Nilsson, 1982), and amnesia (Christianson & Nilsson, 1984). This orientation benefited from the increased availability of neuroimaging techniques in the mid-1990s (e.g., Nyberg, McIntosh, Houle, Nilsson, & Tulving, 1996). A particularly salient example illustrating cross-fertilization between Lars-Göran's research foci is when the action-memory paradigm (a long-standing favourite) was fruitfully adapted in the scanner (Nilsson et al., 2000). A current example on the theme of cross-fertilization is the unique brain-imaging work in the Betula project, where the neural basis of age-related differences in memory operations is examined, profiting from the longitudinal nature of the study along with new developments in molecular genetics (Lind et al., 2006; Persson et al., 2006).

The weakening of traditional disciplinary divides illustrated by this example is also seen at the individual level among the current chapter authors, most of whom would easily fit into any of the three subsections of this volume: general issues in human memory; memory and aging; and memory and the brain. In many, if not most, cases, assigning a particular author to a particular section was indeed an arbitrary task. With this in mind, the introductory section covering general issues in human memory includes chapters by Baddeley; Roediger & Zaromb; Magnussen, Greenlee, Baumann, & Endestad; Mäntylä; and Tulving. The subsequent section, on memory and aging, features texts by Craik & Bialystok; Herlitz, Lovén, Thilers, & Rehnman; Dixon; Lövdén; and Bäckman & Nyberg. The final section, on memory and the brain, includes contributions by Öhman; Brand & Markowitsch; Rönnberg, Rudner, & Foo; Näätänen & Kreegipuu; and Lind & Nyberg.

We hope that the volume will convey some of the excitement we felt during the presentations and discussions at Näsby Castle, and that readers will appreciate this cross-disciplinary summary of current research on human memory.

The conference on which the book is based was supported by grants from the Swedish Council for Working Life and Social Research and from the Bank of Sweden Tercentenary Foundation.

References

Bäckman, L., Nilsson, L.-G., & Chalom, D. (1986). New evidence on the nature of the encoding of action events. *Memory & Cognition, 14*, 339–346.

Christianson, S.-Å., & Nilsson, L.-G. (1984). Functional amnesia as induced by a psychological trauma. *Memory & Cognition, 12*, 142–155.

Lind, J., Persson, J., Ingvar, M., Larson, A., Cruts, M., Van Broeckhoven, C., et al. (2006). Reduced functional brain activity in cognitively intact apolipoprotein E-ε4 carriers. *Brain, 129*, 1240–1248.

Mäntylä, T., & Nilsson, L.-G. (1988). Cue distinctiveness and forgetting: Effectiveness of self-generated retrieval cues in delayed recall. *Journal of Experimental Psychology: Learning, Memory, and Cognition, 14*, 502–509.

Nilsson, L.-G. (1973). *Memory processes and the concept of reinforcement*. Doctoral Dissertation, Uppsala University, Uppsala, Sweden.

Nilsson, L.-G. (1974). Further evidence for organization by modality in immediate free recall. *Journal of Experimental Psychology, 103*, 948–957.

Nilsson, L.-G. (1976). Roles of two types of outcome on storage and retrieval processes in memory. *Quarterly Journal of Experimental Psychology, 28*, 93–104.

Nilsson, L.-G., Adolfsson, R., Bäckman, L., Molander, B., & Nyberg, L. (2004). Betula: A prospective study on memory, health, and aging. *Aging, Neuropsychology, and Cognition, 11*, 134–148.

Nilsson, L.-G., Bäckman, L., Erngrund, K., Nyberg, L., Adolfsson, R., Bucht, G., et al. (1997). The Betula prospective cohort study: Memory, health, and aging. *Aging, Neuropsychology, and Cognition, 4*, 1–32.

Nilsson, L.-G., Christianson, S.-Å., Silfvenius, H., & Blom, S. (1984). Preoperative and postoperative memory testing of epileptic patients. *Acta Neurologica Scandinavica, 69*, 43–56.

Nilsson, L.-G., Law, J., & Tulving, E. (1988). Recognition failure of recallable unique names: Evidence for an empirical law of memory and learning. *Journal of Experimental Psychology: Learning, Memory, and Cognition*, *14*, 266–277.

Nilsson, L.-G., Nyberg, L., Klingberg, T., Åberg, C. S., Persson, J., & Roland, P. E. (2000). Activity in motor areas while remembering action events. *NeuroReport*, *11*, 2199–2201.

Nilsson, L.-G., Wright, E., & Murdock, B. B. (1975). Effects of visual presentation method on single-trial free recall. *Memory & Cognition*, *3*, 427–433.

Nyberg, L., McIntosh, A. R., Houle, S., Nilsson, L.-G., & Tulving, E. (1996). Activation of medial temporal structures during episodic memory retrieval. *Nature*, *380*, 715–717.

Persson, J., Nyberg, L., Lind, J., Larsson, A., Nilsson, L.-G., Ingvar, M., & Buckner, R. L. (2006). Structure-function correlates of cognitive decline in aging. *Cerebral Cortex*, *16*, 907–915.

Rönnberg, J., Öhngren, G., & Nilsson, L.-G. (1982). Hearing deficiency, speechreading, and memory functions. *Scandinavian Audiology*, *11*, 261–268.

Shaps, L. P., & Nilsson, L.-G. (1980). Encoding and retrieval operations in relation to age. *Developmental Psychology*, *16*, 636–643.

Part I

Memory

2 Long-term and working memory

How do they interact?

Alan Baddeley

I have known Lars-Göran Nilsson since we met at an Attention and Performance meeting in Stockholm many years ago. As a local, he proved a knowledgeable guide to the colourful nightlife that characterized Stockholm at the time. We have been friends ever since, and I was delighted to be invited to participate in his Festschrift. Despite being friends, we have never collaborated, my own principal interest being in working memory and Lars-Göran's in long-term memory. It seemed appropriate, therefore, that my contribution to this tribute should concern the interaction between long-term and working memory.

Working memory is assumed to be a system for the temporary storage and manipulation of the information involved in complex cognition; as such it could be regarded as a system that underpins our capacity for coherent sustained thought. As a growing area of study, it receives, from time to time, proposals that working memory should be incorporated within the more established areas of perception and/or long-term memory. Of these takeover bids, the least worrying is that from perception (e.g., Allport, 1984; Jones, Macken, & Nichols, 2004), which tends to be focused on a single component of working memory – namely, the phonological loop – and appears to have little to say about the crucial executive function of working memory (for a response to two of these proposals, see Baddeley & Larsen, 2007; Baddeley & Wilson, 1993).

A more serious alternative to the multicomponent model is presented by the proposal that working memory simply comprises the currently activated portion of long-term memory (LTM), the implication being that if we study LTM, then an understanding of working memory will be provided as a bonus. One version of this was spelled out in an influential article by Melton (1963), which observed that a range of experimental paradigms used to study short-term memory (STM) showed clear evidence of long-term influences, thereby obviating the need for a separate short-term system. In responding to this, Waugh and Norman (1965) pointed out the need to distinguish between experimental paradigms and the concepts that they were intended to investigate. A standard STM paradigm such as digit span does not provide a pure measure of the hypothetical system assumed to underpin performance, hence demonstrating that a long-term component does not invalidate the assumption of a further short-term system. Waugh and Norman (1965) proposed a distinction between STM, defined in terms of an experimental paradigm and the underlying memory systems, one of which, *secondary memory*, was regarded as equivalent to LTM, while *primary memory* was its short-term equivalent. A similar distinction was made by Atkinson and Shiffrin (1968), who distinguished between experimental paradigms, for which they maintained the labels STM and LTM, and the systems that were assumed to underpin them, a *short-term store* (STS) and a *long-term store* (LTS).

For many years this point appeared to have been accepted by the field, but recently the paradigm-concept confusion appears to have returned on the basis of neurobiological and neuroimaging data where the observation that many working memory tasks involve the activation of areas that also underpin LTM is sometimes claimed to obviate the need to assume a separate working memory (e.g., Ruchkin, Grafman, Cameron, & Berndt, 2003). Arguments against the idea of a separate working memory system have also begun to appear in more behaviourally based reviews, such as that of Nairne (2002). In this case, the argument is driven by the observation that a range of phenomena observed in STM tasks cannot be adequately explained by a simplified version of the phonological loop component of working memory, which is described as "the standard model" (Nairne, 2002). I entirely agree, hence the need for a multicomponent system (for a more detailed discussion, see Baddeley, 2007, chap. 3).

A somewhat different version of the activated LTM view is that of Cowan (2001, 2005). Superficially, his views and mine appear to be opposed, but in practice, I regard the differences as principally those of emphasis (Baddeley, 2001, 2007), with Cowan being particularly concerned with the important attentional aspect of working memory, rather than its subsidiary temporary storage systems, although his work has contributed substantially to both areas (Cowan, 1999, 2005). Our one substantial point of disagreement concerns the way in which long-term and working memory interact. I myself propose a separate component of working memory: the episodic buffer, which provides a multidimensional temporary store in which information can be registered and manipulated by the central executive. Cowan prefers to think of the information as remaining in LTM. However, in order to account for the capacity to manipulate such information and combine it in novel ways, he assumes a system that can hold the "addresses" of the locations in LTM. We neither of us can currently think of a way of separating these two but accept that this is an important area that requires further investigation.

So what is my objection to the activated LTM position? I do not think that it is wrong, but I regard it as unhelpful in appearing to provide a simple explanation to a complex question. Working memory does, I agree, involve activated LTM, but it does so in a range of different ways, some of which will be described briefly before going on to discuss recent attempts to further investigate just one of these forms of interaction. They can broadly be divided into two categories, one concerning the way in which working memory influences LTM, and the other the influence of LTM on working memory.

Control of LTM by working memory

Strategic control

Long-term learning is clearly influenced by strategy, which in turn typically depends on working memory (WM). A case in point is that of the use of visual imagery in mnemonics to enhance learning, in which the strategy is controlled by the central executive and temporary storage is provided by the visuospatial sketchpad (Baddeley, Grant, Wight, & Thomson, 1973; Baddeley & Lieberman, 1980).

Exploiting the recency effect

A marked feature of many memory tasks involving both LTM and STM is the enhanced recall of the most recently presented items or events. This ranges from recalling the last items from a list of 20 unrelated words or, indeed, proverbs (Glanzer, 1972) to recalling where you last parked your car (da Costa Pinto & Baddeley, 1991) or the rugby teams that you have played against (Baddeley & Hitch, 1993). The recency effect is regarded as resulting from the use of a powerful but limited strategy, applied to activated representations in any of a range of memory systems. This includes both long- and short-term systems as illustrated by patient PV, who has a phonological storage deficit and shows grossly impaired short-term recency, coupled with normal recency when material is retrieved from long-term storage (Vallar, Papagno, & Baddeley, 1991).

Short-term storage and long-term learning

Short-term storage and long-term learning occurs when temporary storage facilitates long-term learning, a good example being that of the phonological loop facilitating the acquisition of vocabulary. Patients such as PV who have defective phonological storage find it difficult to acquire new phonological forms, such as foreign-language vocabulary. Normal participants also appear to use the phonological loop to help in the acquisition of a second-language vocabulary. Acquisition is disrupted by variables such as articulatory suppression, phonological similarity, and word length that are known to impact on the phonological loop. Such factors have little impact on the capacity to learn pairs of unrelated but familiar words, a task that is known to rely principally upon semantic coding (for a review and discussion, see Baddeley, Gathercole, & Papagno, 1998).

The impact of LTM on working memory

Language habits and serial STM

My final example is one that has concerned my colleagues and I over recent years, and which I shall describe in more detail. Miller (1956) demonstrated that subjects are able to use the redundancy within a sequence of items to facilitate serial recall, an effect that occurs for letter and word sequences, in which recall improves as the sequence conforms more and more closely to the statistical structure of one's native language.

Miller, Bruner, and Postman (1954) reported a study in which they briefly presented sequences of letters that varied in their approximation to English, ranging from random letter strings through letters selected according to their frequency of individual letters or pairs of letters or trigrams, up to known English words. The strings were presented tachistoscopically and resulted in highly lawful results whereby performance was predicted by the information contained in the sequence, as measured by Shannon and Weaver's (1949) information theory. They interpreted their results in terms of a limit on perception, a view that I subsequently challenged by repeating their experiment but ensuring that exposure was long enough for the subject to read out each of the letters, hence demonstrating adequate perceptual performance. The results were clear, with retention increasing with order of approximation to English, showing exactly the same function as had been attributed by Miller et al. (1954) to perceptual limitations.

Our results are of course readily explained in terms of Miller's (1956) concept of chunking, whereby immediate memory span can be expanded by using long-term knowledge to combine lower level components such as letters into a smaller number of higher level chunks. Miller and Selfridge (1950) showed a similar clear relationship in the case of word sequences ranging from random to prose. An elegant study by Tulving and Patkau (1962) using such approximations to English prose showed that, whereas total number of words recalled increased as the word sequences became more redundant and prose-like, the number of chunks remained constant, while the average number of words per chunk increased.

This would not, of course, have surprised Miller (1956), so why is it worth our concern now? The reason is simple; it contains two problems of considerable general importance that still remain to be solved – namely, how serial order is stored and how chunks are formed. Before going on to discuss these issues, it would be useful to give a brief overview of the multicomponent model of working memory that underpins my own view of the field.

Working memory: The multicomponent model

In the 1950s the weight of opinion within experimental psychology favoured a unitary theory of memory comprising a single long-term memory system based on stimulus–response associations. In the late 1950s this was challenged by the demonstration of very rapid forgetting in the apparent absence of interference from similar items (Brown, 1958; Peterson & Peterson, 1959). As mentioned earlier, this view was in turn challenged by Melton (1963), who argued that there was no need to assume a separate short-term system as both interference and long-term effects were present in classic STM paradigms.

This challenge resulted in a search for more convincing empirical evidence. By the late 1960s the balance of evidence appeared to favour a dichotomous view of memory, of which the most influential version was the model developed by Atkinson and Shiffrin (1968), which proposed three types of memory. The first involved brief sensory memories, both auditory (echoic) and visual (iconic), which fed into a limited-capacity short-term store, which served as a working memory. The STS was assumed to be capable of manipulating information and was responsible for feeding information into a long-term store and, in due course, retrieving it from LTS. This was the most influential of several similar multistore models, and it came to be known as the modal model.

Although influential, this model began to encounter problems of two kinds. The first concerned its assumption that learning occurs automatically, with amount learned simply depending on time spent in the STS. This proved not to be the case and resulted in alternative formulations, notably Craik and Lockhart's (1972) Levels of Processing theory. This proposed that amount of learning was a function of depth of processing, with shallow visual processing leading to less learning than with deeper phonological encoding, which in turn was less effective than richer and deeper semantic coding.

A second problem encountered by the Atkinson and Shiffrin model concerned the nature of the STS. A major source of evidence for a dichotomy came from neuropsychological patients. Patients suffering from the classic amnesic syndrome appear to have grossly impaired LTS but preserved STS and, as such, fitted the modal model well (Baddeley & Warrington, 1970). A second type of patient showed the opposite pattern, with impaired digit span and very poor performance on the Peterson task, coupled with excellent LTM (Shallice & Warrington, 1970). Such patients tend to have a digit span of only one or two items, suggesting a grossly impaired STS, again fitting neatly into a multistore model. If that is the case, however, according to the modal model an impaired STS should result in major problems in long-term learning and, indeed, given the assumption that the STS acts as a working memory, ought to result in severe problems in cognition more generally. This was not the case; long-term memory appeared to be normal in such STM patients, who lived perfectly competent lives – one was a secretary, another a taxi driver, while a third ran a shop and a family.

This paradox led to a further investigation in which Baddeley and Hitch (1974) attempted to simulate such patients by using a dual-task methodology to impair the STS capacity of normal participants. This was achieved by requiring them to maintain sequences of digits at the same time as attempting to perform cognitively demanding tasks. These involved reasoning, comprehending, and learning. We assumed that, if the STS indeed acted as a working memory, then the longer the sequence maintained, the less the capacity remaining free, and the greater the decrement in concurrent task performance. All three tasks gave the same result – namely, a consistent decline of performance as digit load increased – but it was an effect that was very far from the catastrophic decline predicted by the modal model. In response to these results Baddeley and Hitch proposed to fractionate the STS, producing a three-component model of working memory; this was comprised of an attentional controller, the *central executive*, assisted by two subsidiary short-term storage systems, one for speech, the *phonological loop*, and the other for imagery, the *visuospatial sketchpad*.

In the years that followed, we explored this framework concentrating initially on the more tractable subsystems and treating the executive simply as a limited-capacity multipurpose system – in effect, a homunculus. As Attneave (1960) pointed out, however, homunculi can be useful as a way of identifying problems that are currently too difficult to solve. To continue to be useful, however, it is important that one analyses the role the homunculus must play, breaking this down into sub-tasks and gradually taking each one and explaining it until eventually all are accounted for, the executive is understood, and the homunculus can retire.

Our first attempt at this retirement plan came with the proposal that, rather than being an all-powerful multipurpose system, we should treat the homunculus as a purely attentional component. A further step was to decide what functions any central executive would need to perform, and what capacities these would require. Four were proposed (Baddeley, 1996), comprising the capacity to focus attention, to divide attention, to switch attention, and to interface with LTM. Some progress was made on the first three (see Baddeley, 2007, chap. 7), but the link to LTM proved more of a problem.

The problem was solved in part by the assumption of a two-way link between the phonological loop and long-term phonological memory. This was principally based on the previously described evidence for a link between the phonological loop and the acquisition of vocabulary, together with evidence that language habits could facilitate immediate serial recall (Baddeley, 1964; Miller et al., 1954). An equivalent link between the sketchpad and long-term visuospatial semantic memory was also proposed, although this issue is currently unexplored.

There remained, however, a whole range of phenomena that did not fit readily into the three-component model. One of these concerned the question of how the phonological and visuospatial systems could interact with each other given that they depended on different and presumably incompatible codes. The second issue comprised the abundant evidence for the importance of existing language structures in working memory. Immediate memory span for unrelated words is about 5 words, whereas memory for sentences tends to comprise 12 or more words, far more than could readily be held in the phonological loop. Given the abandonment of the idea that the executive has storage capacity, where were these maintained?

This issue was presented in a particularly acute form by the demonstration by Daneman and Carpenter (1980) of the predictive power of their working memory span measure. This involves presenting participants with a sequence of sentences, each of which they must process before going on to recall the last word of each. They found that this was an excellent predictor of language comprehension, a result that has been replicated many times (Daneman & Merikle, 1996) and extended to cover a very wide range of other cognitive skills, ranging from the acquisition of computer programming skills (Kyllonen & Stephens, 1990), to performance on standard intelligence tests (Kyllonen & Christal, 1990), and to the capacity to comprehend messages presented in noise (as described by Rönnberg, Rudner, & Foo in chapter 14, this volume). While the predictive capacity of working memory span did a great deal for the credibility of working memory as a practical tool, it was far from clear how such results could be accommodated within the existing model. Driven by these and a range of other findings, I opted to propose a fourth component of working memory: the episodic buffer.

The buffer was assumed to comprise a temporary store that utilizes a multidimensional coding system. This allows it to provide an interface between the subsystems of working memory, perception, and LTM. It is also assumed to be accessible through conscious awareness. In general, the model appears to have been well received, providing as it does a bridge between our multicomponent model, which tends to emphasize separable temporary storage systems, and a range of models that emphasize individual differences in attentional or executive processing (e.g., Cowan, 2005; Engle, 1996; Miyake & Shah, 1999). However, if it is to prove anything other than another homunculus, we clearly need to demonstrate that it is capable of generating tractable questions with relevant answers.

If we were to make any progress, we decided we needed to focus on a limited range of specific questions. We chose to study the role of the episodic buffer in binding information from multiple sources, a function that was central to its inception. We opted to study binding in two very different contexts, one of which was apparently simple and comprised the binding of colour to shape in visual STM. The other, presumably more complex, area concerned the binding that underpins the application of language habits to immediate serial verbal recall.

Redundancy and binding in verbal STM

Our basic approach was to compare the immediate recall of word sequences comprising a meaningful sentence with the recall of the equivalent words in scrambled order. Concurrent tasks were then used to disrupt the component processes of working memory. Our principal question was whether the advantage to be gained from the syntactic and semantic redundancy of the sentences would be reduced as concurrent executive load increased, suggesting an active role for working memory in binding words into chunks, or whether such binding operates automatically.

In our first series of studies, Jefferies, Lambon Ralph, and Baddeley (2004) used a paradigm in which subjects were required to remember a sequence of either short sentences or word strings (e.g., *The boy sold the goldfish; It was a cold and stormy winter* versus *Goldfish boy sold; winter stormy cold*). The first step was to establish immediate memory span for each type of material. This was clearly greater for sequences of sentences, even though successive sentences within each sequence were unrelated. Our first experiment involved sequences of sentences or lists that were 50% greater than span. Baseline performance was then compared to that achieved while carrying out an attentionally demanding secondary task. For this we chose a method that Craik and colleagues had found to have a robust impact on the capacity for learning – namely, a continuous four-choice reaction time task in which each of four keys was associated with one of four lights. When a light came on, the participant pressed the associated key, which immediately produced another stimulus (Craik, Govoni, Naveh-Benjamin, & Anderson, 1996). Finally, each set of sentences or scrambled words was presented and tested over three successive trials to evaluate the effect of the relevant variables on rate of long-term learning.

By varying number of sentences or lists, we were broadly successful in equating overall difficulty across both types of material. Our secondary task also succeeded in impairing performance, although the magnitude of the impairment was considerably less than we anticipated. However, the pattern of the concurrent task effect differed between the two types of material. In the case of the unrelated words, it was absent on Trial 1 and gradually built up over Trials 2 and 3, whereas the opposite pattern occurred for sentences. A second study that included rather longer sequences also broadly replicated this observation of a decline in the effect of concurrent load across trials for sentences, and the opposite for lists.

How should we explain this pattern? One hypothesis concerned the role of binding in determining performance. In the case of the unrelated words, participants on Trial 1 could have relied principally on the phonological loop, only later using semantic coding to bind sequences together into subjective units. Tulving (1962) has shown that a gradual development of clusters over successive learning trials characterizes the acquisition of lists of unrelated words. In the case of the sentences, internal redundancy should provide the necessary *within-sentence* binding, leaving only the need to provide a binding *between* the unrelated sentences. Much of this binding was presumably achieved on the first or second trial, resulting in a diminishing effect of concurrent disruption over trials.

We tested this hypothesis in a third experiment, again using scrambled words and unrelated sentences, but adding a third condition in which the sentences were thematically linked, as in normal prose, hence reducing the demand of between-sentence binding. If our hypothesis were correct, then we would expect this latter condition to show the least impact of our concurrent task. This proved to be the case. The pattern for word lists and for unrelated sentences was broadly equivalent to that obtained across the previous two studies, but, as predicted, the concurrent task had much less effect on the retention and learning of thematically related material.

What are the implications of our results for the episodic buffer model? They are certainly consistent with the assumption that the executive plays some role in binding, but the magnitude of the effect was small and, in the absence of concurrent tasks focusing specifically on the separate components of working memory, difficult to evaluate.

Our next set of studies (Baddeley, Hitch, & Allen, 2009) attempted to avoid these limitations. We chose to use sentences varying in length rather than sequences of related or unrelated sentences. This, however, leads to a methodological problem. Whereas memory span for unrelated words is 5 or 6, span for naturalistic sentences will typically range between 10 and 20 words, depending on the precise nature of the sentence. In order to circumvent this problem we devised a task we termed *constrained sentence span*. This involves repeatedly using a very limited set of nouns, verbs, adjectives, and adverbs. This means that items were continuously being re-paired, a process whereby we hoped that proactive interference would minimize the contribution of LTM and maximize the working memory contribution to inter-word binding. We were successful in reducing both span length and inter-sentence variability, allowing us to use sentences of broadly equivalent difficulty to the scrambled word lists while being only a few items longer, with sentences such as *The old pilot rapidly sold the green bicycle to the blonde lawyer* being approximately equivalent in difficulty to slightly shorter word lists such as *blonde bicycle lawyer old rapidly pilot*.

We carried out a series of experiments in which we systematically explored the influence of sentence-based redundancy on immediate recall, when each of three initial components of working memory was systematically disrupted (Baddeley et al., 2009). In one such study, we presented the sentences auditorily at the same time as requiring subjects to perform a visual or verbal *n*-back task. In the case of the verbal task, a sequence of digits was presented auditorily, and the participant was required either simply to repeat each as it appeared, disrupting the phonological loop, or to repeat the digit that had been presented two items before. This 2-back condition involves the simultaneous storage and manipulation of the digits, a task that depends on the central executive and loads heavily on the operation of the frontal lobes (Owen, McMillan, Laird, & Bullmore, 2005). The visuospatial *n*-back task involved presenting a sequence of 3 × 3 matrices. In each case, one cell was occupied by a dot. The subject was required to touch the occupied cell either immediately in the 0-back condition, or to touch the cell that had been occupied two items before in the 2-back task. Participants were required to recall verbally constrained sentences comprising 8 words, or sequences comprising

6 of the same items in scrambled order, under both baseline control conditions and when performing each of the four concurrent tasks.

We were successful in obtaining a modest but very robust enhancement in recall for our constrained sentences over that of our word lists. Second, our concurrent tasks behaved in an orderly manner. As expected, simple visuospatial suppression had little effect on verbal recall, while some disruption did occur with the 2-back version, which could be expected to place both visuospatial and executive demands on participants. A more substantial disruption occurred with the 0-back verbal task, the well-established effect of articulatory suppression on immediate verbal recall, while the greatest disruption occurred with the 2-back verbal task, which combined articulatory suppression with an executive processing demand.

Of crucial relevance for our hypothesis, however, was the question of whether any of these main effects of concurrent task on recall was accompanied by an interaction with type of sequence. We found no evidence of such an interaction between sequence type and concurrent task. The advantage gained from the sentential form therefore did not appear to depend on the availability of executive resources, although such resources were clearly and systematically involved in determining overall level of performance. In terms of our original hypothesis, these results suggest that the processes responsible for the sentential advantage for spoken sentences is automatic and does not depend on the central executive. The original version of the episodic buffer model hypothesized that binding within the buffer was dependent on the limited-capacity central executive. Were this the case, then disrupting the executive should reduce the sentence advantage. This clearly was not the case.

Our second experiment explored the generality of this finding by using visually presented sentences and lists. The procedure remained the same except that the words were presented visually one after the other. This was incompatible with performing the visual *n*-back task, and we therefore limited ourselves to the verbal concurrent tasks. Again, each of our major variables had a significant effect, but on this occasion we also obtained a significant interaction, such that suppression by digit repetition reduced the impact of sentence-based redundancy on recall, while the 2-back verbal task obliterated it. We were somewhat concerned that our result might simply reflect a floor effect, and the study was therefore repeated using a less demanding 1-back task with broadly equivalent results (Baddeley et al., 2009).

What are the implications of these two sets of experiments for our original hypothesis? First of all, they suggest that with auditory presentation, the contribution of language habits to sequential binding is virtually automatic, whereas this is not the case when the material is read in a word-by-word fashion, presumably a substantially less well practised method of presentation. The fact that such effects of redundancy are obtained robustly and regularly under more naturalistic auditory conditions suggests that we should consider amending our original episodic buffer model and providing direct links between the buffer and sketchpad and loop. This conclusion is broadly supported by a parallel set of studies investigating binding in visual working memory. These will be briefly summarized next.

Binding in visual working memory

A very welcome recent development in the study of working memory has been the increasing convergence of interest between those, like myself, who come from a short-term memory tradition and others whose background is in the study of visual attention. This has led to the development of a very fruitful paradigm focusing on the binding of features such as colour and shape into objects to be retained in visual working memory (Luck & Vogel, 1997; Vogel, Woodman, & Luck, 2001; Wheeler & Treisman, 2002). We chose to use this paradigm to study the influence of executive processes on visual binding as providing a possible contrast with the more complex question of binding in sentence processing. We have so far carried out a range of studies in which participants viewed an array of four coloured shapes and were subsequently probed for retention of colour irrespective of shape, for shape irrespective of colour, or for the binding of shape to colour (Allen, Baddeley, & Hitch, 2006). We accompanied this task by a range of secondary activities ranging from articulatory suppression to counting back in ones or threes, aimed at investigating the role of the phonological loop and central executive in this task.

As is characteristic of this paradigm, articulatory suppression had no impact on performance, suggesting that it is a purely visuospatial task. Our other secondary tasks did impair overall performance to a degree that was broadly commensurate with the probable attentional load involved. Crucially, however, there was no interaction between binding and these concurrent task effects. Our tasks had no greater impact on binding than on maintaining the individual unbound features. However, in a subsequent study in which the coloured shapes were presented and tested *sequentially*, there was evidence to suggest that, despite being acquired apparently automatically, binding between features was more subject to interference from subsequent items than was the retention of its constituent features. This is consistent with earlier work by Wheeler and Treisman (2002), who found binding between features to be vulnerable to the effects of a visual search task.

We have now moved on to study binding under more demanding conditions. So far we have looked at the capacity to bind shape and colour when they are spatially separated, involving, for example, a sequence of four shapes (e.g., square, circle, diamond, chevron) and above them four patches of colour (e.g., red, blue, yellow, green). This is a more demanding task; however, there is still no evidence to suggest that the requirement to bind is differentially susceptible to an attentionally demanding concurrent task (Karlsen, Allen, Baddeley, & Hitch, 2009). Even more surprisingly, we find that the binding of *visually* presented shape with a *spoken* colour is no more disrupted by a concurrent attentional task than is retention of the constituent features (Karlsen et al., 2009).

The role of symmetry in binding

It has been known for many years that symmetrical patterns are easier to remember than are asymmetrical patterns (Attneave, 1960). A series of recent experiments has explored the role of executive processes in this phenomenon (Rossi-Arnaud, Pieroni, & Baddeley, 2006). We used a task that was analogous to the Corsi block tapping test, in which participants see an array of blocks, the tester taps a sequence of the blocks, and the participant attempts to imitate this, resulting in a tapping span that is typically about 5 items. This task is generally assumed to depend on the spatial component of the visuospatial sketchpad (Della Sala, Gray, Baddeley, & Wilson, 1999).

In our modified version of this task, the blocks comprised a regular 5 × 5 array, and the participants' task was to repeat a sequence of taps that could form either a symmetrical or asymmetrical path, in which the symmetry could be vertical, horizontal, or diagonal in its axis. Participants performed this task either with or without performing a concurrent task, which could involve articulatory suppression, tapping in a regular spatial array, or a backward counting task that was assumed to absorb executive resources.

We observed first of all that our participants were able to make use of vertical symmetry but gained little or no advantage from patterns that were symmetrical on a horizontal or diagonal axis. We found no effect on performance of articulatory suppression, a modest disruption from spatial tapping, and a more substantial impact of our central executive task. However, none of these effects interacted with symmetry, suggesting an advantage gained from symmetry that was automatic but was influencing a memory task that itself was far from automatic.

We were unsurprised that vertical symmetry was most effective, since this is known to have a more powerful effect on perception than do other forms of symmetry, but we were surprised that horizontal symmetry did not appear to influence retention. One possible reason might be that given the sequential nature of the presentation, subjects might simply not have been aware of any symmetry other than vertical. We therefore went on to carry out a parallel series of experiments using simultaneous pattern presentation rather than the sequential presentation analogous to the Corsi task. The patterns and concurrent tasks used were essentially the same as in the previous study, except that patterns were presented simultaneously, as in pattern span – a task that is known to load more heavily on the visual than the spatial aspect of the sketchpad (Della Sala et al., 1999). Under these conditions we did obtain an advantage to patterns that were symmetrical about a horizontal though not diagonal axis, although the effect was not as marked as that of vertical symmetry. Performance was again disrupted by our visuospatial and executive secondary tasks, but not by articulatory suppression. Crucially, however, we found no interaction between secondary tasks and the influence of symmetry, again suggesting that the impact of symmetry is automatic and does not depend on general attentional resources.

Implications for the episodic buffer

We began with the assumption that binding is an attentionally demanding activity. We went on to test this in a range of dual-task studies. In the case of visual working memory, the binding of shapes to colours appears to be relatively automatic, in the sense that general information processing resources are not differentially required, even, it would appear, when the colour and shape are separated, or when one is visual or the other auditory. In the case of the sequential binding of linguistic materials, again the process appears to be relatively automatic, provided that the binding is based on overlearned language skills and presentation is auditory, although attention does seem to be required when presentation is visual.

How should binding be conceptualized? I would now suggest the division of binding into a number of separable categories. One category is essentially perceptual, taking advantage of automatic chunking processes. Examples include symmetry, continuation, and other Gestalt principles in vision, and rhythm and prosody in audition. Our results so far suggest that the chunking resulting from these perceptual processes is likely to be automatic rather than attentionally based.

I suggest that a second type of binding occurs through episodic memory, a system that allows us to encode and recollect specific episodes by binding them to their context. Such a mechanism is presumably also automatic, in the sense that we do not need to intentionally commit an episode to mind in order to recollect it subsequently. So where does that leave the role of attention in chunking?

In the case of episodic memory, I assume that although binding is automatic, the likelihood of a firm bond being formed will depend on two features. The first of these involves the existence of prior association or expectation. It is easier to learn to associate the words *bread* and *food* than *bread* and *chair*, for example. The second is a physiological process sometimes referred to as consolidation, which for the sake of simplicity I will refer to as "mnemonic glue". It is this latter capacity that is defective in patients suffering from the classic amnesic syndrome and, to a lesser extent, by all us as we get older. Simple priming effects typically involve existing representations and hence do not depend on this capacity to glue arbitrary events together. For this reason they tend to be preserved in amnesic patients (Squire, 1992).

A recent series of studies on memory and aging by Naveh-Benjamin and his collaborators provides a good example of the distinction between these two factors. They tested the capacity of young and older participants to learn to recognize pairs of words. When the words were paired arbitrarily, the young showed a clear advantage, but this disappeared when semantically associated pairs were used (Naveh-Benjamin, Guez, & Shulman, 2004). Their original hypothesis was that this reflected an attentional or executive deficit in the elderly, a hypothesis they tested by repeating the study but this time comparing young subjects with and without an attentional-demanding concurrent task (Naveh-Benjamin et al., 2004). If the crucial difference between their young and older groups depended on the difference in attentional capacity, then giving young participants a demanding concurrent task should make them behave like the older group and show a marked effect in the low- but not high-association pairs. This was not the case. They found a relatively small impact of attention, concluding that the age difference in learning was likely to be based on mnemonic rather than executive factors. The arbitrary pairings placed a heavy burden on the capacity for new long-term learning in contrast to a modest burden placed by the pairs of words that were already quite highly associated. It was the impaired capacity for new learning that resulted in the age-deficit pattern, not a deficit in attentional capacity or speed of processing.

But if binding is automatic, why should a demanding concurrent task influence learning at all? I suggest there are two reasons, one automatic and one strategic. First, I assume that episodic binding depends on representing the two or more features or items to be bound simultaneously within the episodic buffer. An attentionally demanding task is likely to utilize the buffer for other concurrent activities. These will compete for time and space within the buffer, hence reducing the likelihood of simultaneous maintenance and hence of adequate binding.

A second reason is more strategic in nature and concerns the potential role of the central executive in attempting to optimize the use of any existing associations between the items to be bound. This may operate through explicit mnemonic strategies – as in the case, for example, of classic imagery mnemonics where word sequences are encoded using an existing visual framework (Baddeley & Lieberman, 1980) – or else indirectly through deeper encoding where elaboration links the new material to existing semantic or episodic memory schemata (Craik & Lockhart, 1972).

Such speculation leaves us with a rather different concept of the episodic buffer from that proposed by Baddeley (2000), one in which the link with the central executive is still an important one, but where the process of binding is relatively automatic. The executive can still influence binding but does so indirectly.

So how *does* working memory interact with LTM? In many ways, it does so both implicitly and explicitly. LTM influences working memory performance implicitly through priming and the recency effect, through the influence of language habits at a phonological and syntactic level, and through the role of semantic knowledge in the binding of items into chunks. At an explicit level, LTM influences the choice and use of strategies for the optimal encoding of information in working memory and makes possible the processes known as redintegration, whereby long-term knowledge is used to disambiguate information in working memory and to monitor its overall plausibility. Working memory does, indeed, involve activated LTM, but also much, much more.

References

Allen, R. J., Baddeley, A. D., & Hitch, G. J. (2006). Is the binding of visual features in working memory resource-demanding? *Journal of Experimental Psychology: General, 135*, 298–313.

Allport, D. A. (1984). Auditory-verbal short-term memory and conduction aphasia. In H. Bourna & D. G. Bouwhuis (Eds.), *Attention and Performance X: Control of language processes* (pp. 313–326). Hove, UK: Lawrence Erlbaum Associates.

Atkinson, R. C., & Shiffrin, R. M. (1968). Human memory: A proposed system and its control processes. In K. W. Spence & J. T. Spence (Eds.), *The psychology of learning and motivation: Advances in research and theory* (Vol. 2, pp. 89–195). New York: Academic Press.

Attneave, F. (1960). In defense of homunculi. In W. Rosenblith (Ed.), *Sensory communication* (pp. 777–782). Cambridge, MA: MIT Press.

Baddeley, A. D. (1964). Immediate memory and the "Perception" of letter sequences. *Quarterly Journal of Experimental Psychology, 16*, 364–367.

Baddeley, A. D. (1996). Exploring the central executive. *Quarterly Journal of Experimental Psychology, 49A*, 5–28.

Baddeley, A. D. (2000). The episodic buffer: A new component of working memory? *Trends in Cognitive Sciences, 4*(11), 417–423.

Baddeley, A. D. (2001). Is working memory still working? *American Psychologist, 56*(11), 851–864.

Baddeley, A. D. (2007). *Working memory, thought and action*. Oxford, UK: Oxford University Press.

Baddeley, A. D., Gathercole, S. E., & Papagno, C. (1998). The phonological loop as a language learning device. *Psychological Review, 105*(1), 158–173.

Baddeley, A. D., Grant, S., Wight, E., & Thomson, N. (1973). Imagery and visual working memory. In P. M. A. Rabbitt & S. Dornic (Eds.), *Attention and performance V* (pp. 205–217). London: Academic Press.

Baddeley, A. D., & Hitch, G. J. (1974). Working memory. In G. A. Bower (Ed.), *Recent advances in learning and motivation* (Vol. 8, pp. 47–89). New York: Academic Press.

Baddeley, A. D., & Hitch, G. J. (1993). The recency effect: Implicit learning with explicit retrieval? *Memory and Cognition, 21*, 146–155.

Baddeley, A. D., Hitch, G. J., & Allen, R. J. (2009). *Working memory and binding in sentence recall*. Manuscript submitted for publication.

Baddeley, A. D., & Larsen, J. D. (2007). The phonological loop unmasked? A comment on the evidence for a "perceptual-gestural" alternative. *Quarterly Journal of Experimental Psychology, 60*, 497–504.

Baddeley, A. D., & Lieberman, K. (1980). Spatial working memory. In R. S. Nickerson (Ed.), *Attention and performance VIII* (pp. 521–539). Hillsdale, NJ: Lawrence Erlbaum Associates, Inc.

Baddeley, A. D., & Warrington, E. K. (1970). Amnesia and the distinction between long- and short-term memory. *Journal of Verbal Learning and Verbal Behavior, 9*, 176–189.

Baddeley, A. D., & Wilson, B. A. (1993). A case of word deafness with preserved span: Implications for the structure and function of short-term memory. *Cortex*, *29*, 741–748.

Brown, J. (1958). Some tests of the decay theory of immediate memory. *Quarterly Journal of Experimental Psychology*, *10*, 12–21.

Cowan, N. (1999). An embedded-processes model of working memory. In A. Miyake & P. Shah (Eds.), *Models of working memory* (pp. 62–101). Cambridge, UK: Cambridge University Press.

Cowan, N. (2001). The magical number 4 in short-term memory: A reconsideration of mental storage capacity. *Behavorial and Brain Sciences*, *24*, 87–114; discussion, 114–185.

Cowan, N. (2005). *Working memory capacity*. Hove, UK: Psychology Press.

Craik, F. I. M., Govoni, R., Naveh-Benjamin, M., & Anderson, N. D. (1996). The effects of divided attention on encoding and retrieval processes in human memory. *Journal of Experimental Psychology: General*, *125*(2), 159–180.

Craik, F. I. M., & Lockhart, R. S. (1972). Levels of processing: A framework for memory research. *Journal of Verbal Learning and Verbal Behavior*, *11*, 671–684.

da Costa Pinto, A., & Baddeley, A. D. (1991). Where did you park your car? Analysis of a naturalistic long-term recency effect. *European Journal of Cognitive Psychology*, *3*, 297–313.

Daneman, M., & Carpenter, P. A. (1980). Individual differences in working memory and reading. *Journal of Verbal Learning and Verbal Behaviour*, *19*, 450–466.

Daneman, M., & Merikle, P. M. (1996). Working memory and language comprehension: A meta-analysis. *Psychonomic Bulletin & Review*, *3*, 422–433.

Della Sala, S., Gray, C., Baddeley, A., & Wilson, L. (1999). Pattern span: A tool for unwelding visuo-spatial memory. *Neuropsychologia*, *37*, 1189–1199.

Engle, R. W. (1996). Working memory and retrieval: An inhibition-resource approach. In J. T. E. Richardson, R. W. Engle, L. Hasher, R. H. Logie, E. R. Stoltfus, & R. T. Zacks (Eds.), *Working memory and human cognition* (pp. 89–119). New York: Oxford University Press.

Glanzer, M. (1972). Storage mechanisms in recall. In G. H. Bower (Ed.), *The psychology of learning and motivation: Advances in research and theory* (Vol. 5). New York: Academic Press.

Jefferies, E., Lambon Ralph, M. A., & Baddeley, A. D. (2004). Automatic and controlled processing in sentence recall: The role of long-term and working memory. *Journal of Memory and Language*, *51*, 623–643.

Jones, D. M., Macken, W. J., & Nicholls, A. P. (2004). The phonological store of working memory: Is it phonological and is it a store? *Journal of Experimental Psychology: Learning, Memory, and Cognition*, *30*(3), 656–674.

Karlsen, P., Allen, R. J., Baddeley, A. D., & Hitch, G. J. (2009). *Binding across space and time in visual working memory*. Manuscript submitted for publication.

Kyllonen, P. C., & Christal, R. E. (1990). Reasoning ability is (little more than) working memory capacity. *Intelligence*, *14*, 389–433.

Kyllonen, P. C., & Stephens, D. L. (1990). Cognitive abilities as the determinants of success in acquiring logic skills. *Learning and Individual Differences*, *2*, 129–160.

Luck, S. J., & Vogel, E. K. (1997). The capacity of visual working memory for features and conjunctions. *Nature*, *390*, 279–281.

Melton, A. W. (1963). Implications of short-term memory for a general theory of memory. *Journal of Verbal Learning and Verbal Behavior*, *2*, 1–21.

Miller, G. A. (1956). The magical number seven, plus or minus two: Some limits on our capacity for processing information. *Psychological Review*, *63*, 81–97.

Miller, G. A., Bruner, J. S., & Postman, L. (1954). Familiarity of letter sequences and tachistoscopic identification. *Journal of General Psychology*, *50*, 129–139.

Miller, G. A., & Selfridge, J. A. (1950). Verbal context and the recall of meaningful material. *American Journal of Psychology*, *63*, 176–185.

Miyake, A., & Shah, P. (Eds.). (1999). *Models of working memory: Mechanisms of active maintenance and executive control*. New York: Cambridge University Press.

Nairne, J. S. (2002). Remembering over the short-term: The case against the standard model. *Annual Review of Psychology*, *53*, 53–81.

Naveh-Benjamin, M., Guez, J., & Shulman, S. (2004). Older adults' associative deficit in episodic memory: Assessing the role of decline in attentional resources. *Psychonomic Bulletin and Review*, *11*, 1067–1073.

Owen, A. M., McMillan, K. M., Laird, A. R., & Bullmore, E. (2005). N-Back working memory paradigm: A meta-analysis of normative functional neuroimaging studies. *Human Brain Mapping*, *25*, 46–59.

Peterson, L. R., & Peterson, M. J. (1959). Short-term retention of individual verbal items. *Journal of Experimental Psychology*, *58*, 193–198.

Rossi-Arnaud, C., Pieroni, L., & Baddeley, A. D. (2006). Symmetry and binding in visuo-spatial working memory. *Journal of Cognitive Neuroscience*, *139*, 393–400.

Ruchkin, D. S., Grafman, J., Cameron, K., & Berndt, R. S. (2003). Working memory retention systems: A state of activated long-term memory. *Behavioral and Brain Sciences*, *26*, 709–777.

Shallice, T., & Warrington, E. K. (1970). Independent functioning of verbal memory stores: A neuropsychological study. *Quarterly Journal of Experimental Psychology*, *22*, 261–273.

Shannon, C. E., & Weaver, W. (1949). *The mathematical theory of communication*. Urbana, IL: University of Illinois Press.

Squire, L. R. (1992). Declarative and nondeclarative memory: Multiple brain systems supporting learning and memory. *Journal of Cognitive Neuroscience*, *4*, 232–243.

Tulving, E. (1962). Subjective organisation in free recall of "unrelated" words. *Psychological Review*, *69*, 344–354.

Tulving, E., & Patkau, J. E. (1962). Concurrent effects of contextual constraint and word frequency on immediate recall and learning of verbal material. *Canadian Journal of Psychology*, *16*, 83–95.

Vallar, G., Papagno, C., & Baddeley, A. D. (1991). Long-term recency effects and phonological short-term memory: A neuropsychological case study. *Cortex*, *27*, 323–326.

Vogel, E. K., Woodman, G. F., & Luck, S. J. (2001). Storage of features, conjunctions, and objects in visual working memory. *Journal of Experimental Psychology: Human Perception and Performance*, *27*(1), 92–114.

Waugh, N. C., & Norman, D. A. (1965). Primary memory. *Psychological Review*, *72*, 89–104.

Wheeler, M. E., & Treisman, A. M. (2002). Binding in short-term visual memory. *Journal of Experimental Psychology: General*, *131*, 48–64.

3 Memory for actions

How different?

Henry L. Roediger, III and Franklin M. Zaromb

In the early 1980s, several groups of researchers began research on a topic variously called action memory, the enactment effect, and the subject-performed task effect. We take this as the topic of our chapter for several reasons. First, research by Lars-Göran Nilsson and his colleagues has played an important role in this research arena; second, Nilsson's supervisor, Ronald L. Cohen, was one of the initiators and champions of this line of research until his early death; and third, the effect is quite interesting in its own right and is now a central topic in the field.

The study of action memory arose independently among three different groups of researchers in the early 1980s (Zimmer & Cohen, 2001). The first published report was by Engelkamp and Krumnacker (1980) from Saarland University in Germany. They had subjects listen to a series of instructions that described a series of mini-tasks that could be performed in the lab (e.g., break the toothpick, comb your hair, touch your left ear with your right hand, pick up the toy car). All subjects heard the actions described ("pick up the toy car") with intentional learning instructions, but three different conditions were manipulated within subjects. In one condition, students simply heard the commands, in a second condition they heard them and were asked to imagine performing the action described, and in a third condition they were instructed to actually perform the action. During a later test, they were instructed to recall the actions by writing down the phrases that had been presented. The results are presented in the left panel of Figure 3.1. Recall was best after performing the action, next best after imagining performance of the action, and worst when the command had simply been heard. Engelkamp and Krumnacker referred to the superiority of recall following performance of the relevant action as the enactment effect.

At roughly the same time, Ronald Cohen (1981), then working at Glendon College, York University in Toronto, developed a similar procedure. His subjects studied four lists of action phrases either under instructions to listen to them or to perform the actions. He called the experimental condition one of using subject-performed tasks, or SPTs. His finding was perfectly consistent with that of Engelkamp and Krumnacker (1980), as subjects recalled the subject-performed tasks better than those that were merely heard (see the

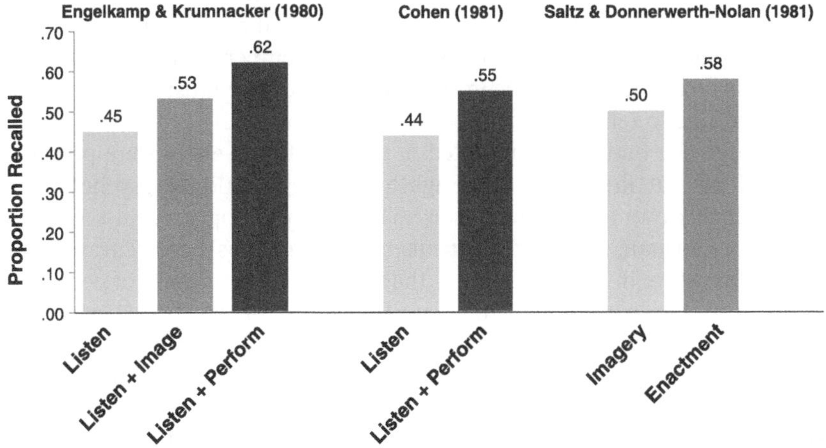

Figure 3.1 Data from three reports in 1980–1981 showing the enactment effect. The bar on the right of each panel shows retention after enactment, whereas the bars on the left show retention after either listening to the commands or listening to and imagining them. (Data adapted from selected conditions of the original papers listed in the figure.)

second panel in Figure 3.1). He called the effect the subject-performed task effect or SPT-effect.

Also in 1981, Saltz and Donnerwerth-Nolan, working at Wayne State University in Detroit, had students remember action statements presented as subject–verb–object sentences (e.g., “The dentist NAILED the sign on the WALL”). For some sentences students actually acted out the stated action, whereas for other sentences the students imagined the experimenter performing the action. (The nature of a secondary task was also manipulated; we report data from only one of two conditions here.) Once again, the basic finding was that when subjects enacted the command stated in the sentence, they remembered the sentence better on a later test than if they imagined the experimenter performing it. (See the right-hand panel of Figure 3.1.) Prior research by Paris and Lindauer (1976) had also shown that children remembered sentences better when acting them out, especially if cued by the implied object of the sentence that had to be inferred, such as *broom* in the case of “The boy swept the floor.”

These three studies in the early 1980s were impressive in showing that actions were well remembered relative to verbal statements describing the action. Even more impressively, actions were even well remembered compared to imagined actions, either imaginings of the subjects themselves performing the action or of the experimenter doing so. Imagery has long been encouraged as a beneficial encoding strategy for mnemonic success (e.g., Bower, 1972; Paivio, 1969), so finding that actions speak as loudly as, or even louder than, images and words in terms of mnemonic benefit is especially noteworthy. In addition, using the subject-performed task or action memory paradigm brought more than a whiff of ecological validity to the enterprise of studying human memory. Humans hardly evolved to remember lists of words, tractable as this technique might be in the lab, but surely we must have evolved in part to be able to remember actions we have performed.

Although the findings represented in the enactment effect were powerful, they did not, at first, take the English-speaking world of psychology by storm. Engelkamp and Krumnacker's (1980) paper appeared in a German journal in German, and English speakers are notoriously recalcitrant about reading literature in languages other than their own (although, of course, we expect everyone in the world to know English). Cohen's (1981) paper was published in the *Scandinavian Journal of Psychology* (in English), but again the English and American psychological audience did not (and does not) routinely run across this journal. The Saltz and Donnerwerth-Nolan (1981) paper was published in the *Journal of Verbal Learning and Verbal Behavior*, then and now (under a new name) a dominant North American journal, but they cast their paper as about motor imagery in language (which it was), so their reporting of data showing an enactment effect was not made the central focus. The first author of this chapter was fortunate to hear about the action memory research while on sabbatical at the University of Toronto in 1981–1982, when Ronald Cohen gave a provocative Ebbinghaus Empire presentation on his work. Roediger foresaw a bright future for this research area, because it was new and interesting and the basic technique was easy to carry out (although he did not himself use it until much later; Goff & Roediger, 1998).

Of course, with time, this whole picture changed and action memory became a central focus of study for many people. The study of action memory (or SPT events) became a frequently used paradigm, adding to the arsenal of methodologies that psychologists used to conduct research on learning and memory. Although some researchers saw the paradigm as another useful technique, Cohen (1981) made much stronger claims. In this first paper he asked if principles derived from action memory experiments obeyed the same laws of memory as with standard (mostly verbal) materials. The answer he provided was, by and large, no. Although immediate free recall of SPTs showed a normal recency effect, the primacy effect was absent. In addition, a levels-of-processing manipulation (Craik & Tulving, 1975) did not affect recall of SPT events, unlike with word lists. In brief, Cohen argued that action memory tasks obeyed different laws of memory from those obtained with normal verbal tasks such as word lists.

Since Cohen's original experiments raising this issue, research on action memory has often revolved around the issue of the extent to which the laws of memory are different for subject-performed tasks and, as a corollary, whether the study of action memory is not more ecologically valid than research using nonsense words, words, sentences, prose passages, and the like. We continue this debate in our chapter.

The purpose of this chapter is to review selectively the literature on memory for enacted events and to address the question of generality of findings. Our chapter has several parts. We first outline conditions necessary to establish laws of memory (or any other phenomenon): What characteristics should laws have? Second, we introduce Jenkins's (1979) framework for understanding memory experiments as a useful heuristic to aid our asking whether laws of memory exist. Following Roediger (2008), we conclude that laws of memory have thus far proved elusive and that the claims for laws of memory early in the history of psychology have vanished over time as we have learned more. Rather, findings in human memory (and practically all of psychology) turn out to be highly context dependent. After setting this stage, the main section of our chapter examines research on action memory using the lens of Jenkins's model of memory experiments. Are findings from action memory experiments consistently different from those obtained with other materials? Are there laws of action memory, even if not for more traditional materials? After answering these questions, we briefly consider theories of action memory.

Laws of nature

Philosophers and scientists have written volumes on proper understanding of the laws of nature and what properties a law should have. We will not add much to this verbiage but will cut to what we see as the heart of the matter, using Teigen's (2002) excellent summary (see Cohen, 1985, too). Teigen proposed five criteria for the establishment of a law in science. The first is validity, or the fact of a well-established regularity in nature through many observations. A deterministic law should have no exceptions, whereas a probabilistic law should permit few exceptions. The second is universality, with a law being independent of time and place. Third, true laws take priority over observations – that is, when observations appear to conflict with a law, we tend to doubt the observations. Fourth, the law should have explanatory power by being connected to other general principles. The final property is that the law should have autonomy by being self-contained. It should be encapsulated in a brief description, often a mathematical one.

If we accept Teigen's definition of a scientific law (and we do), then the question becomes: Has the scientific study of human memory produced any laws that meet these criteria? Has the subfield of action memory research produced law-like statements? We turn next to Jenkins's (1979) framework to help us in answering these questions.

Jenkins' model of memory experiments

In 1979 James J. Jenkins wrote a chapter for a volume entitled *Levels of Processing in Human Memory* edited by Cermak and Craik. It was a brief chapter, tucked in towards the end of a long book, and it was a commentary chapter on other chapters in the volume. Despite its somewhat obscure origin, now 30 years in the past, we believe the content of the chapter represents a seminal contribution to the field (see Roediger, 2008). Briefly, Jenkins proposed not a model for memory (we have plenty – probably too many – of those) but, rather, a model for memory experiments. He proposed that the typical memory experiment can be conceived as a constellation of four sets of factors, as portrayed here in Figure 3.2 (which is adapted from Jenkins, 1979). The sets of factors are the types of subjects tested (college students, fifth grade students, older adults, etc.), the types of events that are to be remembered (pictures, prose passages, lists of words), the study or encoding task put to the subject (instructional set, strategies given, settings), and finally the way memory is tested, or retrieval factors (free recall, cued recall, forced-choice recognition testing, and many more).

In a typical memory experiment, Jenkins argued, the researcher is usually only concerned with manipulating one or two factors in this whole constellation. For example, imagine that the researcher is interested in comparing retention of pictures and words (the verbal labels of the pictures) on tests of free recall and yes/no recognition (e.g., Madigan, 1983; Paivio, 1969). Interestingly, the test mode in these experiments is almost always verbal – that is, in free recall, subjects recall the names of the pictures and the verbal labels they saw – whereas in recognition they see the word *elephant* at test regardless of whether they studied its verbal or pictorial representation during study. This basic sort of experiment then would represent at least a 2 × 2 design,

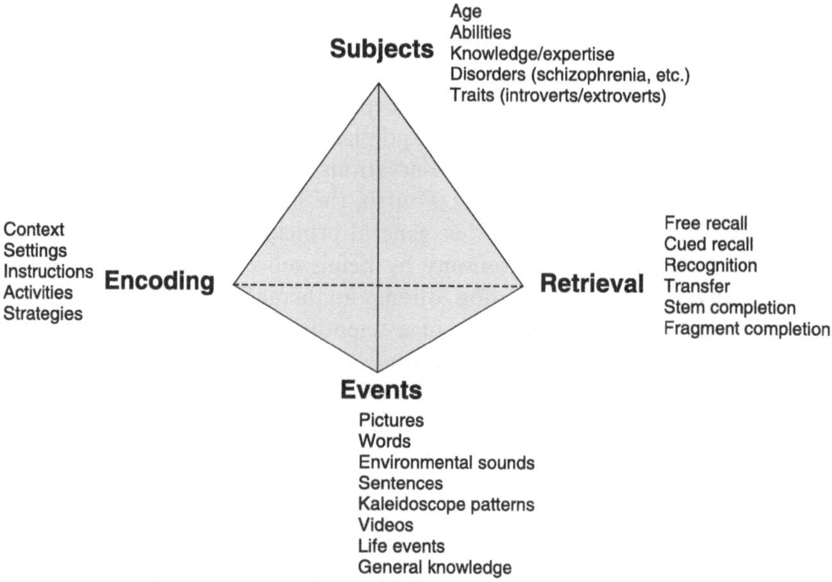

Figure 3.2 Jenkins's (1979) model of memory experiments in which at least four sets of factors are considered. In a typical experiment, only one or two factors are manipulated and retention is usually assessed using a single measure. Many other factors are held constant or allowed to randomly vary. (Adapted from Jenkins, 1979.)

with one factor being type of material (pictures/words) and the other factor being type of test (free recall/recognition). In the typical experiment, the other factors would be held constant or, in the lingo of experimental psychologists, would be control variables. College students are typically used as subjects, and the students are typically given intentional learning instructions before the material is presented.

The outcome of this particular experiment is also well known: pictures are both recalled and recognized better than words, even when the response mode in the recall test is verbal (producing names of pictures and words) and even if the test items on the recognition test are also verbal. That is, even when a nearly exact match occurs between word encoding and recognition testing item (a copy cue: study *elephant*, test with *elephant*), performance is worse than when the pictures are encoded and the test item is the verbal label (study a picture of an elephant, recognize the word elephant). Data from recall and recognition experiments following this basic form are shown in Figure 3.3. The punchline is that the picture superiority effect occurs on both recall and recognition tests with verbal tests. (A thought question for the reader: Can these results be reconciled with ideas of encoding specificity or transfer-appropriate processing? How? Shouldn't arguments favouring a match between encoding and retrieval predict suprior performance in the study word/test word condition relative to the study picture/test word condition?)

Because the picture superiority effect seems to occur with any subjects who

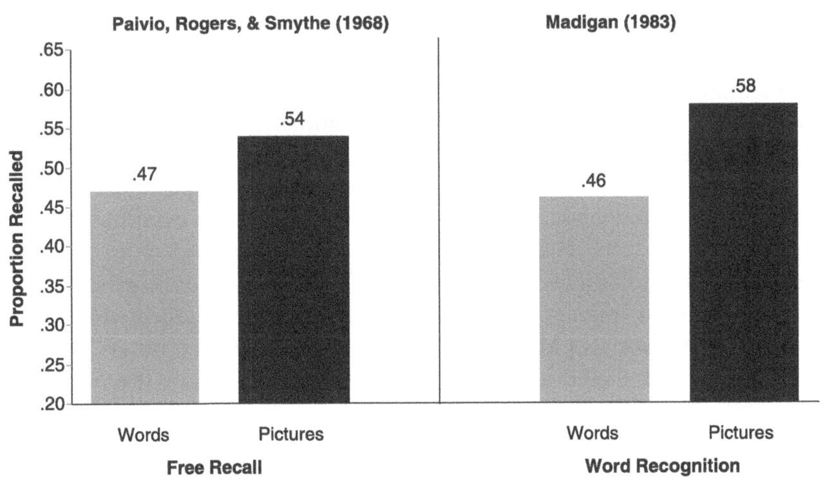

Figure 3.3 The picture superiority effect in recall and recognition experiments. Subjects study easily named pictures or words (the labels of the pictures). They are then tested in free recall (write the names of the pictures and words in any order) or in verbal recognition (recognize the words that represented pictures or words in the study phase). Despite the use of verbal coding on the test, pictures are better recalled and recognized than are words. (Data are adapted from the original reports listed in the figure.)

are fluent in their language and with intentional and incidental learning instructions, it might be thought to be a general law of memory: Pictures are better retained than words. The effect also occurs in between-subject designs (students study and recall or recognize only pictures or only words) as well as within-subjects designs (for one example of a between-subjects experiment showing the picture superiority effect, see Erdelyi & Becker, 1974).

Nonetheless, any idea of a general law of pictorial materials being universally better retained than verbal materials can be quickly dashed when a factor held constant in the typical experiment outlined above is manipulated. That factor is the nature of the test and cues used on the test. Although the picture superiority effect generally holds in both recall and recognition tests (and, as noted above, even when the test mode is verbal), these are both explicit or episodic memory tests, ones that ask the subject to mentally travel back in recent time and retrieve episodes of pictorial and verbal elements (Schacter, 1987; Tulving, 1972). The pattern can change dramatically when one uses certain types of implicit memory tests. In one class of implicit memory test – data-driven or perceptual implicit memory tests (Roediger & Blaxton, 1987; Tulving & Schacter, 1990) – subjects study words and pictures as in the typical experiment, but then they are tested in a different manner. They are given implicit memory instructions telling them that when they see a test stimulus they should respond with the first item that comes to mind to that cue. (Nothing about conscious recollection is mentioned in the instructions, and researchers often go to some length to disguise the test so as to discourage conscious recollection.) Subjects can be given either word fragments or picture fragments with these implicit instructions to say the first thing that comes to mind to the cue. The measure of interest is priming, or the facilitation of performance on the tested fragments from having studied a relevant picture or word relative to the completion rate in the absence of recent prior study of the element.

In general, results from this type of experiment using perceptual implicit memory tests show exquisite modality specificity, unlike experiments using explicit memory tests. That is, study of pictures produces priming on picture fragments but not on word fragments, whereas study of words produces priming on word fragments but not much on picture fragments (Weldon & Roediger, 1987; see also McDermott & Roediger, 1994; Rajaram & Roediger, 1993). The picture superiority effect disappears – it actually reverses – on a verbal perceptual implicit memory test.

The data shown in Figure 3.4 come from selected conditions of McDermott and Roediger (1994, Expt. 4), where the data shown are priming from pictures or words (i.e., a baseline completion rate of guessing the fragments' identities when they had not been studied has been subtracted out). As can be seen, the picture superiority effect holds on an implicit test with picture fragments, but completely reverses on the primed word fragment completion test. On the word fragment completion test, words produced greater priming than did pictures, in line with the transfer-appropriate processing account of task

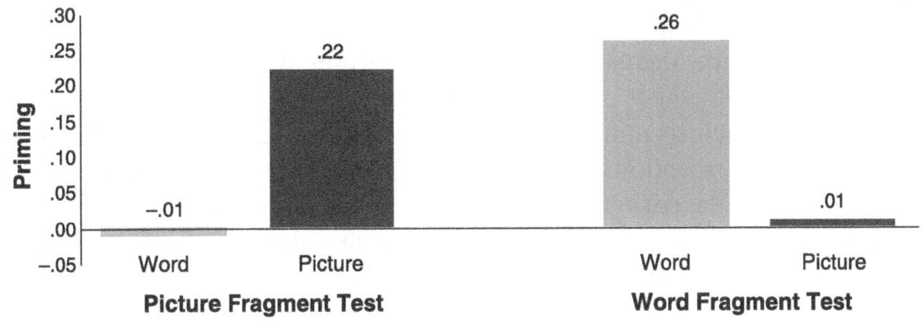

Figure 3.4 Priming on verbal and pictorial implicit memory tests after study of words and pictures. The pattern of priming shows specificity of modality: Prior study of pictures primes picture fragment naming but not word fragment completion, whereas prior study of words has the reverse effect. Baseline (non-studied) completion rates have been subtracted, so the data are priming scores. (Data are adapted from selected conditions in McDermott & Roediger, 1994, Expt. 4.)

dissociations (see Roediger & Srinivas, 1993). One might think that pictures are automatically named when they are presented, but if so this type of verbalization does not lead to priming on the verbal implicit test. (When McDermott and Roediger explicitly told subjects during study to imagine the form of the stimulus – that is, to imagine the written word or the image of the appropriate object – then some priming did occur on the task-appropriate test.) This test-appropriate pattern of results on perceptual implicit memory tests as shown in Figure 3.4 holds with both intentional and incidental learning instructions (Roediger, Weldon, Stadler, & Riegler, 1992) and on a variety of verbal implicit memory tests (Rajaram & Roediger, 1993).

In short, we can confidently say that the picture superiority effect reverses on verbal implicit memory tests. This outcome violates the idea of a general law that pictures are retained better than words. Rather, whether pictures are retained better than words, or the reverse, depends on the combination of study and test conditions used to examine the effect. In this case, the type of test used is critical, but other examples exist. Paivio and Csapo (1973) showed how the picture superiority effect can be reversed even on an explicit test, by manipulating study conditions.

Roediger (2008) examined the issue of whether *any* laws of learning and memory exist. As scientific psychology developed in the late nineteenth and early twentieth century, researchers sought to provide general laws of behaviour that would be like the famous laws of physics and chemistry. Thus, within the realm of learning and memory, Thorndike boldly proclaimed in 1911 that "Two laws explain all of learning." These were the law of effect and the law of exercise. Roediger examined 8 candidate variables that have been said to (or might be expected to) provide lawful relations with retention within the field of the cognitive/behavioural study of human memory. These variables included the effects of repetition, study time, distribution and spacing of practice, generation, retention over time (forgetting), as well as the mirror effect and the picture superiority effect. All these variables have been claimed to provide regular relations with certain types of retention tests. However, when Roediger examined them through the lens of Jenkins's tetrahedral model, each seemingly regular effect of these variables was shown to have important exceptions when other variables were manipulated, as just demonstrated in the paragraphs above with the picture superiority effect.

Roediger (2008) noted that most phenomena studied in human learning and memory are actually highly reliable; perform the same experiment the same way and the same outcome will (by and large) be obtained. The problem for the field in claiming laws is one of generality across the dimensions of Jenkins's (1979) tetrahedron. A highly replicable finding in one set of circumstances will lose its robustness when examined across the four corners of the model (subjects, encoding activities, materials, and types of test). In fact, if anything, Jenkins's model omits one critical variable that greatly matters in learning and memory experiments, as well as in all sorts of cognitive psychology experiments: the nature of the experimental design used (between-subjects or within-subjects). McDaniel and Bugg (2008) have reviewed five important memory phenomena in which results differ depending on the type of design used. Often an experimental effect (e.g., the generation effect, the word frequency effect) will be revealed in a within-subjects design, but the effect may evaporate (word frequency) or even reverse (generation) in a between-subjects design. This design feature is not embedded in Jenkins's framework, but it often matters in experiments, as Poulton (1963) also showed with reaction time experiments (see also, in the realm of animal learning, Bower, 1961). We will discuss the issue of type of design further in the context of action memory experiments.

Are there laws of action memory?

Cohen (1981) argued that laws for the enactment effect, or SPT tasks, were different from those based on standard verbal or pictorial materials. Of course, if Roediger (2008) and, for that matter, Cohen himself a bit later (1985) are right, there may be no general laws of memory to which principles of action memory would represent an exception. However, the enactment effect was not one that Roediger (2008) considered at length in his chapter. We aim to remedy that oversight in the remainder of this chapter by applying Jenkins's model of memory experiments to the enactment effect (see also Nilsson, 2000; Zimmer et al., 2001).

The enactment effect can often be quite substantial, typically ranging from 20–30% (Nyberg & Nilsson, 1995), and, as we will discuss, this effect generalizes across a wide range of subject populations and experimental conditions. Therefore, it seems a good candidate to examine for robustness across other variables. Another purpose of our chapter is to suggest modifications of Jenkins's (1979) model. We have already noted that type of design is one important factor omitted from Jenkins's model. In addition, we suggest that enactment tasks in memory experiments may themselves constitute an independent factor. That is, task enactment does not always fit squarely into the category of either a study/encoding manipulation or an event (materials) factor – it has features of both. When the to-be-learned items are action verbs or phrases, and when subjects are instructed to physically perform the actions or merely to listen to the instruction, this manipulation seems to fit squarely in Jenkins's framework as a study or encoding factor. On the other hand, when subjects are asked to perform actions with real objects provided by the experimenter (e.g., fill a glass), task enactment in this case creates the to-be-learned event, so it seems more like a type of material. Furthermore, in studies that require subjects to perform the to-be-learned actions during both the study and test phases (e.g., Engelkamp, Zimmer, Mohr, & Sellen, 1994; Kormi-Nouri, Nyberg, & Nilsson, 1994; Mulligan & Hornstein, 2003; Saltz & Dixon, 1982), enactment can simultaneously serve as an encoding/event factor as well as a retrieval factor.

A final justification for treating task enactment as an independent factor has to do with the types of interactions that occur when enactment is manipulated in conjunction with other encoding and/or retrieval variables. As we will discuss, task enactment – for reasons that are still unknown – has been shown to eliminate, or in the very least greatly reduce, the mnemonic effects of manipulating levels-of-processing (Craik & Lockhart, 1972) and item generation (Jacoby, 1978; Slamecka & Graf, 1978). This seems counterintuitive, because a reasonable assumption is that a combination of recall-enhancing encoding tasks (e.g., generating plus performing) should yield positive (perhaps even additive) benefits to retention or, at the very least, should not harm performance. These counteractive effects, therefore, underscore the notion that task enactment can play an important independent role in memory experiments.

We turn now to consider the four prongs of Jenkins's (1979) model, with a focus on action memory experiments. As we shall see, no robust laws of action memory seem to be validated.

Subjects

The enactment effect, which has been primarily demonstrated in young adults, has been also observed in a variety of other subject populations. These include healthy groups of children (Cohen & Stewart, 1982), older adults (e.g., Bäckman & Nilsson, 1984, 1985; Freeman & Ellis, 2003; Rönnlund, Nyberg, Bäckman, & Nilsson, 2003), deaf (von Essen & Nilsson, 2003; Zimmer & Engelkamp, 2003), blind (Kormi-Nouri, 2000), and mentally retarded subjects (Cohen & Bean, 1983).

Since performance on tests of explicit memory (e.g., recall or recognition) for verbally encoded materials is typically impaired for children, older adults, and mentally retarded subjects compared to young adults, these data have been interpreted to reflect fundamental differences between action and verbal memory (Cohen, 1981, 1983; Nilsson, 2000). Nevertheless, there has been some discrepancy in the literature as to whether the memorial benefit of task enactment remains intact or changes with age.

For instance, whereas Cohen and Stewart (1982) reported no differences in recall performance for subject-performed tasks among 9-, 11-, and 13-year-old children, other researchers have observed significant improvements in recall with age (e.g., Foley & Johnson, 1985; Foley & Ratner, 2001). At the other end of the life cycle, Cohen, Sandler, and Schroeder (1987) as well as Brooks and Gardiner (1994) observed that, after subjects performed to-be-learned lists of action phrases, older adults recalled as much as younger adults when tested with short study lists but not with long lists. By contrast, several studies reported age-related declines in memory for performed actions using comparable shorter study lists and tests of free or cued recall (Dijkstra & Kaschak, 2006; Knopf, 1991; Rönnlund, Nyberg, Bäckman, & Nilsson, 2003). Knopf and Neidhardt (1989) observed age-related differences in free recall of subject-performed actions, but when given a recognition test, which typically minimizes self-initiated retrieval demands relative to tests of free or cued recall, performance was similar for young and older adults. These data provide support for the notion that verbal and task enactment encoding involve fundamentally similar cognitive processes (e.g., Bäckman & Nilsson, 1985; Kormi-Nouri & Nilsson, 2001). Consistent with Jenkins's (1979) model, these various and seemingly contradictory findings underscore the notion that the effects of aging on the enactment effect are themselves influenced by interactions with other factors such as types of materials (e.g., list length) or tests (e.g., recall vs. recognition).

More surprising demonstrations of generalization have been shown in patients suffering from amnestic mild cognitive impairment (aMCI; Karantzoulis, Rich, & Mangels, 2006), Alzheimer's disease (Karlsson et al., 1989), frontal-lobe dysfunction related to epileptic surgery (McAndrews & Milner, 1991), Korsakoff's syndrome (Mimura et al., 1998), and even Parkinson's disease (Knopf, Mack, Lenel, & Ferrante, 2005). Taken together, these findings demonstrate just how extensively the superiority of remembering previously performed actions over information that was verbally encoded generalizes across subject populations, especially among subject populations that exhibit marked deficits in episodic verbal memory tasks and motor functioning.

This statement must be qualified, however, by noting cases where task enactment does not appear to enhance memory performance. Gardiner, Brandt, Vargha-Khadem, Baddeley, and Mishkin (2006) recently reported a series of experiments conducted with a developmental amnesic patient that showed no benefit of task enactment at study on subsequent recognition memory performance relative to verbal encoding. This single study is particularly striking, because in separate experiments, the same patient did exhibit both levels-of-processing and bizarreness effects (enhanced memory for bizarre compared to ordinary items) in tests of recognition memory. The authors suggest, however, that the levels-of-processing and bizarreness effects were not pure, in that they most likely reflected contributions from semantic memory and not a clean dissociation between verbal episodic and action memory task performance.

In addition, some evidence indicates that schizophrenic patients show little or no benefit of task enactment (Daprati, Nico, Saimpont, Franck, & Sirigu, 2005). Similarly, patients suffering from frontal lobe syndrome, which primarily affects action-related planning processes, do not show an enactment effect (Knopf et al., 2005). Nyberg, Persson, and Nilsson (2002) analysed individual differences among participants in a longitudinal aging study and tentatively concluded that specific biological and neuropsychological factors related to motor system dysfunction, which are more prevalent in older adults, may impair one's ability to benefit from task enactment. Still, more research is necessary to specify what aspects of motor planning, encoding, and episodic integration contribute to the enactment effect, and which of these, in turn, may be differentially affected by developmental and age-related processes, brain damage, sensory impairments, or other neurological disorders.

In sum, when healthy subjects are tested in action memory experiments, virtually all groups reveal an enactment effect. However, some neurologically impaired groups do not show the effect, probably due to impairments affecting the motor system.

Events

The memorial benefit of task enactment has been demonstrated with a variety of study materials and types of actions. These include verbs, phrases, and sentences, actions performed or observed with real or imagined objects, and even the use of sign language (for reviews, see Engelkamp & Zimmer, 1994; Nilsson, 2000; Zimmer et al., 2001). Yet there is a great deal of debate in the literature as to whether these various types of materials and actions directly influence the magnitude of enactment effect.

For example, in the early studies of the enactment effect, researchers asked whether it is better to perform actions such as "to fill a glass", with the use of a real glass and liquid, or whether simply pretending to fill a glass yields a comparable enactment effect. Whereas some researchers tended to use real objects in their experiments, because the experience of engaging with the objects was presumed to play an important role during enactment encoding (e.g., Bäckman, Nilsson, & Chalom, 1986; Kormi-Nouri & Nilsson, 1999; Nilsson & Bäckman, 1989), others have argued that it was necessary to only use imagined objects, because only the bare motor component was critical to producing enactment effects (e.g., Engelkamp & Zimmer, 1983, 1996). Engelkamp and Zimmer (1983, 1996) demonstrated that both task enactment and the use of real objects to perform the to-be-learned actions enhance memory performance, but independently of one another. However, more recently, Kormi-Nouri (2000) reported two experiments that systematically varied task enactment encoding with verbal encoding; the use of real or imaginary objects; and the use of real or imagined actions. Furthermore, Kormi-Nouri (2000) compared performance for sighted subjects with groups of blindfolded and blind subjects. Across all groups and conditions, subject-performed tasks were better recalled than verbally encoded items. There were also no differences in recall performance between the subject groups, with the exception that blind subjects demonstrated worse recall for subject-performed tasks that were both imagined and, further, involved imaginary objects. Enhanced recall for subject-performed tasks occurred regardless of whether subjects actually performed or only imagined the to-be-learned actions, or whether they used real objects or simply imagined using the objects. Therefore, Kormi-Nouri (2000) argued that the enactment effect does not depend on either motor movements or the use of real objects, a striking conclusion.

Another question that dates back to the early days of action memory research is whether it is better to actually perform the to-be-learned action descriptions, or whether observing someone else (i.e., the experimenter) perform the to-be-learned actions produces comparable memory performance. For instance, Cohen (1981) in his pioneering study reported no difference between these two encoding conditions (performing vs. observing), and Steffens (2007) has more recently made the same observation. However, Engelkamp and Zimmer (1983, 1997) demonstrated superior memory for subject-performed actions relative to actions that subjects only observed. Although it is unclear what specific factors determine the relative memorial advantage of performing over observing actions, two factors appear to play decisive roles – list length and experimental design. For longer lists of to-be-learned actions (e.g., 24–48 items), or for randomly mixed lists of actions that are to be either performed or observed in a within-subjects design, performing is superior to observing the actions. However, when the lists are relatively short (e.g., 12 or fewer items) or the conditions are blocked within-subjects or distributed between-subjects, performing the actions results in memory test performance similar to observing the actions. Later, we will discuss in greater detail the influence of experimental design on the enactment effect.

Among the various types of study materials and actions that have been shown to elicit enactment effects, it also remains unclear whether the organization of the study items influences the magnitude of the effect. Numerous studies dating back to the early 1950s have examined the relationship between organization and learning by measuring the extent to which subjects recollect similar responses together, or in clusters, in tests of free recall. The similarity of the responses within each cluster may be based on semantics, temporal contiguity, or other psychological dimensions (e.g., Bousfield, 1953; Deese, 1959; Jenkins & Russell, 1952; Mandler, 1967; Miller, 1956; Tulving, 1962).

On the one hand, several studies conducted by Engelkamp and colleagues (e.g., Engelkamp & Zimmer, 1990; Engelkamp, Zimmer, & Mohr, 1990; Zimmer, 1991; Zimmer & Engelkamp, 1989) have demonstrated that organizational scores for recall protocols do not benefit from task enactment. By contrast, Bäckman and colleagues (Bäckman & Nilsson, 1984, 1985; Bäckman et al., 1986; Kormi-Nouri & Nilsson, 1999) have reported higher organizational scores for recall of actions that were performed during study. That is, task enactment may have enabled subjects to benefit more from the relational structure of the study list to aid recall. In a more recent study, Koriat and Pearlman-Avnion (2003) showed that task enactment influences the specific type of mental organization that occurs during encoding and retrieval. Specifically, they found that when subjects performed to-be-learned actions, they tended to cluster their recall responses based on motor movement similarities among list items. However, when subjects verbally encoded the described actions, they tended to cluster their responses based on inter-item semantic associations.

Aside from the organization of the study materials or subjects' recall protocols, do particular types of items tend to be remembered better than others following task enactment? The answer is yes. For instance, studies conducted by Kormi-Nouri (1995) and Kormi-Nouri and Nilsson (1998) have shown that pre-experimental semantic associations among verbs and nouns used to create individual action phrases modulated the memorial benefit of task enactment such that items with well-established pre-experimental semantic associations (e.g., "read the book") tend to benefit more from task enactment than items whose elements are weakly associated (e.g., "look at the stone"). Similarly, Engelkamp and Jahn (2003) observed that under task enactment study conditions, action phrases with highly associated objects and verbs were better recalled than phrases with weakly associated objects and verbs.

One type of study material that may not benefit from task enactment is the learning of paired associates. Engelkamp (1986) reported that paired-associate learning was surprisingly worse following enactment than following verbal encoding. Subjects studied unrelated pairs of verbs, either under standard verbal encoding conditions or by performing the described actions. Using a test of free recall, task enactment improved memory performance compared to verbal encoding. However, using a test of cued recall in which subjects were presented with one verb from each pair and asked to recall the verb-associate, recall after verbal encoding was superior to that after task enactment. This and related findings have been taken as evidence to support the notion that while performing to-be-learned actions enhances memory for the particular actions (item-specific processing), it does not enhance memory for relations among associated pairs of actions (relational processing), especially if the actions appear to be unrelated.

In order to fully address the question of whether the enactment effect generalizes across all types of study materials and actions, more research is needed to examine whether stimuli that do not directly lend themselves to active performance can benefit from some form of related enactment. Do all types of actions and activities benefit from task-enactment encoding? It is interesting to note that Cohen (1981) originally included a wide variety of tasks such as "fold your arms", "sharpen the pencil", "yawn", "read the

Xmas card", "spell COLD", and "add 2 + 3", some of which emphasized bodily movements, the use of objects, or distinct mental operations. Curiously, the performance of tasks such as the last three item examples probably involves the same sorts of perceptual and cognitive processing instructed of subjects when they perform verbal learning levels-of-processing and generation tasks, and yet, surprisingly, levels-of-processing and generation effects do not robustly occur under task enactment encoding conditions.

Another limit to the generalization of the enactment effect may be the complexity of the to-be-learned materials. The vast majority of studies that have examined the memorial consequences of task performance have employed lists of simple, discrete actions. Due to the simplicity of the actions, it remains unclear whether the memorial benefit of task enactment extends to more complex sequences of actions or goal-oriented activities that are more representative of everyday actions (for a detailed discussion of these issues, see Foley & Ratner, 2001).

In sum, although the enactment effect occurs with a wide variety of materials, there are clearly conditions in which the effect does not occur, such as with short lists of materials or in paired-associate recall.

Encoding

The memorial benefit of enactment has been demonstrated using several different encoding manipulations, including, but not limited to, instructing subjects to perform actions with either real or imaginary objects (e.g., Engelkamp & Zimmer, 1983, 1994); with intentional or incidental learning instructions (e.g., Zimmer & Engelkamp, 1984); by performing the target actions while blindfolded (Engelkamp, Zimmer, & Biegelmann, 1993; Kormi-Nouri, 2000); or in using sign language to enact the target actions (von Essen & Nilsson, 2003; Zimmer & Engelkamp, 2003).

However, a number of encoding variations that have been shown to greatly impact memory for verbally encoded stimuli do not appear to influence memory for actions. For instance, numerous studies have shown that the levels-of-processing effect (Craik & Lockhart, 1972; Craik & Tulving, 1975) does not occur, or at the very least is greatly reduced, when subjects were instructed to perform the study items (Cohen, 1981; Cohen & Bryant, 1991; Nilsson & Cohen, 1988; Nilsson & Craik, 1990; Zimmer & Engelkamp, 1999). The generation effect (Jacoby, 1978; Slamecka & Graf, 1978), in which there is a memorial advantage for information that is generated by subjects compared to information that is passively heard or read, was not obtained when items were encoded through enactment (Nilsson & Cohen, 1988).

Additional factors that are known to have significant influence on memory for verbally encoded stimuli, but little to no influence on subject-performed actions, include varying the study time interval (Cohen, 1985); the amount of item elaboration (Helstrup, 1987); whether the to-be-learned stimuli are bizarre or ordinary actions (Engelkamp et al., 1993; Knopf, 1991); and instructing subjects to study items under conditions of divided attention (e.g., Bäckman, Nilsson, Herlitz, Nyberg, & Stigsdotter, 1991; Bäckman, Nilsson, & Kormi-Nouri, 1993; Bäckman et al., 1986).

In sum, the strongest case to be made that action events differ systematically in memorability relative to verbal events comes from these different effects of encoding manipulations in the two domains.

Retrieval

The enactment effect has also been demonstrated in performance on different tests of memory, including free recall, cued recall, and recognition, with the effect generally being more pronounced on tests of recognition than in recall (e.g., Mohr, Engelkamp, & Zimmer, 1989). In addition, task enactment enhances the accessibility of items in priming on conceptual implicit memory tests. For instance, when subjects were instructed to generate category instances, previously enacted actions were generated more frequently than were actions previously studied with verbal encoding or non-studied actions (Zimmer, 1991). However, as noted above, the enactment effect does not occur in paired associate learning (Engelkamp, 1986).

The memorial benefit of task enactment has also been observed using the classic release from proactive interference (PI) paradigm (Wickens, 1970). In this paradigm, subjects typically study and attempt to recall individual triads of verbal stimuli (i.e., letters or words) on successive trials. Between study and test, subjects might be asked to perform a simple counting or arithmetic task to minimize rehearsal for a number of seconds (i.e., 20 s). The typical finding is that recall performance decreases sharply across trials, which can be described as a build-up of proactive interference. However, when there is a shift in the symbolic representation or taxonomic class of the triad on a later trial, there is a marked increase in recall performance, known as the release from PI. Nilsson and Bäckman (1991) applied the PI-release paradigm to studies of task enactment and demonstrated increased release from PI for previously performed actions relative to that for actions studied under verbal encoding.

Several studies have examined the effects of task enactment on hypermnesia, the improvement in recall across repeated tests (Erdelyi & Becker, 1974). In these experiments, subjects were given several successive recall tests after receiving lists of action descriptions that were either performed or verbally encoded during the study phase. Interestingly, these studies have shown that task enactment during study led both to more item gains (recall of additional study items that were not recalled on previous recall attempts) over repeated test trials as well as item losses (forgetting of items that were successfully recalled on previous recall attempts) relative to verbal events (Engelkamp & Seiler, 2003; Engelkamp, Seiler, & Zimmer, 2004).

Another line of research has investigated whether task enactment at retrieval in addition to study further enhances memory performance. Engelkamp and colleagues conducted a series of studies that demonstrated a benefit on recognition test performance when subjects enacted to-be-learned tasks during both study and test phases (e.g., Engelkamp & Zimmer, 1995; Engelkamp et al., 1994). Likewise, other recent studies have shown that having subjects perform to-be-learned actions during both encoding and retrieval increased the recall advantage of enactment relative to task enactment during study alone (Koriat & Pearlman-Anvion, 2003; Mulligan & Hornstein, 2003; Steffens, Buchner, & Wender, 2003). Indeed, these findings are consistent with theories such as the encoding specificity principle (Tulving & Thomson, 1973) and the transfer-appropriate processing framework (Bransford, Franks, Morris, & Stein, 1979), which posit that memory performance depends on the extent of overlap between recall and study conditions.

On the other hand, several types of memory tests and retrieval conditions do not appear to benefit from enactment. For instance, if subjects studied a list of items and were later instructed to recall the items in the correct order (serial recall) or to rearrange the items in their correct order, enactment encoding was no better than verbal encoding (Olofsson, 1996). Moreover, enactment does not appear to enhance retention of source information or one's ability to monitor learning. Several studies have showed no improvements in memory for the spatial or temporal context in which actions were originally studied compared to items that were verbally encoded (Cornoldi, Corti, & Helstrup, 1994; Koriat, Ben-Zur, & Cruch, 1991; Zimmer, 1994). Other researchers reported that subjects were worse in predicting their performance in a subsequent recall test following enactment encoding than they were following verbal encoding (Cohen, 1983, 1988, 1989; Cohen & Bryant, 1991; Engelkamp & Cohen, 1991).

In sum, although many retrieval tasks reveal an enactment effect, some popular tests, such as serial and paired-associate recall, do not. Free recall and recognition procedures do typically reveal the enactment effect.

Experimental design

In addition to the four sets of factors that Jenkins proposed in his model, experimental design is another factor that has been shown to directly influence a substantial number of mnemonic effects that are widely believed to be stable (for a review, see McDaniel & Bugg, 2008). Consider the generation effect. When list items that subjects are instructed to generate are randomly mixed with items that subjects are instructed to passively read, generated items are better remembered than are read items (e.g., Jacoby, 1978; Slamecka & Graf, 1978). However, when generated and read items are distributed between-subjects such that one group of subjects only generates study items and another group only reads study items, then recall performance is usually found to be equivalent in both conditions (Slamecka & Katsaiti, 1987). Comparable recall performance for generated and read items has also been reported in within-subjects designs when the two types of items are presented in homogeneous blocks (Begg & Snider, 1987; Hirshman & Bjork, 1988; Slamecka & Katsaiti, 1987).

The memorial advantage of performing to-be-learned actions over standard verbal encoding instructions does generalize across various experimental designs. However, as discussed above, if one compares recall for actions that were performed by subjects themselves versus actions that subjects observed others (such as the experimenter) perform, different patterns emerge, depending on the experimental design. Engelkamp and Zimmer (1997) reported that when subject-performed and experimenter-performed actions are randomly distributed within-subjects, subject-performed actions were recalled the best. However, this benefit of task enactment disappeared when the encoding conditions were distributed between-subjects (see also, Cohen, 1981, 1983).

To explain these discrepancies, Engelkamp and Zimmer (1997) suggested that whereas performing actions during encoding enhances processing of the features of the individual actions themselves (item-specific processing), observing the actions enhances processing of the temporal or semantic associations among actions in the study list (relational processing). Furthermore, when the encoding conditions are randomly distributed within-subjects, the enhanced item-specific processing for subject-enacted tasks detracts from the enhanced relational processing enjoyed by observing task enactment, thereby yielding superior recall performance in the subject-performance condition. By contrast, with the two conditions distributed between-subjects, recall should be equivalent because the enhanced item-specific processing of one condition will more or less match the enhanced relational processing of the other condition.

An alternative account of these findings is provided by the item-order theoretical framework, in which subjects make use of both item-specific and temporal-order information to guide retrieval (McDaniel & Bugg, 2008; Nairne, Riegler, & Serra, 1991; Serra & Nairne, 1993). The item-order account maintains that enhanced item-specific processing occurs at the expense of encoding temporal or order information about item presentation within the study list. In a within-subjects design, memory for order information is equivalent across all encoding conditions (performing vs. observing actions), because enactment would disrupt the encoding of order information throughout the list of described actions whereas item-specific processing of the individual actions would be enhanced in the subject-enactment condition. By contrast, in the between-subjects design, order memory would be enhanced for experimenter-enacted items at study, whereas order memory would remain diminished for subject-enacted items, thereby potentially reducing the difference between the two conditions (performed or observed).

McDaniel and Bugg (2008) recently reviewed studies of the generation effect, as well as the word-frequency effect (high-frequency words are recalled better than low-frequency words), the perceptual interference effect (perceptually masked words are recalled better than unmasked words), the bizarreness effect (items conceived in a bizarre scenario are better recalled than items conceived in an ordinary scenario), and the enactment effect (subject-performed tasks are better recalled than experimenter-performed tasks), in order to examine whether the puzzling influence of experimental design may be adequately explained in terms of a unifying theoretical framework. Indeed, they argued that the item-order theoretical framework can at present account for the collective findings related to each of these five effects (Nairne et al., 1991; Serra & Nairne, 1993).

For our purposes, McDaniel and Bugg (2008) cited data from studies conducted by Engelkamp and Dehn (2000) and Golly-Häring and Engelkamp (2003) that provide support for the predictions of the item-order theoretical framework. Engelkamp and Dehn observed that whereas free-recall performance varied with experimental design – that is, subject-performed actions were recalled better in within- but not in between-subjects designs – recognition of subject-performed actions was superior in both types of designs. The latter finding is consistent with the notion that item-specific processing enhances recognition test performance (and processing of order information is not particularly critical). Furthermore, when subjects attempted to reconstruct the presentation order of the study items, predictions of the item-order account were fulfilled. That is, order reconstruction scores were superior for experimenter-performed actions compared to subject-performed actions in the between-subjects design and were intermediate for actions studied in the within-subjects design. In a more recent study, Golly-Häring and Engelkamp (2003) provided further support for the item-order account by demonstrating that when the study lists are composed of categorically related items, subject-performed actions are better recalled than experimenter-performed actions, regardless of experimental design. They argued that this outcome occurred because subjects can effectively encode and make use of these inter-item associations to aid recall and compensate for deficits in order information encoding incurred through task enactment.

To conclude this section, action memory effects respond to design features of an experiment (within- or between-subjects designs) in a similar way to other well-known effects such as the generation effect and the word-frequency effect. In this case, action memory effects behave like other behavioural effects. However, it should be borne in mind that the effects due to changing designs discussed above refer to a comparison between subject-performed tasks and observing someone else perform the task. The advantage of subject-performed tasks to verbal tasks (hearing the instruction) survives design changes, similar to the picture superiority effect and the levels of processing effect. Why some study or encoding manipulations are affected by design changes and others are not remains an interesting target for future research.

Theory

The various ways that subject-performed tasks can be instantiated in memory experiments also highlights fundamental distinctions among the theories proposed to explain the benefit of task enactment. That is, each theory predicts that the manipulation of certain factors will be important in determining the presence and magnitude of enactment effects, while variations among other factors will have a negligible influence.

Cohen (e.g., 1981, 1983) proposed that, in contrast to standard verbal learning task conditions in which subjects may strategically rehearse, mentally organize, or form associations among to-be-learned items during study, subject performance of to-be-learned actions is a non-strategic form of encoding that is automatic and highly efficient. Task enactment represents an optimal form of encoding and, as such, is superior to verbal encoding. Therefore, experimental factors that either impair or minimize the use of "strategic" encoding and/or retrieval processes should lead to a memorial advantage for task enactment. As we will discuss later, some of these factors include subject factors such as age, intelligence, brain damage, and other neurological disorders.

Furthermore, the non-strategic encoding view does not specify the types of actions that may or may not benefit from subject performance. In fact, as already mentioned, Cohen (1981) originally included a wide variety of tasks such as "fold your arms", "sharpen the pencil", "yawn", "read the Xmas card", "spell COLD", and "add 2 + 3", some of which emphasize bodily movements, the use of objects, or distinct mental operations. It seems that a further prediction of the non-strategic encoding view is that the enactment effect should generalize across all types of subject-performed activities.

Bäckman and Nilsson (1984, 1985) argued that subject task performance involves both strategic and non-strategic forms of encoding (see also Bäckman et al., 1986). That is, when subjects perform to-be-learned actions, the action descriptions may be strategically encoded as verbal information, whereas the physical aspects of task enactment are encoded non-strategically (Bäckman et al., 1991, 1993). According to this dual encoding theory and in contrast to the non-strategic encoding view, factors that impair the use of strategic processes can reduce or eliminate the enactment effect. On the other hand, the inclusion of more physical components (e.g., real objects) to the study tasks should produce or increase the magnitude of the enactment effect.

An alternative proposal, by Engelkamp and Zimmer (e.g., 1983, 1984, 1985), was that the independent encoding of motor information during task performance produces the enactment effect. According to their theory, motor, verbal, and visual information are encoding independently in distinct mental codes or representations. More importantly, motor encoding is assumed to be more efficient than verbal and visual encoding. One methodological implication of these theoretical assumptions is that the enactment effect depends on the interaction between encoding activities and types of materials. Specifically, memory performance will be enhanced to the extent that either the encoding instructions or to-be-learned actions include a motor activation component (e.g., "raise your arm"). This requirement of a motor component suggests both extensions and limitations to the generalization of the enactment effect. In contrast to Cohen's (1981, 1983) approach, the enactment effect would depend on whether subjects are instructed to perform a physical activity. In contrast to the dual encoding account, Engelkamp and Zimmer further argued that the enactment effect does not depend on subjects' physical interactions with the environment (e.g., objects). An additional prediction is that task enactment during retrieval can either facilitate or interfere with memory performance depending on the similarity of the motor movements done at study and test.

In a radical departure from the above-mentioned accounts, Kormi-Nouri (1995) and Kormi-Nouri and Nilsson (2001) have argued that task enactment encoding is purely strategic and that there is little distinction between verbal and motor encoding. Rather, when subjects are asked to learn and perform lists of described actions, consistent with Tulving's (1983) conception of episodic memory, task enactment enhances subjects' experience and awareness of the learning episode as compared to standard verbal encoding conditions. Kormi-Nouri and Nilsson proposed that memory performance will be enhanced to the extent that task performance facilitates "episodic integration" of the to-be-learned information (e.g., verbs, objects) into a cohesive, distinct memory trace (Kormi-Nouri & Nilsson, 2001). This theoretical approach implies, for instance, that factors that impair episodic memory performance in general will likewise impair memory for previously performed actions.

The current status of theories of the enactment effect is one of ferment, with contending theories having both strengths and weaknesses in accounting for the huge body of empirical data. We have covered the action memory research somewhat selectively in this review, so a more thorough assessment would probably uncover even more problems for extant theories.

Conclusions

In the past 30 years, research on action memory (or the enactment effect or subject-performed tasks) has reached a state of scientific maturity in that a large body of research has been published on it. Cohen's (1981) proclamation that different laws of memory might underlie action memory relative to verbal memory seems, in its boldest form, to be wrong. There are no "laws of memory" using the criteria Teigen (2002) proposed, either in action memory or anywhere else in our field. On the other hand, if we soften the claim to one of "different principles" or "different patterns of effect", then we can see some evidence that Cohen (1981) was right. For example, the review of encoding effects above indicated that variables that commonly affect verbal memory tasks often have a different effect (or no effect) on action memory tasks. Nonetheless, surveying this body of literature and trying to reach firm conclusions about the effect of enactment as a variable usually leads us to such statements as "Self-performed tasks are better retained than watching another person perform a task, but this effect depends on the type of materials used, the method of measuring retention, the type of experimental design, using neurologically intact subjects in the experiment, and so on." As seemingly occurs with all memory phenomena, the answer to almost any question is "it depends" (Roediger, 2008). Our textbooks may tell pat stories for the instructors' and students' convenience, but scientists at the forefront of studying some phenomenon know that these are usually "just so" stories because the truth would demoralize students (and their instructors). "It depends" is just not a satisfying answer to questions, even though it usually represents the true state of affairs.

Interestingly, Lars-Göran Nilsson drew conclusions much like our own in an essay that appeared the year before the dawn of action memory research. In 1979 he published an edited volume of important essays to honour the 500th anniversary of Uppsala University. We think it is fitting to conclude our chapter in his honour with his prescient words from the introductory chapter he wrote 30 years ago:

> Apparently, there is no general theory in the making, and there are no single findings terminating any research pursuits. Certain discoveries may of course answer specific questions, but beyond those there are always still more challenging questions that require further study. Thus, as it now stands, there is no real hope for a final general theory in memory research. The general-theory view of science is of course more common among people in general than among scientists. However, even scientists often hope for a general theory that will be the salvation for a given field; and one might wonder how this view has become so popular. One very likely reason is the way undergraduate courses are usually taught. When we teach courses, we often seek to present the material in such a general and coherent form that it commonly violates scientific reality. If we would present the material in a way that more exactly reflects the diverging state of affairs in the memory area, it would probably leave the students in a state of bewilderment. Simplification and other pedagogical tricks may be necessary to avoid this state, but it is important to keep in mind that they are made for educational and not for scientific purposes.

Acknowledgements

This research was supported by a grant from the James S. McDonnell Foundation.

References

Bäckman, L., & Nilsson, L.-G. (1984). Aging effects in free recall: An exception to the rule. *Human Learning*, *3*, 53–69.

Bäckman, L., & Nilsson, L.-G. (1985). Prerequisites for lack of age differences in memory performance. *Experimental Aging Research, 11*, 67–73.

Bäckman, L., Nilsson, L.-G., & Chalom, D. (1986). New evidence on the nature of the encoding of action events. *Memory & Cognition, 14*, 339–346.

Bäckman, L., Nilsson, L.-G., Herlitz, A., Nyberg, L., & Stigsdotter, A. (1991). A dual conception of the encoding of action events. *Scandinavian Journal of Psychology, 32*, 289–299.

Bäckman, L., Nilsson, L.-G., & Kormi-Nouri, R. (1993). Attentional demands and recall of verbal and color information in action events. *Scandinavian Journal of Psychology, 34*, 246–254..

Begg, I., & Snider, A. (1987). The generation effect: Evidence for generalized inhibition. *Journal of Experimental Psychology: Learning, Memory, and Cognition, 13*, 553–563.

Bousfield, W. A. (1953). The occurrence of clustering in the recall of randomly arranged associates. *Journal of General Psychology, 49*, 229–240.

Bower, G. H. (1961). A contrast effect in differential encoding. *Journal of Experimental Psychology, 62*, 196–199.

Bower, G. H. (1972). Mental imagery and associative learning. In L. W. Gregg (Ed.), *Cognition in learning and memory* (pp. 51–88). New York: Wiley.

Bransford, J. D., Franks, J. J., Morris, C. D., & Stein, B. S. (1979). Some constraints on learning and memory research. In L. S. Cermak & F. I. M. Craik (Eds.), *Levels of processing and human memory* (pp. 331–354). Hillsdale, NJ: Lawrence Erlbaum Associates, Inc.

Brooks, B. M., & Gardiner, J. M. (1994). Age differences in memory for prospective compared with retrospective subject-performed tasks. *Memory & Cognition, 22*, 27–33.

Cohen, R. L. (1981). On the generality of some memory laws. *Scandinavian Journal of Psychology, 22*, 267–281.

Cohen, R. L. (1983). The effect of encoding variables on the free recall of words and action events. *Memory & Cognition, 11*, 573–582.

Cohen, R. L. (1985). On the generality of the laws of memory. In L.-G. Nilsson & T. Archer (Eds.), *Perspectives on learning and memory* (pp. 247–277). Hillsdale, NJ: Lawrence Erlbaum Associates, Inc.

Cohen, R. L. (1988). Metamemory for words and enacted instructions: Predicting which items will be recalled. *Memory & Cognition, 16*, 452–460.

Cohen, R. L. (1989). Memory for action events: The power of enactment. *Educational Psychology Review, 1*, 57–80.

Cohen, R. L., & Bean, G. (1983). Memory in educable mentally retarded adults: Deficit in subject or experimenter? *Intelligence, 7*, 287–298.

Cohen, R. L., & Bryant, S. (1991). The role of duration in memory and metamemory of enacted instructions (SPTs). *Psychological Research, 53*, 183–187.

Cohen, R. L., Sandler, S. P., & Schroeder, K. (1987). Aging and memory for words and action events: Effects of item repetition and list length. *Psychology and Aging, 2*, 280–285.

Cohen, R. L., & Stewart, M. (1982). How to avoid developmental effects in free recall. *Scandinavian Journal of Psychology, 23*, 9–16.

Cornoldi, C., Corti, M. T., & Helstrup, T. (1994). Do you remember what you imagined you would do in that place? The motor encoding cue-failure effect in sighted and blind people. *Quarterly Journal of Experimental Psychology, 47A*, 311–329.

Craik, F. I. M., & Lockhart, R. S. (1972). Levels of processing: A framework for memory research. *Journal of Verbal Learning and Verbal Behavior*, *11*, 671–684.

Craik, F. I. M., & Tulving, E. (1975). Depth of processing and the retention of words in episodic memory. *Journal of Experimental Psychology: General*, *104*, 268–294.

Daprati, E., Nico, D., Saimpont, A., Franck, N., & Sirigu, A. (2005). Memory and action: An experimental study on normal subjects and schizophrenic patients. *Neuropsychologica*, *43*, 281–293.

Deese, J. (1959). Influence of inter-item associative strength upon immediate free recall. *Psychological Reports*, *5*, 305–312.

Dijkstra, K., & Kaschak, M. P. (2006). Encoding in verbal, enacted and autobiographical tasks in young and older adults. *Quarterly Journal of Experimental Psychology*, *59*, 1338–1345.

Engelkamp, J. (1986). Differences between imaginal and motor encoding. In F. Klix & H. Hagendorf (Eds.), *Human memory and cognitive capabilities*. Amsterdam: Elsevier, North-Holland.

Engelkamp, J., & Cohen, R. L. (1991). Current issues in memory of action events. *Psychological Research*, *53*, 175–182.

Engelkamp, J., & Dehn, D. M. (2000). Item and order information in subject-performed tasks and experimenter-performed tasks. *Journal of Experimental Psychology: Learning, Memory, and Cognition*, 26, 671–682.

Engelkamp, J., & Jahn, P. (2003). Lexical, conceptual and motor information in memory for action phrases: A multi-system account. *Acta Psychologica*, *113*, 147–165.

Engelkamp, J., & Krumnacker, H. (1980). Imagery and motor processes in the retention of verbal materials. *Zeitschrift für experimentelle und angewandte Psychologie*, *27*, 511–533.

Engelkamp, J., & Seiler, K. H. (2003). Gains and losses in action memory. *Quarterly Journal of Experimental Psychology*, *56A*, 829–848.

Engelkamp, J., Seiler, K. H., & Zimmer, H. D. (2004). Memory for actions: Item and relational information in categorized lists. *Psychological Research*, *69*, 1–10.

Engelkamp, J., & Zimmer, H. D. (1983). Zum Einfluβ von Wahrnehmen und Tun auf das Behalten von Verb-Objekt-Phrasen. *Sprache & Kognition*, *2*, 117–127.

Engelkamp, J., & Zimmer, H. D. (1984). Motor program information as a separable memory unit. *Psychological Research*, *46*, 283–299.

Engelkamp, J., & Zimmer, H. D. (1985). Motor programs and their relation to semantic memory. *General Journal of Psychology*, *9*, 239–254.

Engelkamp, J., & Zimmer, H. D. (1990). Zur Architektur des Gedächtnisses. *Magazin Forschung*, *1*, 2–7.

Engelkamp, J., & Zimmer, H. D. (1994). *The human memory: A multimodal approach*. Seattle: Hogrefe.

Engelkamp, J., & Zimmer, H. D. (1995). Similarity of movement in recognition of self-performed tasks and of verbal tasks. *British Journal of Psychology*, *86*, 241–252.

Engelkamp, J., & Zimmer, H. D. (1996). Organisation and recall in verbal tasks and subject-performed tasks. *European Journal of Cognitive Psychology*, *8*, 257–273.

Engelkamp, J., & Zimmer, H. D. (1997). Sensory factors in memory for subject-performed tasks. *Acta Psychologica*, *96*, 43–60.

Engelkamp, J., Zimmer, H. D., & Biegelmann, U. E. (1993). Bizarreness effects in verbal tasks and subject-performed tasks. *European Journal of Cognitive Psychology*, *5*, 393–415.

Engelkamp, J., Zimmer, H. D., & Mohr, G. (1990). Differential effects of concrete nouns and action verbs. *Zeitschrift für Psychologie, 198*, 189–216.

Engelkamp, J., Zimmer, H. D., Mohr, G., & Sellen, O. (1994). Memory for self-performed tasks: Self-performing during recognition. *Memory & Cognition, 22*, 34–39.

Erdelyi, M. H., & Becker, J. (1974). Hypermnesia for pictures: Incremental memory for pictures but not words in multiple recall trials. *Cognitive Psychology, 6*, 159–171.

Foley, M. A., & Johnson, M. K. (1985). Confusions between memories for performed and imagined actions: A developmental comparison. *Child Development, 54*, 51–60.

Foley, M. A., & Ratner, H. H. (2001). The role of action-based structures in activity memory. In H. D. Zimmer, R. L. Cohen, M. J. Guynn, J. Engelkamp, R. Kormi-Nouri, & M. A. Foley (Eds.), *Memory for action: A distinct form of episodic memory?* (pp. 112–135). Oxford, UK: Oxford University Press.

Freeman, J. E., & Ellis, J. A. (2003). Aging and the accessibility of performed and to-be-performed actions. *Aging Neuropsychology and Cognition, 10*, 298–309.

Gardiner, J. M., Brandt, K. R., Vargha-Khadem, F., Baddeley, A., & Mishkin, M. (2006). Effects of level of processing but not of task enactment on recognition memory in a case of developmental amnesia. *Cognitive Neuropsychology, 23*, 930–948.

Goff, L. M., & Roediger, H. L. III. (1998). Imagination inflation for action events: Repeated imaginings lead to illusory recollections. *Memory & Cognition, 26*, 20–33.

Golly-Häring, C., & Engelkamp, J. (2003). Categorical-relational and order-relational information in memory for subject-performed and experimenter-performed actions. *Journal of Experimental Psychology: Learning, Memory, and Cognition, 29*, 965–975.

Helstrup, T. (1987). One, two, or three memories? A problem-solving approach to memory for performed acts. *Acta Psychologica, 66*, 37–68.

Hirshman, E., & Bjork, R. A. (1988). The generation effect: Support for a two-factor theory. *Journal of Experimental Psychology: Learning, Memory, and Cognition, 14*, 484–494.

Jacoby, L. L. (1978). On interpreting the effects of repetition: Solving a problem versus remembering a solution. *Journal of Verbal Learning and Verbal Behavior, 17*, 649–667.

Jenkins, J. J. (1979). Four points to remember: A tetrahedral model of memory experiments. In L. S. Cermak & F. I. M. Craik (Eds.), *Levels of processing in human memory* (pp. 429–446). Hillsdale, NJ: Lawrence Erlbaum Associates, Inc.

Jenkins, J. J., & Russell, W. A. (1952). Associative clustering during recall. *Journal of Abnormal and Social Psychology, 47*, 818–821.

Karantzoulis, S., Rich, J. B., & Mangels, J. A. (2006). Subject-performed tasks improve associative learning in amnestic mild cognitive impairment. *Journal of the International Neuropsychological Society, 12*, 493–501.

Karlsson, T., Bäckman, L., Herlitz, A., Nilsson, L. G., Winblad, B., & Österlind, P. O. (1989). Memory improvement at different stages of Alzheimer's disease. *Neuropsychologia, 27*, 737–742.

Knopf, M. (1991). Having shaved a kiwi fruit: Memory of unfamiliar subject-performed actions. *Psychological Research, 53*, 203–211.

Knopf, M., Mack, W., Lenel, A., & Ferrante, S. (2005). Memory for action events: Findings in neurological patients. *Scandinavian Journal of Psychology, 46*, 11–19.

Knopf, M., & Neidhardt, E. (1989). Gedächtnis für Handlungen unterschiedlicher Vertrautheit-Hinweise aus entwicklungspsychologischen Studien. *Sprache & Kognition, 1*, 203–215.

Koriat, A., Ben-Zur, H., & Druch, A. (1991). The contextualization of input and output events in memory. *Psychological Research, 53*, 260–270.

Koriat, A., & Pearlman-Avnion, S. (2003). Memory organization of action events and its relationship to memory performance. *Journal of Experimental Psychology: General, 132*, 435–454.

Kormi-Nouri, R. (1995). The nature of memory for action events: An episodic integration view. *European Journal of Cognitive Psychology, 7*, 337–363.

Kormi-Nouri, R. (2000). The roles of movement and object in action memory: A comparative study between blind, blindfolded and sighted subjects. *Scandinavian Journal of Psychology, 41*, 71–75.

Kormi-Nouri, R., & Nilsson, L.-G. (1998). The role of integration in recognition failure and action memory. *Memory & Cognition, 26*, 681–691.

Kormi-Nouri, R., & Nilsson, L.-G. (1999). Negative cueing effects with weak and strong intralist cues. *European Journal of Cognitive Psychology, 11*, 199–218.

Kormi-Nouri, R., & Nilsson, L.-G. (2001). The motor component is not crucial! In H. D. Zimmer, R. L. Cohen, M. J. Guynn, J. Engelkamp, R. Kormi-Nouri, & M. A. Foley (Eds.), *Memory for action: A distinct form of episodic memory?* (pp. 97–111). Oxford, UK: Oxford University Press.

Kormi-Nouri, R., Nyberg, L., & Nilsson, L.-G. (1994). The effect of retrieval enactment on recall of subject-performed tasks and verbal tasks. *Memory & Cognition, 22*, 723–728.

Madigan, S. (1983). Picture memory. In J. C. Yuille (Ed.), *Imagery, memory and cognition* (pp. 65–89). Hillsdale, NJ: Lawrence Erlbaum Associates, Inc.

Mandler, G. (1967). Organization and memory. In K. W. Spence & J. T. Spence (Eds.), *The psychology of learning and motivation* (Vol. 1, pp. 327–372). New York: Academic Press.

McAndrews, M. P., & Milner, B. (1991). The frontal-cortex and memory for temporal-order. *Neuropsychologia, 29*, 849–859.

McDaniel, M. A., & Bugg, J. M. (2008). Instability in memory phenomena: A common puzzle and a unifying explanation. *Psychonomic Bulletin & Review, 15*, 237–255.

McDermott, K. B., & Roediger, H. L. (1994). Effects of imagery on perceptual implicit memory tests. *Journal of Experimental Psychology: Learning, Memory, and Cognition, 20*, 1379–1390.

Miller, G. A. (1956). The magical number seven plus or minus two: Some limits on our capacity for processing information. *Psychological Review, 63*, 81–97.

Mimura, M., Komatsu, S., Kato, M., Yashimasu, H., Wakamatsu, N., & Kashima, H. (1998). Memory for subject performed tasks in patients with Korsakoff syndrome. *Cortex, 34*, 297–303.

Mohr, G., Engelkamp, J., & Zimmer, H. D. (1989). Recall and recognition of self-performed acts. *Psychological Research, 51*, 181–187.

Mulligan, N. W., & Hornstein, S. L. (2003). Memory for actions: Self-performed tasks and the reenactment effect. *Memory & Cognition, 31*, 412–421.

Nairne, J. S., Riegler, G. L., & Serra, M. (1991). Dissociative effects of generation on item and order information. *Journal of Experimental Psychology: Learning, Memory, and Cognition, 17*, 702–709.

Nilsson, L.-G. (1979). Functions of memory. In L.-G. Nilsson (Ed.), *Perspectives on memory research: Essays in honor of Uppsala University's 500th anniversary* (pp. 3–15). Hillsdale, NJ: Lawrence Erlbaum Associates, Inc.
Nilsson, L.-G. (2000). Remembering actions and words. In E. Tulving & F. I. M. Craik (Eds.), *The Oxford handbook of memory* (pp.137–148). Oxford: Oxford University Press.
Nilsson, L.-G., & Bäckman, L. (1989). Implicit memory and the enactment of verbal instructions. In S. Lewandowksy, J. Dunn, & K. Kirsner (Eds.), *Implicit memory: Theoretical issues* (pp. 173–183). Hillsdale, NJ: Lawrence Erlbaum Associates, Inc.
Nilsson, L.-G., & Bäckman, L. (1991). Encoding dimensions of subject-performed tasks. *Psychological Research, 53*, 212–218.
Nilsson, L.-G., & Cohen, R. L. (1988). Enrichment and generation in the recall of enacted and non-enacted instructions. In M. M. Gruneberg, P. E. Morris, & R. N. Sykes (Eds.), *Practical aspects of memory: Current research and issues* (Vol. 1, pp. 427–432). Chichester, UK: Wiley.
Nilsson, L.-G., & Craik, F. I. M. (1990). Additive and interactive effects in memory for subject-performed tasks. *European Journal of Cognitive Psychology, 2*, 305–324.
Nyberg, L., & Nilsson, L.-G. (1995). The role of enactment in implicit and explicit memory. *Psychological Research, 57*, 215–219.
Nyberg, L., Persson, J., & Nilsson, L.-G. (2002). Individual differences in memory enhancement by encoding enactment: Relationships to adult age and biological factors. *Neuroscience and Biobehavioral Reviews, 26*, 835–839.
Olofsson, U. (1996). The effect of motor enactment on memory for order. *Psychological Research, 59*, 75–79.
Paivio, A. (1969). Mental imagery in associative learning and memory. *Psychological Review, 76*, 241–263.
Paivio, A., & Csapo, K. (1973). Picture superiority in free recall: Imagery or dual coding? *Cognitive Psychology, 80*, 279–285.
Paivio, A., Rogers, T. B., & Smythe, P. C. (1968). Why are pictures easier to recall than words? *Psychonomic Science, 11*, 1–2.
Paris, S. G., & Lindauer, B. (1976). The role of inference in children's comprehension and memory for sentences. *Cognitive Psychology, 8*, 217–227.
Poulton, E. C. (1963). Compensatory tracking with differentiating and integrating control systems. *Journal of Applied Psychology, 47*, 398–402.
Rajaram, S., & Roediger, H. L. (1993). Direct comparison of four implicit memory tests. *Journal of Experimental Psychology: Learning, Memory, and Cognition, 19*, 765–776.
Roediger, H. L. (2008). Relativity of remembering: Why the laws of memory vanished. *Annual Review of Psychology, 59*, 225–254.
Roediger, H. L., & Blaxton, T. A. (1987). Retrieval modes produce dissociations in memory for surface information. In D. S. Gorfein & R. R. Hoffman (Eds.), *Memory and learning: The Ebbinghaus centennial conference* (pp. 349–379). Hillsdale, NJ: Lawrence Erlbaum Associates, Inc.
Roediger, H. L., & Srinivas, K. (1993). Specificity of operations in perceptual priming. In P. Graf & M. E. J. Masson (Eds.), *Implicit memory: New directions in cognition, development and neuropsychology* (pp. 17–48). Hillsdale, NJ: Lawrence Erlbaum Associates, Inc.
Roediger, H. L., Weldon, M. S., Stadler, M. L., & Riegler, G. L. (1992). Direct comparison of two implicit memory tests: Word fragment and word stem completion.

Journal of Experimental Psychology: Learning, Memory, and Cognition, 18, 1251–1269.

Rönnlund, M., Nyberg, L., Bäckman, L., & Nilsson, L.-G. (2003). Recall of subject-performed tasks, verbal tasks, and cognitive activities across the adult life span: Parallel age-related deficits. *Aging, Neuropsychology and Cognition, 10*, 182–201.

Saltz, E., & Dixon, D. (1982). Let's pretend: The role of motoric imagery in memory for sentences and words. *Journal of Experimental Child Psychology, 34*, 77–92.

Saltz, E., & Donnerwerth-Nolan, S. (1981). Does motoric imagery facilitate memory for sentences? A selective interference test. *Journal of Verbal Learning and Verbal Behavior, 20*, 322–332.

Schacter, D. L. (1987). Implicit memory: History and current status. *Journal of Experimental Psychology: Learning, Memory, and Cognition, 13*, 501–518.

Serra, M., & Nairne, J. S. (1993). Design controversies and the generation effect: Support for an item-order hypothesis. *Memory & Cognition, 21*, 34–40.

Slamecka, N. J., & Graf, P. (1978). The generation effect: Delineation of a phenomenon. *Journal of Experimental Psychology, 26*, 589–607.

Slamecka, N. J., & Katsaiti, L. T. (1987). The generation effect as an artifact of selective displaced rehearsal. *Journal of Memory and Language, 26*, 589–607.

Steffens, M. C. (2007). Memory for goal-directed sequences of actions: Is doing better than seeing? *Psychonomic Bulletin & Review, 14*, 1194–1198.

Steffens, M. C., Buchner, A., & Wender, K. F. (2003). Quite ordinary retrieval cues may determine free recall of actions. *Journal of Memory and Language, 48*, 399–415.

Teigen, K. H. (2002). One hundred years of laws in psychology. *American Journal of Psychology, 115*, 103–118.

Thorndike, E. L. (1911). *Animal intelligence: Experimental studies.* Lewiston, NY: Macmillan.

Tulving, E. (1962). Subjective organization in free recall of "unrelated" words. *Psychological Review, 69*, 219–237.

Tulving, E. (1972). Episodic and semantic memory. In E. Tulving & W. Donaldson (Eds.), *Organization and memory* (pp. 381–403). New York: Academic Press.

Tulving, E. (1983). *Elements of episodic memory*. New York: Oxford University Press.

Tulving, E., & Schacter, D. L. (1990). Priming and human memory systems. *Science, 247*, 301–306.

Tulving, E., & Thomson, D. M. (1973). Encoding specificity and retrieval processes in episodic memory. *Psychological Review, 80*, 352–373.

Von Essen, J. D., & Nilsson, L.-G. (2003). Memory effects of motor activation in subject-performed tasks and sign language. *Psychonomic Bulletin & Review, 10*, 445–449.

Weldon, M. S., & Roediger, H. L. (1987). Altering retrieval demands reverses the picture superiority effect. *Memory & Cognition, 15*, 269–280.

Wickens, D. D. (1970). Encoding categories of words: An empirical approach to meaning. *Psychological Review, 77*, 1–15.

Zimmer, H. D. (1991). Memory after motoric encoding in a generation-recognition model. *Psychological Research, 53*, 226–231.

Zimmer, H. D. (1994). Representation and processing of the spatial layout of objects with verbal and nonverbal input. In W. Schnotz & R. W. Kulhavy (Eds.), *Comprehension and graphics* (pp. 97–112). Amsterdam: Elsevier, North Holland.

Zimmer, H. D., & Cohen (2001). Remembering actions: A specific type of memory? In H.D. Zimmer, R. L. Cohen, M. J. Guynn, J. Engelkamp, R. Kormi-Nouri, &

M. A. Foley (Eds.), *Memory for action: A distinct form of episodic memory?* (pp. 3–24). Oxford, UK: Oxford University Press.

Zimmer, H. D., Cohen, R. L., Guynn, M. J., Engelkamp, J., Kormi-Nouri, R., & Foley, M. A. (2001). *Memory for action: A distinct form of episodic memory?* Oxford, UK: Oxford University Press.

Zimmer, H. D., & Engelkamp, J. (1984). Planungs- und ausführungsanteile motorischer gedächtniskomponenten und ihre wikrung auf das behalten ihrer verbalen bezeichnungen. *Zeitschrift für Psychologie*, *192*, 379–402.

Zimmer, H. D., & Engelkamp, J. (1989). Does motor encoding enhance relational information? *Psychological Research*, *51*, 158–167.

Zimmer, H. D., & Engelkamp, J. (1999). Levels of processing effects in subject-performed tasks. *Memory & Cognition*, *27*, 907–914.

Zimmer, H. D., & Engelkamp, J. (2003). Signing enhances memory like performing actions. *Psychonomic Bulletin & Review*, *10*, 450–454.

4 Visual perceptual memory – *anno* 2008

Svein Magnussen, Mark W. Greenlee, Oliver Baumann, and Tor Endestad

Introduction

The concept of perceptual memory refers to the neural and cognitive processes underlying the storage of sensory information along such basic stimulus dimensions as spatial frequency, orientation, and motion (Magnussen, 2000; Magnussen & Greenlee, 1999). The concept is related to, but not identical with, the concept of visual working memory (Baddeley, 2003). In perceptual memory experiments, memory is assessed in terms of the precision by which stimulus information is retained in memory, rather than in terms of the number of visual items or categories that can be retained; with a research strategy, that is closer to the correspondence metaphor of memory than it is to the storehouse metaphor (Koriat, Goldsmith, & Pansky, 2000).

Research on visual perceptual memory has a long scientific history, beginning with a paper by Fredrich Hegelmaier in 1852 on the memory for line length, in which he, prior to Fechner (1860), introduced the psychophysical method of constant stimuli and published the first experimental data on perceptual memory (Laming & Laming, 1992). Hegelmaier's paper was quickly forgotten – if indeed ever noticed – and the study of memory took a different course, largely owing to the impact of another German scientist, Herman Ebbinghaus. However, the study of perceptual memory survived in psychophysics (Laming & Scheiwiller, 1985) and was revived two decades ago, when it grew out of research on the mechanisms of visual processing (Magnussen, Greenlee, Asplund, & Dyrnes, 1990; Regan, 1985), a context in which it has remained, separated from mainstream memory research. The programme of modern perceptual memory research as formulated by Magnussen et al. (1990) has aimed to bridge the gap between perception and memory, noting that even if the simplest perceptual process involves the linking of online sensory signals with stored representations, perception and memory research progressed along parallel, isolated paths. Traditional research on visual memory employed alphanumeric stimuli or pictures of meaningful scenes that invited higher level categorical coding; thus, little could be concluded from these experiments regarding the perceptual component of visual memory. The strategy chosen by perceptual memory researchers was to start by investigating the storage of those elemental attributes of the visual stimulus that electrophysiological experiments on animal models and psychophysical studies on humans strongly indicated were the building blocks of visual perception – spatial frequency, orientation, motion, and colour (DeValois & DeValois, 1990; Pasternak, Bisley, & Valkins, 2003) – and from there to move on to more complex visual patterns and realistic pictures. The idea that visual memory recruited processes involved in online perceptual processing was not new (e.g., see Damasio, 1989), and several more recent brain imaging studies confirm the recruitment of early areas of visual analysis in visual imagery (Ganis, Thompson, & Kosslyn, 2004; Kosslyn & Thompson, 2003; Slotnick, Thompson, & Kosslyn, 2005). The new aspect in the study of visual perceptual memory was the use of experimental methods borrowed from psychophysics and theoretical models taken from research on spatial vision.

The basic experiment

Figure 4.1 illustrates the basic design of a visual perceptual memory experiment using the classic tool of vision research – sinusoidal gratings – which are computer-generated patterns where the luminance is modulated in a sinusoidal fashion. The grating may vary in spatial frequency (defined as the number of light–dark cycles per unit visual angle) or in contrast and orientation, and it may be stationary, flickering, or moving, varying in direction and speed of movement. The space-average luminance of the grating equals

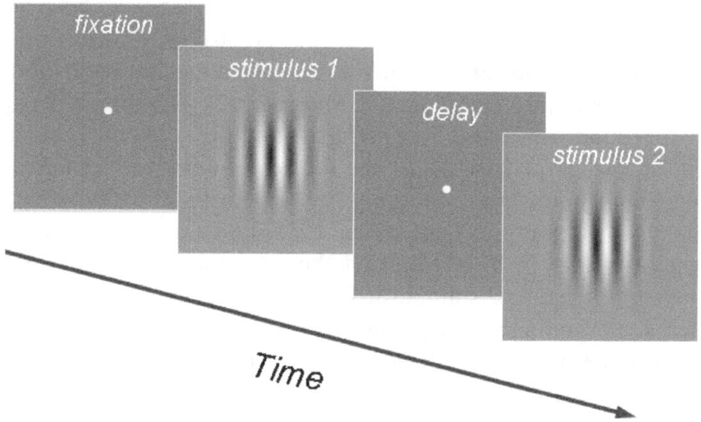

Figure 4.1 Illustrating the delayed discrimination experiment to explore visual perceptual memory with sinusoidal gratings modulated by a Gaussian envelope. In a two-alternative forced-choice task, the observer decides which of two gratings, Stimulus 1 or Stimulus 2, has the higher (or lower) spatial frequency. The gratings are separated by variable inter-stimulus intervals, and discrimination thresholds (or some equivalent measure) index the precision of perceptual storage of S1.

the background luminance, and in most modern experiments the grating is modulated by a Gaussian envelope to avoid external cues to discrimination (e.g., Baumann, Endestad, Magnussen, & Greenlee, 2008; Lalonde & Chaudhuri, 2002). Such simple patterns allow direct measurement of perceptual discriminations of spatial frequency (or size), orientation, contrast, and motion, which are the main features to which neurons in the primary visual cortex, area V1, are tuned (DeValois & DeValois, 1990; Pasternak et al., 2003). This chapter will limit the discussion to the features of spatial frequency and motion.

In a perceptual memory experiment, memory is measured in a delayed discrimination task with a variable interval between the two stimuli to be compared. The observer fixates a blank computer screen, a reference grating is briefly flashed, followed by an inter-stimulus interval of 1–60 s, and a brief presentation of a test grating of higher or lower value in, for example, spatial frequency, and the observer's task is to decide which of the two gratings had the higher value. With adaptive procedures, the computer algorithm selects two new stimuli whose spatial frequencies depend on whether the answer on the previous trial was correct or incorrect, whereas in other experimental designs a large range of stimulus pairs with preset values are presented in random order; in both cases, the reference spatial frequency is jittered so that the observer is never confronted with the exact same stimulus twice and, in order to solve the task, has to remember the spatial frequency of a novel reference grating on each trial. Such trial-by-trial jitter of the reference frequency is an important control in perceptual memory experiments to avoid forming permanent long-term representations of a particular spatial frequency. Several authors have also pointed out the possible danger of testing regimes such as the method of constant stimuli, in which observers may form a representation of an imaginary "reference" by repeated exposure to a range of testing frequencies alone (Lages & Treisman, 1998) and no short-term memory of the individual reference grating is required to yield a psychometric function and discrimination threshold. In light of these precautions, memory for spatial frequency (or orientation, contrast, motion) is measured by the delayed discrimination threshold, $\Delta F/F$, or some equivalent measure, and the time course of memory decay can be tracked by varying the time interval between the two stimuli (ISI). Memory decay is indexed by changes in the discrimination threshold as the representation of the reference grating fades over time.

Somewhat surprisingly, the results of a number of experiments showed that at least for some basic attributes, such as spatial frequency and motion, discrimination thresholds did not change across intervals of 30–60 s, suggesting little or no decay in the precision of perceptual information in short-term memory (Bennett & Cortese, 1996; Blake, Cepeda, & Hiris, 1997; Lalonde & Chaudhuri, 2002; Magnussen & Greenlee, 1992; Magnussen et al., 1990). Furthermore, in many of the experiments, delayed spatial frequency discrimination thresholds were in the hyper-acuity range, with thresholds below the value expected based on cone spacing of the retina (Magnussen, 2000; Magnussen & Greenlee, 1999). Thus, sensory representations of the spatial frequency and the speed of a moving grating is maintained in short-term memory for periods exceeding 10 s with the same fidelity of simultaneous comparisons of test and reference stimulus pairs. Figure 4.2a illustrates this point, plotting some representative data for the memory of spatial frequency and motion. For other attributes, such as orientation, a slight decay is reported (Magnussen, Idås, & Holst Myhre, 1998), whereas memory for the contrast of gratings shows pronounced decay in short-term memory (Magnussen, Greenlee, & Thomas, 1996). The difference in decay across various attributes suggests different types of neural representations (Greenlee, Magnusssen, & Thomas, 1991).

A close association between mechanisms of perceptual discrimination and memory does not imply that they represent the same processes; most concepts of memory assume a process that is distinct from online perceptual analysis, in the sense that information is transformed into a memory code. In psychophysical and cognitive research, memory is defined operationally by the time factor – memory starts when the stimulus goes off – rather than in terms of separate brain processes. The measure of accuracy of memory performance indexes the final outcome of the memory process and cannot distinguish between intermediate processes. However, measurements of the time spent on the decision in delayed discrimination might indicate the time of transfer from a perceptual code to a memory code, on the logic that if information is transferred to a memory code and later retrieved, the process of retrieving information would be added to the discrimination task in the memory condition. Thus, the observer should spend more time on the decision in the delayed compared to the simultaneous discrimination task, and the retention interval at which response times starts to increase should be an indicator of the time of transfer from a perceptual mode to a memory mode (Magnussen, 2000; Magnussen & Greenlee, 1999).

The results of several experiments confirmed that choice reaction times were prolonged in delayed discrimination tasks (Baumann et al., 2008; Greenlee, Koessler, Cornelissen, & Mergner, 1997; Reinvang, Magnussen, & Greenlee, 2002; Reinvang, Magnussen, Greenlee, & Larsson, 1998; Rothmayr et al., 2007). A systematic study of the short-term memory for spatial frequency and orientation (Magnussen et al., 1998) showed, first, that this increase was not the result of increased uncertainty in predicting the arrival of the test grating at longer ISIs, and, second, that the transfer from a perceptual mode to a memory mode occurred after 3–4 s following termination of the reference grating. The shape of this function is illustrated in Figure 4.2b, which plots results from several unpublished experiments from our laboratory, probing a series of spatial frequencies and ISIs. Choice RTs start to rise after about 4 s, then increase with retention time in the short-term interval of 10 s. These results suggest that during the first 3 to 4 s following termination of a visual stimulus, information of elemental attributes of the visual stimulus

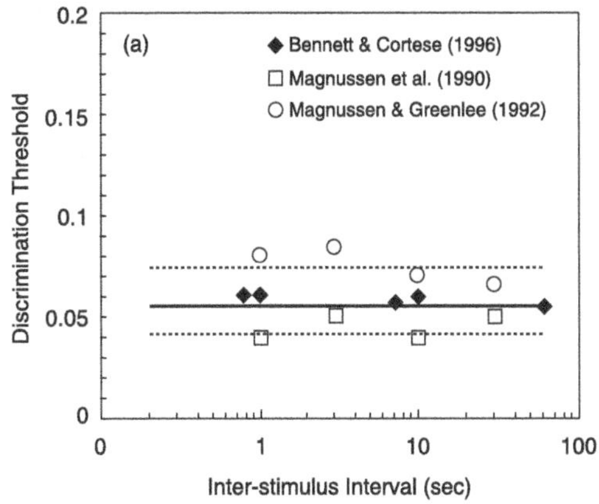

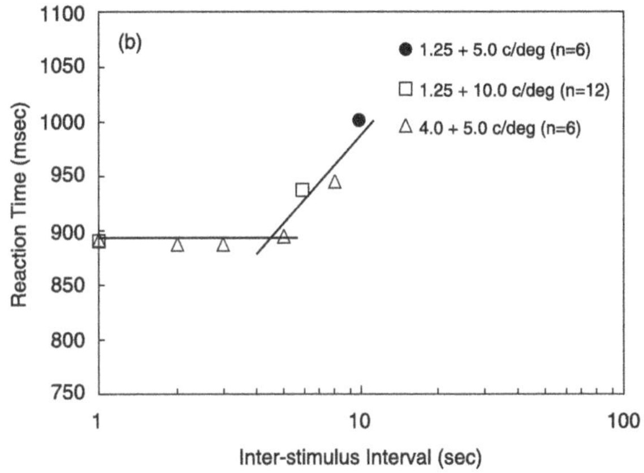

Figure 4.2 (a) Delayed discriminations thresholds for spatial frequency and motion as a function of inter-stimulus interval. Results for spatial frequency are single-subject data re-plotted from Magnussen et al. (1990, Fig. 4) and Bennett and Cortese (1996, Fig. 1); results for motion are re-plotted from Magnussen and Greenlee (1992, Fig. 2), representing the average of two observers. (b) Choice reaction times in a delayed discrimination of spatial frequency as a function of inter-stimulus interval (ISI). Results are pooled from a number of experiments testing different spatial frequencies and ISIs, normalized to a common RT value for ISI = 1 s.

is maintained in a real-time-like form, as accessible as online representations, before the transformation from a perceptual-type representation to a memory-type representation takes place. Furthermore, the physiological representation of spatial frequency (and motion) is maintained in short-term memory with a fidelity that matches the real-time physiological image. Thus, the transfer from a sensory representation to a short-term memory representation does not imply a loss of resolution of the spatial frequency or motion signals.

In describing this memory feat, we use the term "perceptual short-term memory" rather than the currently more popular "working memory concept" (Baddeley, 2003), chiefly because the memory performance in these experiments cannot be understood as an expression of episodic memory. Obviously, in most situations, including the experimental situations probing perceptual memory, several memory systems are activated in parallel, and the resulting performance may be supported by several systems (Tulving, 2002). In these experiments episodic memory is activated as the observer remembers seeing a grating and perhaps whether stripes were thick or thin, but the memory performance in delayed discriminations with a spatial resolution in the hyperacuity range only turns up in forced choice experiments and does not have a conscious counterpart. On the contrary, the observer often has the feeling of just guessing, but also a feeling of guessing correctly. From these observations we conclude that the high-fidelity memory performance in delayed discrimination experiments is based on an implicit or non-declarative type of memory (Schacter, Wagner, & Buckner, 2000), rather than on explicit or declarative memory. Consistent with this interpretation, Tanaka and Sagi (1998a, 1998b) found evidence for sub-threshold priming of detection of Gabor patterns in the short-term memory range, and the priming effect was selective for features of the visual stimulus such as spatial frequency and orientation. Additional support for the hypothesis that visual perceptual memory performance is based on implicit memory is the finding that the performance on this memory task is similar for young and elderly subjects (Bennett, Sekuler, McIntosh, & Della-Maggiore, 2001; Della-Maggiore et al., 2000). Several studies of memory and aging have shown that indicators of implicit memory, such as priming, are not affected by age whereas tests of explicit memory performances exhibit age decline (Bäckman, Small, & Wahlin, 2001; Nilsson, 2003).

Perceptual short-term memory is robust

Visual perceptual short-term memory is astonishingly robust, with memory decay being resistant to a number of factors that affect spatial frequency or motion discrimination performance. The absence of age effects has already been noted, and several studies of patients with focal brain damage show intact short-term memory performance, albeit overall impaired discrimination performances. Greenlee, Rischewski, Mergner, and Seeger (1993) tested patients with focal lesions in the infero-temporal (IT) and superior temporal (ST) cortex on delayed spatial frequency discrimination and found that both groups were impaired in spatial frequency discrimination compared to normal controls, but that there were no significant effects of memory delay (1–10 s) – that is, discrimination performance is impaired but the subsequent course of memory is not affected – and the short-term memory functions for the patient and control participants were comparable. A similar pattern of results was reported by Greenlee, Lang, Mergner, and Seeger (1995) in a study of delayed velocity discrimination, with impaired velocity discrimination, but the overall effect of memory delay in the patients with lesions in ST, IT, or lateral parietal cortex (LP) was only significant for the ST region. Greenlee et al. (1997) tested patients with lesions in the occipito-temporal (OT), ST, and frontal cortex for the short-term memory of block patterns, and again they observed no additional impairment of the discrimination performance (assessed by *d′*) across memory delay.

Some factors that might be expected to affect spatial frequency or motion discrimination do not act either on thresholds in simultaneous discrimination or on the subsequent memory function as indexed by delayed discrimination. For example, delayed spatial frequency discriminations are not affected by the relative orientation of reference and test gratings (Magnussen et al., 1990, 1998) and, in a similar fashion, delayed orientation discriminations are not affected by the relative spatial frequency of the gratings (Magnussen et al., 1998). Discrimination thresholds of single components of complex gratings are similar to those of simple gratings, and with no memory decay (Magnussen & Greenlee, 1999). The contrast of the gratings may be varied randomly across trials without affecting spatial frequency discrimination thresholds or the decay function, and in delayed discrimination of spatial frequency and contrast in a dual-task design, neither thresholds nor the subsequent course of memory are affected for either component, when the effect of stimulus uncertainty is factored out (Magnussen et al., 1996; Thomas, Magnussen, & Greenlee, 2000). Similar results were obtained for dual judgments of two contrast components (Magnussen et al., 1996); thus, even if contrast information declines, the slope of the decay function appears to be quite resistant to interference.

A number of experimental factors that degrade the perceptual discrimination process leave the memory function intact. Magnussen et al. (1990) found that thresholds increased as the contrast of the test and reference grating increased, but the decay functions were parallel for low- and high-contrast gratings. Similar results were reported for velocity discrimination of gratings with low and high velocities; thresholds were higher for high-velocity gratings, but the short-term memory functions were parallel (Magnussen & Greenlee, 1992). When observers are required to remember more than one spatial frequency or spatial frequency combinations, thresholds increase or accuracy scores decline, but the subsequent memory function is uncorrupted (Kahana & Sekuler, 2002; Magnussen & Greenlee, 1997, 1999). Similar results were reported by Blake et al. (1997) for motion. When the task load was increased by having the observer remember several directions of motion presented in sequence, the discrimination performance decreased in proportion to the number of motion components that had to be remembered, but this task load factor did not interact with retention time on memory performance.

Taken together, these findings are consistent with the recent hypothesis that decay in perceptual memory is deterministic rather than the result of random perturbations of visual representations as time goes by (Gold, Murray, Sekuler, Bennett, & Sekuler, 2005). The course of memory decay is remarkably unaffected by subject factors and by experimental manipulations that impair the over-all level of discrimination performance. So far, two exceptions to this general rule have been reported. First, Ben-Yehudah and Ahissar (2004) have found that delayed as compared with simultaneous spatial frequency discrimination is consistently impaired among adult dyslectics, suggesting that a deficit in perceptual short-term memory may be involved. Second, Magnussen et al. (1996) showed that when participants had to keep track of spatial frequency information in a design where the absolute spatial frequency of the reference grating varied across a wide spatial frequency range, the short-term memory for spatial frequency started to decay. Similarly, the decay of memory for grating contrast was more pronounced with large variations in reference contrast.

A model of perceptual memory

Based on the psychophysical results, we proposed a model of perceptual discrimination and memory that assumes that information about elementary stimulus attributes is processed in a network of independent special-purpose memory stores, each devoted to a particular attribute or dimension of the visual stimulus. Each attribute or dimension is represented by an array of memory elements that extract information about one dimension (e.g., spatial frequency) across other dimensions (e.g., orientation). It is further assumed that each individual element in an array represents a limited range along a given stimulus dimension and that elements are linked in a lateral inhibitory network. This arrangement allows inhibition within but not between dimensions. It is further assumed that the special-purpose memory stores draw on independent attentional resources.

The model assumes that discrimination and memory are based on representations that are located at an early stage in the visual process, but beyond visual area V1; this higher order processing stage combines information from V1-type neural representations that are tuned to multiple dimensions of the visual stimulus (DeValois & DeValois, 1990; Pasternak et al., 2003). Results of Magnussen et al. (1998) suggest that this extraction process is performed in terms of a "cortical search" of low-level (V1) representations. They found that when, in delayed spatial frequency discrimination, the relative orientation difference of the reference and test gratings was altered, discrimination thresholds remained unaffected but choice reaction times increased linearly with the separation angle of the reference and test gratings. Likewise, changing the relative spatial frequencies of the gratings in an orientation discrimination task did not affect discrimination accuracy but increased choice RTs. For both conditions the increase in RT added linearly to the increase in choice RT produced by changing the memory delay. The effect is analogous to mental rotation and size transformation (Bundesen, Larsen, & Farrell, 1981), except that it is not accompanied by a conscious strategy of rotation. Rather, it appears as if the brain performs a search across multiple representations in an arrangement of multiple-tuned channels where the functional distance between units coding neighbouring spatial frequencies is greater for units that simultaneously code very different orientations than for units that code neighbouring spatial frequencies and similar or neighbouring orientations. The functional organization in orientation columns and spatial frequency rows of multiple-tuned neurons of V1 proposed by Maffei and Fiorentini (1977) and DeValois and DeValois (1990) would be ideally suited for such a systematic search, but more recent results indicate that this very orderly anatomical organization is probably too simple (Everson et al., 1998; Sirovich & Uglesich, 2004). However, the precise functional organization map of orientation and spatial frequency coding is not critical to the theory.

Thus, the important assumptions of the models are, first, that perceptual short-term memory is based on dimension-specific neural representations beyond V1 that extracts information from multiple-tuned early (V1) representations, and, second, that memory representations are separate from perceptual representations, with a transfer between representational modes after 3–4 s following termination of a stimulus.

Psychophysical evidence

This model fits most of the psychophysical data. First, discrimination and memory of one attribute are not affected by variations along an irrelevant dimension (Magnussen et al., 1998). Second, dual-judgment experiments comparing discrimination and short-term memory for two simultaneously processed stimulus components show that different dimensions (e.g., contrast and spatial frequency) are processed in parallel, but the task of keeping track of two components on the same dimension (e.g., two spatial frequencies or two contrasts) leads to strong interference and substantial increase in discrimination thresholds (Magnussen & Greenlee, 1997; Magnussen et al., 1996; Thomas et al., 2000); however, the memory functions remain unaffected. Third, manipulations of stimulus complexity by varying one dimension of the stimulus acts on the discrimination threshold of that dimension but leaves discrimination and memory for simultaneously processed other dimensions unaffected (Magnussen et al., 1996).

Fourth, the most powerful psychophysical evidence for the model comes from experiments on so-called memory masking. Memory masking, originally demonstrated by Magnussen, Greenlee, Asplund, and Dyrnes (1991) and confirmed in a number of studies of the memory for spatial frequency (Bennett & Cortese, 1996; Lalonde & Chaudhuri, 2002) and motion (Magnussen & Greenlee, 1992; McKeefry, Burton, & Vakrou, 2007), refers to the detrimental effect on delayed discrimination thresholds produced by a masker stimulus presented briefly during the interval between reference and test. The basic phenomenon is illustrated in Figure 4.3, re-plotting results from experiments on spatial frequency and motion.

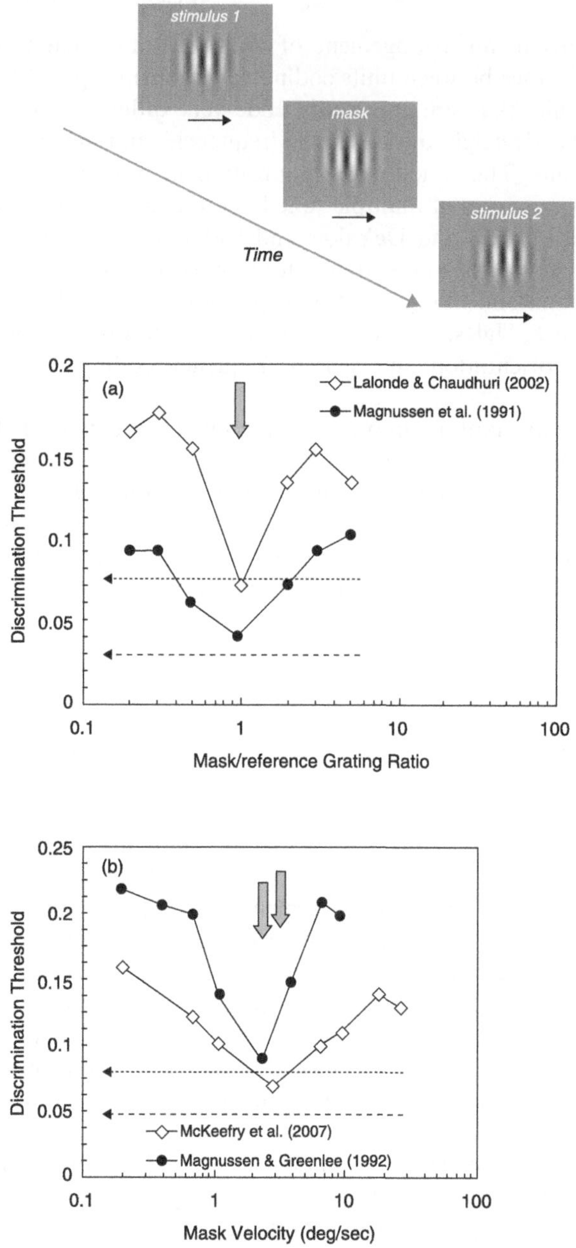

Figure 4.3 Memory masking. (a) Results for spatial frequency, re-plotted from Magnussen et al. (1991, Fig. 2, average of two observers) and Lalonde and Chaudhuri (2002, Fig. 2, average of three observers). Horizontal dashed lines indicate discrimination thresholds in the absence of a masker. (b) Memory masking of motion thresholds. Results are re-plotted from Magnussen and Greenlee (1992, Fig. 3c, average of two observers) and McKeefry et al. (2007, Fig. 2, average of three observers).

Basically, in a memory masking experiment, a masker stimulus is presented during a 10-s ISI, at a point in time during the ISI that is well out of reach of conventional sensory masking in both forward and backward directions (Ogmen, Breitmeyer, & Melvin, 2003). The masking effect is precisely the opposite of sensory masking, in which maximal masking effect is observed with identical test and masker stimuli and the masking effect decreases when the masker moves away from the test stimulus in spatial frequency or orientation. In memory masking of spatial frequency, no masking effect is observed when the spatial frequency of the test/reference and masker gratings are similar, and the masking effect increases as the masker frequency moves away from the reference/test frequency in both directions and reaches a maximum value of a difference of approximately ±1 octave; beyond this value there is evidence for a gradual return to baseline. The size of the masking effect is about a doubling in delayed discrimination thresholds in the various experiments (Bennett & Cortese, 1996; Lalonde & Chaudhuri, 2002; Magnussen et al., 1991; McKeefry et al., 2007). The stimulus selectivity of the memory masking effect fits the hypothesis of inhibition between channels, as the selectivity of the masking effects agrees well with the results of classical psychophysical studies of channel width by masking and spatial adaptation, which is believed to reflect the selectivity of V1 neurons (Blakemore & Campbell, 1969; Greenlee & Magnussen, 1988; Greenlee, Magnussen, & Nordby, 1988). However, memory masking is selective to the *perceived* spatial frequency rather than to the retinal spatial frequency, suggesting that the mechanism of masking is located at a level in the processing stream at which size and shape constancies are computed (Bennett & Cortese, 1996).

Further evidence for a location of the perceptual memory mechanism beyond VI is the observation that, in contrast to sensory masking, memory masking is selective to interference along the dimension on which perceptual discrimination is required but not along other dimensions. Thus, in delayed discrimination of spatial frequency, interference is observed when masker frequency is varied but the discrimination performance is insensitive to changes in the orientation of the masker (Magnussen et al., 1991), and, conversely, changing the spatial frequency of the masker does not affect orientation discrimination (Lalonde & Chaudhuri, 2002). Likewise, memory masking of motion is selective to the speed of the masker grating, but not to the direction of motion (Magnussen & Greenlee, 1992), nor to the spatial/temporal frequency of the grating (McKeefry et al., 2007). Direct evidence for the involvement of cortical areas beyond V1 in the perceptual memory was provided by Campana, Cowey, and Walsh (2002), who showed that transcranial magnetic stimulation (TMS) applied to area V5/MT disrupted perceptual priming of speed discrimination, whereas stimulation to V1 or posterior parietal cortex (PPC) had no effect. Furthermore, TMS applied to V5/MT selectively affected priming of motion, leaving priming of colour discrimination intact. In a follow-up study, Campana, Cowey, and Walsh (2006) found that disruption of V5/MT activity is also inefficient in disturbing memory for spatial position.

Lalonde and Chaudhuri (2002) tested the hypothesis of a two-stage mechanism of perceptual memory, taking advantage of the memory masking effect. They reasoned that if perceptual representations and memory representations were different, the effect of a masker grating required that the masker and the stimulus on which it acted had to be in the same representational mode. They performed two experiments. In the first experiment the masker was presented 3 s or 10 s before the reference grating, which was followed by the test grating after 6 s. Thus, when representation of the masker stimulus was in a perceptual mode (3-s interval; see Figure 4.2), memory masking would be normal, but when the masker representation had transferred to a memory mode, it would not affect a subsequently presented reference grating and no masking would be observed. The results confirmed the prediction. However, the results of the second experiment modified this conclusion. In this experiment, information about the masker stimulus had to be kept alive, because the subject had to perform a second (and easier) discrimination task on the same trials, where the masker had to be compared to a fourth grating presented after the principal discrimination task had been completed. The results now showed normal memory masker functions for both 3-s and 10-s masker-reference intervals. This suggests that some form of attentional control of information, perhaps through a refreshing mechanism similar to the visuospatial sketchpad (Baddeley, 2003), is necessary. These findings suggest either that information may be maintained in a perceptual mode by the refreshing mechanism or, if transferred to a short-term memory representation, that there is interference between spatial frequencies at the level of short-term memory representation. This question remains unsettled.

Brain imaging of perceptual memory

All experimental tasks requiring focal attention and conscious perception recruit a common set of overlapping brain regions (Naghavi & Nyberg, 2005). In visual perceptual memory experiments, conventional visual working memory mechanisms are obviously activated in parallel with the memory mechanisms responsible for the high-fidelity perceptual memory performance. This parallel activation of memory systems makes it difficult to isolate the perceptual memory component of the activation patterns.

A limited set of brain areas have been identified as the neural correlates of visual short-term memory by means of PET (Bennett et al., 2001; Cornette, Dupont, & Orban, 2002; Della-Maggiore et al., 2000), ERP (Reinvang et al., 1998), and fMRI (Pessoa, Gutierrez, Bandettini, & Ungerleider, 2002; Rothmayr et al., 2007). Among these is posterior parietal cortex, which may reflect the neural capacity limit of visual working memory (Todd & Marois, 2004). Using a multiple-stimulus display to test the capacity of visual working memory, Xu and Chun (2006) have proposed that the inferior intraparietal sulcus (IPS), the superior IPS, and the lateral occipital cortex (LOC) work in parallel to support visual memory encoding and maintenance. They suggest that representations in inferior IPS may be limited to a fixed number of objects, whereas capacity in LOC and superior IPS is limited by object complexity. LOC and superior IPS may thus participate in storing detailed representations of stimuli in visual working memory. In addition, various striate and extra-striate areas of the occipital cortex have been identified as visual perceptual memory correlates (Greenlee, Magnussen, & Reinvang, 2000). Interestingly, relatively early visual areas beyond V1, which have previously only been associated with visual perception, are also active during visual memory delays (for a review, see Pasternak & Greenlee, 2005). Most studies that investigated visual memory found activity in the prefrontal cortex (PFC). The dorsolateral prefrontal cortex (DLPFC; BA 46/9) seems to play a crucial role in working memory-related processes (e.g., Fuster, 2001; Goldman-Rakic, 1995; Zhang, Leung, & Johnson, 2003). DLPFC activity has foremost been found in studies that required the manipulation of relevant items in working memory (e.g., Baumann, Frank, Rutschmann, & Greenlee, 2007b; Cornette, Dupont, Bormans, Mortelmans, & Orban, 2001). Many of these studies have used *n*-back tasks in which the subject has to remember an item presented *n* trials ago and match it to the present item. Delayed discrimination tasks, on the other hand, show less DLPFC activity (e.g., Faillenot, Sunaert, Van Hecke, & Orban, 2001). Contrary to working memory tasks, delayed discrimination tasks only require the maintenance of an item and not its manipulation. A role for DLPFC in the active manipulation of material in visual working memory has been shown (Cabeza & Nyberg, 2000), and DLPFC appears to be involved also in the storage of visual information for several objects (Leung, Gore, & Goldman-Rakic, 2002). Dorsolateral prefrontal cortex, posterior parietal cortex, and regions in the occipital cortex thus appear to work together, and their exact interactions will depend on task demands.

In an attempt to highlight the perceptual memory process, we recently used fMRI to explore the neural correlates of the delayed discrimination of Gabor stimuli differing in spatial frequency (Baumann, Endestad, Magnussen, & Greenlee, 2007a). Fifteen subjects were instructed to code the spatial frequency with retention periods of 6-s duration. Participants had to decide whether two Gabor stimuli, which were presented sequentially and separated by a delay period, had the same or a different spatial frequency. There were two different difficulty levels of the task: one involving Gabor stimuli with very low spatial frequency that were easily coded by counting the dark bars of the Gabor grating, the second involving Gabor stimuli with a high spatial frequency where the first strategy could not be employed. To prepare the subjects for an upcoming trial, a central prompt was presented 2 s before the appearance of the reference stimuli, indicating also whether it would be an easy or a difficult trial. Since the activation pattern for both conditions were highly similar, we report the average of both conditions (see Figure 4.4).

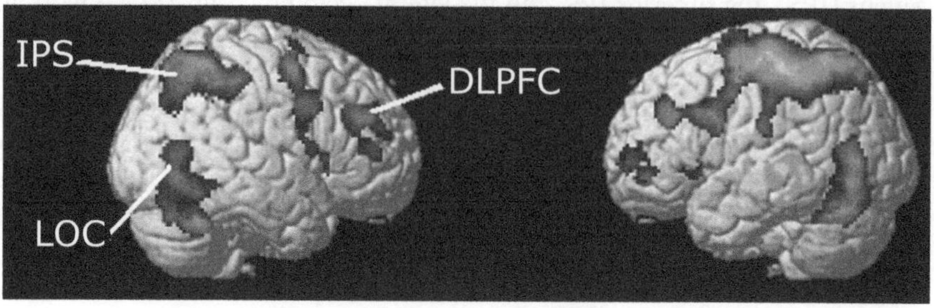

Figure 4.4 Group activation map illustrating significant activity associated with the 6-s retention period. The fMRI data was processed and analysed using Statistical Parametric Mapping SPM 2 (SPM2, Wellcome Department of Cognitive Neurology, London, UK; http://www.fil.ion.ucl.ac.uk/spm/) implemented in MATLAB (The MathWorks, Inc.). In a random-effects group analysis using the general linear model we found the expected activation pattern: DLPFC, superior and inferior parietal cortex, and lateral occipital cortex were clearly activated during the retention period of 6 s. (This figure is published in colour at http://www.cognitiveneurosciencearena.com/brain-scans/.)

A region of interest (ROI) analysis was conducted using "Marsbar" (Brett, Anton, Valabregue, & Poline, 2002). We defined the DLPFC, the superior intraparietal sulcus (sIPS), the inferior intraparietal sulcus (iIPS), and the LOC as regions of interest (see Figures 4.4 and 4.5). The regions were activated in our group random-effects analysis, and the coordinates were congruent with the literature (Volle et al., 2005; Xu & Chun, 2006). The blood oxygen level dependent (BOLD) signal of the voxels for each of these regions was averaged, and the relative change of the BOLD signal during the retention period was computed in comparison to the average activity in these ROIs for the entire fMRI measurement. The BOLD signal in the LOC and sIPS showed separate peaks for the presentation of the prompt and the reference stimulus, whereby the amplitude related to the reference stimulus was much higher. In contrast, the BOLD response of the iIPS to the prompt was sustained until the presentation of the reference stimulus. Compared to the LOC and sIPS, the response in the iIPS to the test stimulus also exhibited a somewhat delayed and more enduring response. These findings suggest that the activation patterns of sIPS and LOC indicate their involvement in the encoding and retrieval processes for the Gabor stimuli, while the activity in the inferior IPS seems to be related to a more general attentional component.

The DLPFC shows a left/right dissociation, with the left DLPFC activated during the encoding period and the right DLPFC during the retrieval period. This pattern is in concordance with the hemispheric encoding/retrieval asymmetry (HERA) model (Habib, Nyberg, & Tulving 2003). Virtually all studies that investigated visual working memory found activity in the

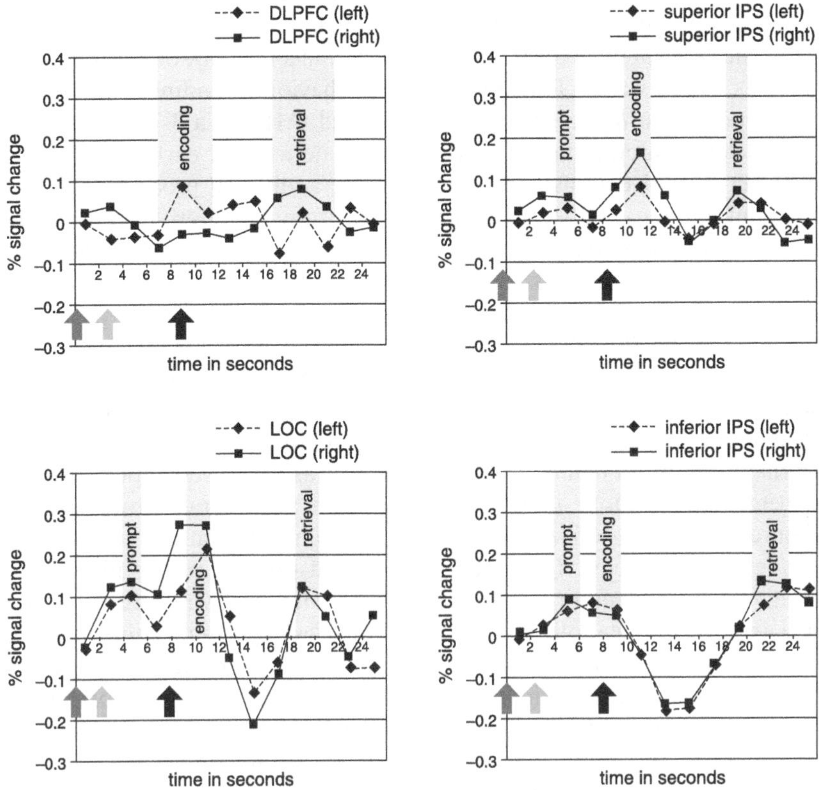

Figure 4.5 Time course of percent BOLD signal change for the four regions of interest. The dark-grey arrow indicates the appearance of the prompt at 0 s, the light-grey arrow the appearance of the reference stimuli at 2 s (subject had to encode the spatial frequency of a Gabor stimulus), and the black arrow with the test stimuli at 8 s (subject had to judge whether the test and the reference grating had the same spatial frequency). The grey-shaded areas indicate onset and duration of hypothetical cognitive processes associated with changes in the BOLD signal.

prefrontal cortex. DLPFC activity has foremost been reported in studies that required the manipulation of relevant items in memory (e.g., Baumann et al., 2007b; Cornette et al., 2001). Delayed discrimination tasks, on the other hand, show less DLPFC activity (Faillenot et al., 2001), and the present results are consistent with this finding.

The results of this experiment shows that the activity pattern evoked in a perceptual memory experiment is basically similar to the activity pattern evoked by conventional visual working memory experiments (Naghavi & Nyberg, 2005), except for a generally lower DLPFC activity, which is to be expected as the experimental task itself must activate working memory mechanisms. In a further attempt to isolate a perceptual memory component, we recently conducted an fMRI experiment (Baumann et al., 2008) designed to test the concept of cortical serial search within a network of multiple-tuned channels, which was so far only based on behavioural findings (Magnussen, 2000; Magnussen & Greenlee, 1999). We used fMRI in a 3-T head scanner and a delayed discrimination task to investigate whether early visual cortex, or higher cognitive areas, are involved in the additional processing of task-irrelevant stimulus properties indicated, for example, by prolonged reaction times for the discrimination of spatial frequencies with large orientation differences. Subjects were asked to remember for 8 s the spatial frequency of centrally presented Gabor stimuli that had either the same or a different orientation. The BOLD fMRI revealed significantly elevated bilateral activity in visual areas V1 and V2 (BA 17 and BA 18) when the gratings to be compared had an orthogonal orientation, compared to when they had the same orientation. The activation of low-level visual areas and the additional finding that no prefrontal and parietal activation was observed supports a model of perceptual memory in which task-relevant information from low-level resources for dimensions like spatial frequency and orientation is extracted by high-level components. It further suggests that the retrieval of high-fidelity visual information requires activation of different stores, which requires more time and higher metabolic costs even if an irrelevant stimulus dimension has been changed. The differential contrast between the activations evoked by the conditions in which stimuli had the same or the orthogonal orientation eliminates any non-specific activations related to the general nature of the memory task. Therefore, these results point to an automatic "cortical search" process that compares information for one stimulus dimension (e.g., spatial frequency) over all other possible stimulus dimensions (e.g., orientation). The results of this study imply that the perceptual memory representations studied in delayed discrimination of orientation and spatial frequency are located quite early in the cortical processing streams.

What are the functions of perceptual memory?

Two decades of research on visual perceptual memory have provided solid evidence for a separate perceptual memory mechanism, closely associated with mechanisms of visual discrimination and located early in the processing stream and organized in terms of a set of parallel, independent domain-specific storage mechanisms. The model outlined above is consistent with most of the available experimental evidence. What is the function of this memory mechanism? One possibility is that it is a memory mechanism with a limited temporal operating range that assists the formation of high-precision long-term memories of structurally coherent images and meaningful patterns (Magnussen, 2000). According to this hypothesis, it is a supporting component of the perceptual representation system (PRS), located before the level of object descriptions (Tulving & Schacter, 1990). The supporting role of low-level storage of visual attributes may not be limited to a short-term memory range, as the consolidation process in long-term memory may proceed for weeks, even months.

A second possibility is that the perceptual memory represents a separate, parallel, implicit long-term memory mechanism storing high-precision information about the elemental visual dimensions and supporting pictorial memory and memory for visual scenes. Tulving (2002) reminds us that memory performances may be supported by several memory systems. The accuracy of episodic memory may be enhanced by the operation of implicit memory systems. According to this view one might expect high-fidelity long-term memory not only for pictures (Standing, 1973) but for specific values along V1 dimensions. However, the existence of long-term memory for elemental dimensions such as spatial frequency is debated. Lages and Treisman (1998) have pointed out methodological weaknesses in the early demonstrations of high-fidelity long-term memory of spatial frequency (Magnussen & Dyrnes, 1994) and have shown that the method of constant stimuli used in that study might produce an artificial short-term reference against which the test gratings might be compared. In a more recent study (Magnussen, Greenlee, Aslaksen, & Kildebo, 2003), this problem was solved by having a large number of observers view a single test grating and decide whether the spatial frequency of the test grating was higher or lower than the spatial frequency of the reference grating presented on a previous occasion, with different groups of participants tested with different spatial frequencies. The resulting group psychometric functions were identical for immediate testing and a 24-hour test interval, suggesting high-precision storage of spatial frequency. However, a recent report failed to replicate the results, showing shallower psychometric functions for long intervals (Lages & Paul, 2006). Thus, the question of a high-fidelity long-term store for spatial frequency is not settled.

Indirect evidence for long-term storage of visual details was reported in a recent study by Vogt and Magnussen (2007), who showed that the long-term memory of naturalistic pictures – *in casu* pictures of doors – was substantially impaired by removing minor pictorial details that remained largely undetected by the participants (examples of the stimuli are shown in Figure 4.6). In that experiment, participants were presented with a study set of 400 pictures, each presented for 5 s, and were subsequently tested for recognition memory with samples consisting of 50 old and 50 new pictures, across an interval of 9 days. The results of the experiment showed that when pictorial details were removed, memory performance dropped by about 20% and the decay function followed a parallel, shallow slope. These results are in line with several other recent studies (e.g., Castelhano & Henderson, 2005; Hollingworth, 2005) and suggest that implicit memory may support explicit memory performance and also that the memory for perceptual details may be more important in memory for naturalistic scenes than was previously realized.

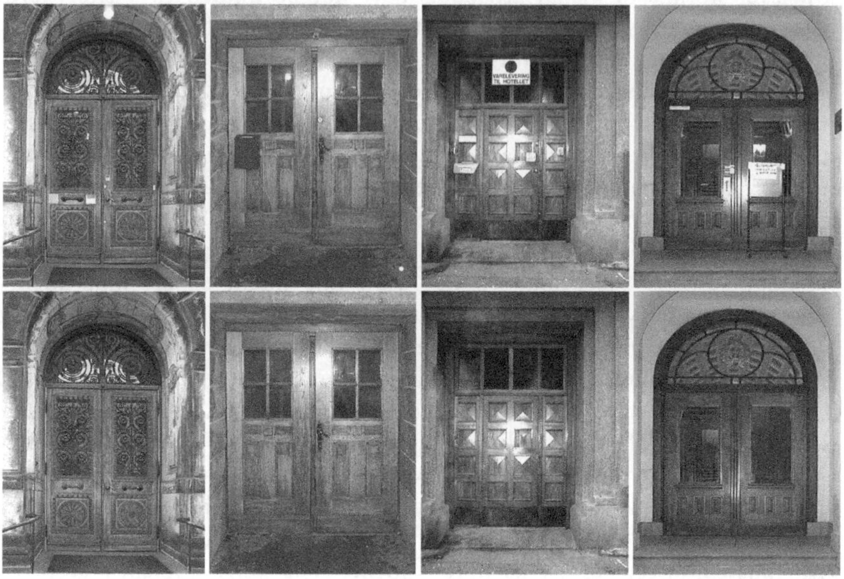

Figure 4.6 Examples of the stimuli used by Vogt and Magnussen (2007) in a study of long-term memory for a single category of objects: doors. The upper row shows the original photographs; the lower row shows the same photographs edited by removing minor details. This manipulation of the pictures caused the memory performance to drop by 20%. (This figure is published in colour at http://www.cognitiveneurosciencearena.com/brain-scans/.)

Acknowledgements

The preparation of this chapter was supported by a grant from the Norwegian Research Council (MH) to SM. Correspondence should be directed to S. Magnussen, Center for the Study of Human Cognition, Department of Psychology, University of Oslo, Box 1094 Blindern, 0317 Oslo, Norway. E-mail: svein.magnussen@psykologi.uio.no

We thank Lars-Göran Nilsson for his "midwife" role in this research. After listening to a conference talk by one of us (SM), outlining the findings of the initial experiments, Lars-Göran, who was then the chief editor of the *European Journal of Cognitive Psychology*, asked us to submit the first paper to that journal. This we did. Within a couple of weeks, we received a reply from the editor informing us that he had read the paper, briefly consulted a colleague in memory research, and accepted the paper without further review. We wish there were more editors like that.

References

Bäckman, L., Small, B. J., & Wahlin, Å. (2001). Ageing and memory: Cognitive and biological processes. In J. E. Birren & K. W. Schaie (Eds.), *Handbook of the psychology of ageing* (5th ed., pp. 349–377). New York: Academic Press.

Baddeley, A. D. (2003). Working memory: Looking back and looking forward. *Nature Neuroscience Reviews*, *4*, 829–839.

Baumann, O., Endestad, T., Magnussen, S., & Greenlee, M. W. (2007a). [Cortical activation during delayed discrimination of Gabor stimuli differing in spatial frequency]. Unpublished raw data.

Baumann, O., Endestad, T., Magnussen, S., & Greenlee, M. W. (2008). Delayed discrimination of spatial frequency for gratings of different orientation: Behavioral and fMRI evidence for low-level perceptual memory stores in early visual cortex. *Experimental Brain Research*, *188*, 363–369.

Baumann, O., Frank, G., Rutschmann R. M., & Greenlee, M. W. (2007b). Cortical activation during sequences of memory-guided saccades: A functional MRI study. *NeuroReport*, *18*, 451–455.

Bennett, P. J., & Cortese, F. (1996). Masking of spatial frequency in visual memory depends on distal, not retinal frequency. *Vision Research*, *36*, 233–238.

Bennett, P. J., Sekuler, A. B., McIntosh, A. R., & Della-Maggiore, V. (2001). The effects of ageing on visual memory: Evidence for functional reorganization of cortical networks. *Acta Psychologica*, *197*, 249–273.

Ben-Yehudah, G., & Ahissar, M. (2004). Sequential spatial frequency discrimination is consistently impaired among adult dyslectics. *Vision Research*, *44*, 1047–1063.

Blake, R., Cepeda, N., & Hiris, E. (1997). Memory for visual motion. *Journal of Experimental Psychology: Human Perception and Performance*, *22*, 353–369.

Blakemore, C., & Campbell, F. W. (1969). On the existence of neurons in the human visual system selectively sensitive to the orientation and size of retinal images. *Journal of Physiology*, *203*, 237–260.

Brett, M., Anton, J. L., Valabregue, R., & Poline J. P. (2002). Region of interest analysis using an SPM toolbox. *NeuroImage*, *16*, 497.

Bundesen, C., Larsen, A., & Farrell, J. E. (1981). Mental transformation of size and orientation. In J. Long & A. Baddeley (Eds.), *Attention and Performance IX* (pp. 279–294). Hillsdale, NJ: Lawrence Erlbaum Associates, Inc.

Cabeza, R., & Nyberg, L. (2000). Imaging cognition II: An empirical review of 275 PET and fMRI studies. *Journal of Cognitive Neuroscience*, *12*, 1–47.

Campana, G., Cowey, A., & Walsh, V. (2002). Priming of motion direction and area V5/MT: A test of perceptual memory. *Cerebral Cortex*, *12*, 663–669.

Campana, G., Cowey, A., & Walsh, V. (2006). Visual area V5/MT remembers "what" but not "where". *Cerebral Cortex*, *16*, 1766–1770.

Castelhano, M. S., & Henderson, J. M. (2005). Incidental visual memory for objects in scenes. *Visual Cognition*, *12*, 1017–1040.

Cornette, L., Dupont, P., Bormans, G., Mortelmans, L., & Orban, G. A. (2001). Separate neural correlates for the mnemonic components of successive discrimination and working memory tasks. *Cerebral Cortex*, *1*, 59–72.

Cornette, L., Dupont, P., & Orban, G. A. (2002). The neural substrate of orientation short-term memory and resistance to distractor items. *European Journal of Neuroscience*, *15*, 165–175.

Damasio, A. R. (1989). Time-locked multiregional activation: A systems-level approach. *Cognition, 33*, 25–62.

Della-Maggiore, V., Sekuler, A. B., Grady, C. L., Bennett, P. J., Sekuler, R., & McIntosh, A. R. (2000). Corticolimbic interactions associated with performance on a short-term memory task are modified by age. *Journal of Neuroscience, 20*, 8410–8416.

DeValois, R. L., & DeValois, K. K. (1990). *Spatial vision.* Oxford, UK: Oxford University Press.

Everson, R. M., Prashanth, A. K., Gabbay, M., Knight, B. W., Sirovich, L., & Kaplan, E. (1998). Representation of spatial frequency and orientation in the visual cortex. *Proceedings of the National Academy of Science USA, 95*, 8334–8338.

Faillenot, I., Sunaert, S., Van Hecke, P., & Orban, G. A. (2001). Orientation discrimination of objects and gratings compared: An fMRI study. *European Journal of Neuroscience, 13*, 585–596.

Fechner, G. T. (1860). *Elemente der Psychophysik.* Leipzig: Breitkopf & Härtel.

Fuster, J. M. (2001). The prefrontal cortex – an update: Time is of the essence. *Neuron, 30*, 319–333.

Ganis, G., Thompson, W. L., & Kosslyn, S. M. (2004). Brain areas underlying visual mental imagery and visual perception: An fMRI study. *Cognitive Brain Research, 20*, 226–241.

Gold, J. M., Murray, R. F., Sekuler, A. B., Bennett, P. J., & Sekuler, R. (2005). Visual memory decay is deterministic. *Psychological Science, 16*, 769–774.

Goldman-Rakic, P. S. (1995). Architecture of the prefrontal cortex and the central executive. *Annals of the New York Academy of Science, 769*, 71–83.

Greenlee, M. W., Koessler, M., Cornelissen, F., & Mergner, T. (1997). Visual discrimination and short-term memory for random dot patterns in patients with a focal cortical lesion. *Cerebral Cortex, 7*, 253–267.

Greenlee, M. W., Lang, H.-J., Mergner, T., & Seeger, W. (1995). Visual short-term memory of stimulus velocity in patients with unilateral posterior brain damage. *Journal of Neuroscience, 15*, 2287–2300.

Greenlee, M. W., & Magnussen, S. (1988). Interactions among orientation and spatial frequency channels adapted concurrently. *Vision Research, 28*, 1303–1309.

Greenlee, M. W., Magnussen, S., & Nordby, K. (1988). Spatial vision of the achromat: Spatial frequency and orientation-specific adaptation. *Journal of Physiology, 395*, 661–678.

Greenlee, M. W., Magnussen, S., & Reinvang, I. (2000). Brain regions involved in spatial frequency discrimination: Evidence from fMRI. *Experimental Brain Research, 132*, 399–403.

Greenlee, M. W., Magnussen, S., & Thomas, J. P. (1991). Different neural codes for spatial frequency and contrast. In A. Valberg & B. B. Lee (Eds.), *From pigments to perception: Advances in understanding visual processes* (pp. 451–454). New York: Plenum Press.

Greenlee. M. W., Rischewski, J., Mergner, T., & Seeger, W. (1993). Delayed pattern discrimination in patients with unilateral temporal lobe damage. *Journal of Neuroscience, 13*, 2565–2574.

Habib, R., Nyberg L., & Tulving E. (2003). Hemispheric asymmetries of memory: The HERA model revisited. *Trends in Cognitive Sciences, 7*, 241–245.

Hollingworth, A. (2005). The relation between on-line visual representation of a scene and long-term scene memory. *Journal of Experimental Psychology: Learning, Memory, and Cognition, 31*, 396–411.

Kahana, M. J., & Sekuler, R. (2002). Recognizing spatial patterns: A noisy exemplar approach. *Vision Research, 42*, 2177–2192.

Koriat, A., Goldsmith, M., & Pansky, A. (2000). Toward a psychology of memory accuracy. *Annual Review of Psychology, 51*, 481–537.

Kosslyn, S. M., & Thompson, W. L. (2003). When is early visual cortex activated during visual mental imagery? *Psychological Bulletin, 129*, 723–746.

Lages, M., & Paul, A. (2006). Visual long-term memory for spatial frequency? *Psychonomic Bulletin & Review, 13*, 486–492.

Lages, M., & Treisman, M. (1998). Spatial frequency discrimination: Visual long-term memory or criterion setting? *Vision Research, 38*, 557–572.

Lalonde, J., & Chaudhuri, A. (2002). Task-dependent transfer of perceptual to memory representations during delayed spatial frequency discrimination. *Vision Research, 42*, 1759–1769.

Laming, D., & Laming, J. (1992). F. Hegelmaier: On memory for the length of a line. *Psychological Research, 54*, 233–239.

Laming, D., & Scheiwiller, P. (1985). Retention in perceptual memory: A review of models and data. *Perception & Psychophysics, 37*, 189–197.

Leung, H. C., Gore, J C., & Goldman-Rakic, P. S. (2002). Sustained mnemonic response in the human middle frontal gyrus during the on-line storage of spatial memoranda. *Journal of Cognitive Neuroscience, 14*, 659–671.

Maffei, L., & Fiorentini, A. (1977). Spatial frequency rows in the striate visual cortex. *Vision Research, 17*, 257–264.

Magnussen, S. (2000). Low-level memory processes in vision. *Trends in Neurosciences, 23*, 247–251.

Magnussen, S., & Dyrnes, S. (1994). High-fidelity perceptual long-term memory. *Psychological Science, 5*, 99–102.

Magnussen, S., & Greenlee, M. W. (1992). Retention and disruption of motion information in visual short-term memory. *Journal of Experimental Psychology: Learning, Memory, and Cognition, 18*, 151–156.

Magnussen, S., & Greenlee, M. W. (1997). Competition and sharing of processing resources in visual discrimination. *Journal of Experimental Psychology: Human Perception and Performance, 22*, 1603–1616.

Magnussen, S., & Greenlee, M. W. (1999). The psychophysics of perceptual memory. *Psychological Research, 62*, 81–92.

Magnussen, S., Greenlee, M. W., Aslaksen, P. M., & Kildebo, O. Ø. (2003). High-fidelity long-term memory for spatial frequency revisited – and confirmed. *Psychological Science, 14*, 74–76.

Magnussen, S., Greenlee, M. W., Asplund, R., & Dyrnes, S. (1990). Perfect visual short-term memory for periodic patterns. *European Journal of Cognitive Psychology, 4*, 345–362.

Magnussen, S., Greenlee, M. W., Asplund, R., & Dyrnes, S. (1991). Stimulus-specific mechanisms of visual short-term memory. *Vision Research, 31*, 1213–1219.

Magnussen, S., Greenlee, M. W., & Thomas, J. P. (1996). Parallel processing in visual short-term memory. *Journal of Experimental Psychology: Human Perception and Performance, 22*, 202–212.

Magnussen, S., Idås, E., & Holst Myhre, S. (1998). Representation of orientation and spatial frequency in perception and memory: A choice reaction-time analysis. *Journal of Experimental Psychology: Human Perception and Performance, 24*, 707–718.

McKeefry, D. J., Burton, M. P., & Vakrou, C. (2007). Speed selectivity in visual short-term memory for motion. *Vision Research, 47*, 2418–2425.

Naghavi, H. R., & Nyberg, L. (2005). Common fronto-parietal activity in attention, memory, and consciousness: Shared demands on integration? *Consciousness and Cognition, 14*, 390–425.

Nilsson, L.-G. (2003). Memory function in normal ageing. *Acta Neurologica Scandinavia, 107* (suppl. 179), 7–13.

Ogmen, H., Breitmeyer, B. G., & Melvin, R. (2003). The what and where in visual masking. *Vision Research, 43*, 1337–1350.

Pasternak, T., Bisley, J. W., & Valkins, D. (2003). Visual information processing in the primate brain. In M. Gallagher & R. J. Nelson (Eds.), *Biological psychology* (pp. 130–185). New York: Wiley.

Pasternak, T., & Greenlee, M. W. (2005). Working memory in primate sensory systems. *Nature Reviews Neuroscience, 6*, 97–107.

Pessoa, L., Gutierrez, E., Bandettini, P. A., & Ungerleider, L. (2002). Neural correlates of visual working memory: fMRI amplitude predicts task performance. *Neuron, 35*, 975–987.

Regan, D. (1985). Storage of spatial frequency information and spatial-frequency discrimination. *Journal of the Optical Society of America, A2*, 619–621.

Reinvang, I., Magnussen, S., & Greenlee, M. W. (2002). Hemispheric asymmetry in visual discrimination and memory: ERP-evidence for the spatial frequency hypothesis. *Experimental Brain Research, 144*, 483–495.

Reinvang, I., Magnussen, S., Greenlee, M. W., & Larsson, P. G. (1998). Electrophysiological localization of cortical regions involved in perceptual memory. *Experimental Brain Research, 123*, 481–484.

Rothmayr, C., Baumann, O., Endestad, T., Rutschmann, R. M., Magnussen, S., & Greenlee M. W. (2007). Dissociation of neural correlates of verbal and non-verbal visual working memory with different delays. *Behavioral Brain Functions, 3*, 56, doi: 10.1186/1744-9081-3-56.

Schacter, D. L., Wagner, A. D., & Buckner, R. L. (2000). Memory systems of 1999. In E. Tulving & F. I. M. Craik (Eds.), *The Oxford handbook of memory* (pp. 627–643). Oxford, UK: Oxford University Press.

Sirovich, L., & Uglesich, R. (2004). The organization of orientation and spatial frequency in primary visual cortex. *Proceedings of the National Academy of Sciences USA, 101*, 16941–16946.

Slotnick, S. D., Thompson, W. L., & Kosslyn, S. M. (2005). Visual mental imagery induces retinotopically organized activation of early visual areas. *Cerebral Cortex, 15*, 1570–1583.

Standing, L. (1973). Remembering 10,000 pictures. *Quarterly Journal of Experimental Psychology, 25*, 207–222.

Tanaka, Y., & Sagi, D. (1998a). A perceptual memory for low-contrast signals. *Proceedings of the National Academy of Sciences USA, 95*, 12729–12733.

Tanaka, Y., & Sagi, D. (1998b). Long-lasting, long-range detection facilitation. *Vision Research, 38*, 2591–2599.

Thomas, J. P., Magnussen, S., & Greenlee, M. W. (2000). What limits simultaneous discrimination accuracy? *Vision Research, 40*, 3169–3172.

Todd, J. J., & Marois, R. (2004). Capacity limit of visual short-term memory in human posterior parietal cortex. *Nature*, *428*, 751–754.

Tulving, E. (2002). Episodic memory: From mind to brain. *Annual Review of Psychology*, *53*, 1–25.

Tulving, E. & Schacter, D. L. (1990). Priming and human memory systems. *Science*, 247, 301–306.

Vogt, S. E., & Magnussen, S. (2007). Long-term memory for 400 pictures on a common theme. *Experimental Psychology*, *54*, 298–303.

Volle, E., Pochon, J. B., Lehéricy, S., Pillon, B., Dubois, B., & Levy, R. (2005). Specific cerebral networks for maintenance and response organization within working memory as evidenced by the "double delay/double response" paradigm. *Cerebral Cortex*, *15*, 1064–1074.

Xu, Y., & Chun, M. M. (2006). Dissociable neural mechanisms supporting visual short-term memory for objects. *Nature*, *440*, 91–95.

Zhang, J. X., Leung, H. C., & Johnson, M. K. (2003). Frontal activations associated with accessing and evaluating information in working memory: An fMRI study. *NeuroImage*, *20*, 1531–1539.

5 Remembering in time

Cognitive control of time keeping

Timo Mäntylä

The aim of this chapter is to examine cognitive mechanisms of temporal information processing in children and adults. The starting point of the chapter is the assertion that temporal information processing is involved in a variety of cognitive constructs, including autobiographic memory, prospective memory, theory of mind, and executive control functions and that sense of time is a prerequisite to different goal-directed activities, such as planning, scheduling, monitoring, and task coordination (Fuster, 1993, 2002; Ingvar, 1985). For example, Fuster proposed a general theory of prefrontal functioning in which temporal organization and integration of cognition and behaviour plays a central role: "The enactment of a goal-directed sequence of actions is a continuous process of temporal integration. At the root of this process is the mediation of cross-temporal contingencies between the action plan, the goal, and the acts leading to the goal" (Fuster, 2002, p. 96).

Consistent with this view, patient studies, brain imaging studies, and neuropharmacological evidence suggest that cognitively controlled timing is related to prefrontally mediated executive functions (e.g., Barkley, Koplowitz, Anderson, & McMurray, 1997; Della Sala, Laiacona, Spinnler, & Rivelli, 1993; Janowsky, Shimamura, & Squire, 1989; Kerns, McInerney, & Wilde, 2001; Klein, Loftus, & Kihlstrom, 2002). For example, Barkley et al. (1997) found that children with attention difficulties show problems in time orientation, as measured by the psychophysical methods of time estimation and time reproduction. In their study, school-aged children with attention deficit/hyperactivity disorder (ADHD) were asked to reproduce varying stimulus durations. Specifically, participants first observed a red light between 12 s and 60 s and then reproduced its duration by means of a flashlight. Barkley et al. (1997) observed that children with ADHD reproduced stimulus durations less accurately and more variably than healthy children. These findings were consistent with Barkley's (1997) model of ADHD and suggest that ADHD-related problems in executive functioning are related to biases in time perception (see also Toplak, Dockstader, & Tannock, 2006).

A general implication of these patient studies is that individual and developmental differences in executive functions should be related to sense of time regardless of aetiology. In other words, healthy individuals with low performance in executive functioning tasks should also make greater timing errors than better functioning individuals. Furthermore, it is important to examine these issues in healthy children and adults, because "empirical findings and methodological issues challenge the etiologic primacy of inhibitory and executive deficits in ADHD" (Castellanos, Sonuga-Barke, Milham, & Tannock, 2006, p. 117).

These studies are consistent with clinical observations suggesting that frontal lobe patients and individuals with ADHD have marked difficulties in time management in everyday activities (e.g., Maté, 1999). It should be noted that such observations and anecdotes appear to refer to very different time frames and contexts from those involved in psychophysical methods of interval timing. Thus, although some individuals show difficulties in, for example, time reproduction, these differences do not necessarily justify the conclusion that the same individuals would have problems in everyday tasks involving temporal information processing. Similarly, individuals with difficulties in executive/frontal functioning tasks might show unimpaired performance in psychophysical tasks of interval timing, but their performance might be compromised in task conditions that reflect temporal complexities of everyday cognition (cf. multitasking or remembering multiple intentions).

Carelli, Forman, and Mäntylä (2008) examined the relation between executive functioning and temporal information processing in healthy adults (university students) and school-aged children. In their study, children and adult participants completed a set of executive functioning tasks and a duration judgment task in which they reproduced stimulus durations between 4 s and 32 s. Furthermore, the adult participants completed the time reproduction under varying task loads (i.e., counting backwards during study or test). Individual and developmental differences in executive functioning were assessed by six experimental tasks that were assumed to reflect one of the three target executive functions of shifting, updating, or inhibition (for similar latent variable approaches, see also Miyake et al., 2000; Salthouse, Atkinson, & Berish, 2003).

The main finding of the study was that individual differences in executive functioning were only weakly related to time reproduction performance in healthy children and adults. Specifically, children with low performance in the updating and inhibition tasks of executive functioning, but not in mental shifting, made somewhat greater errors for longer durations (≥ 24 s) than did children with better updating and inhibition functions. Furthermore, these selective effects were observed for absolute timing errors only (i.e., children with high and low executive functioning made similar under- and overestimations). Adult participants showed a similar pattern of results in that individual differences in executive functions were not related to time reproduction performance under the no-load and test-load conditions. These findings suggest that difficulties in temporal information processing, as measured by the time reproduction task, are *not* closely related to prefrontal-mediated executive functions in healthy children and adults.

One possible reason for the discrepancy between past patient studies and that of Carelli et al. (2008) is that our individual difference approach was not sufficiently powerful to detect a covariation between duration judgments and executive functioning in healthy participants. Another reasonable explanation is that the assessment of cognitive timing should not be based on (or limited to) psychophysical methods of interval timing (e.g., time estimation and reproduction). Alternative strategies for evaluating the hypothesis that individual differences in executive functioning mediate temporal information processing might be (a) to consider time management in everyday life as a cognitive control problem, rather than as a problem of "time perception", and (b) to examine executive functioning in relation to more complex tasks of temporal processing than those used in traditional methods of interval timing. Both hypotheses will be examined in more detail in the following sections of the chapter.

Cognitive control of time keeping

During an ordinary day most of us have a series of tasks to remember and complete. Typically, these tasks are not serial in the sense that they follow a sequential timeline. Instead, most activities are partially overlapping, with different onset and offset times, and their completion also requires monitoring and updating of plans and intentions. For example, one needs to remember to take medication before breakfast while preparing coffee, boiling eggs for some minutes, and later having a meeting with a colleague who reminds you that the meeting at 2 p.m. was postponed two hours, after which you are reminded that you should meet another colleague after the meeting.

Temporal information processing of these kinds of parallel and dynamic activities is not easily handled by the existing models of interval timing. According to the attentional-gate model (Block & Zakay, 1996; Zakay & Block, 1996; see also Block & Zakay, 2006), prospective duration judgments depend on attention-demanding processes that occur concurrently with the processing of non-temporal information. To the extent that a person's attentional resources are limited, fewer resources can be allocated to temporal information, and fewer time signals accumulate in the cognitive counter. Duration judgments are assumed to reflect the total number of accumulated signals, and experienced durations decrease as the difficulty of the secondary task increases (Zakay & Block, 2004; see also Block & Zakay, 1997).

The attentional-gate model makes a good job in predicting performance in task situations that require estimation or reproduction of a discrete (and relatively short) stimulus duration (such as warming a glass of milk in a microwave), but it is not designed for time keeping in more complex situations (e.g., preparing a dinner). Timing models with multiple pacemakers or neural oscillators (Church & Broadbent, 1990; Matell & Meck, 2004; see also Staddon & Higa, 1996) might be used to register separate durations, but even these parallel timers would have limitations and processing costs in complex everyday situations. For example, using the breakfast task as an example, one might argue that the activities of boiling an egg and preparing coffee etcetera could be "time tagged" by a bank of oscillators, and that these time codes could be used to date past episodes and to time the completion of planned activities in the future.

However, one limitation is that these models have been applied to relatively short time intervals. More important, although parallel activities with different onset and offset times can be timed with multiple clocks and pacemakers, having separate timers for each goal-directed task and intention is an inefficient solution in complex tasks. How many timers? How and when to start and stop the timers when completing, updating, or postponing goal-directed activities with independent temporal trajectories? Whether subjective experience of time is based on a pacemaker-accumulator model or some other metaphor of cognitive timing, temporal information processing in complex goal-directed tasks requires some form of coordination and monitoring.

Time monitoring in children and adults

Time keeping in goal-directed tasks can be considered as a cognitive control problem in that temporal coordination of complex activities (such as multitasking and remembering multiple intentions) reflects individual differences in monitoring functions, rather than in time perception per se, and in most everyday situations this strategy must balance the cost of monitoring against the cost of having inaccurate information about the environment.

In general terms, monitoring can be seen as a process in which an agent assesses its environments for the purposes of goal-directed activities (Atkin & Cohen, 1996; Cohen, Atkin, & Hansen, 1994; Harris & Wilkins, 1982). Monitoring means seeing how plans are progressing, checking how much progress has been made, finding out what time it is, updating one's location, looking for obstacles, making sure that nothing has changed unexpectedly, and so on.

A distinction is frequently made between *sensing* and *monitoring* (Atkin & Cohen, 1996; McDermott, 1978). Sensing refers to the typically low-level data acquisition mechanisms needed to keep a representation or a world model up to date (cf. internal clocks and oscillators), and monitoring refers to a meta-level functions in that it involves querying this model. Monitoring involves a strategy or scheme by which monitoring actions are scheduled (i.e., deciding when to ask for the information the sensors provide).

Although monitoring is a necessary task for any agent, including humans, insects, and robots, few studies have investigated how these agents actually behave while the goal or deadline is approaching. Yet the monitoring concept has close connections to several areas, including operant conditioning (e.g., Ferster & Skinner, 1957), process control (Moray, 1986), foraging behaviour in ethology (Pyke, 1984), and some areas of the AI domain. For example, early work on reinforcement schedules is closely related to monitoring problems. In the fixed interval (FI) schedules, the subject receives reinforcement for its first response occurring at more than *T* time units since its previous reinforcement. A typical finding is that the subject waits a certain period of time *T* before responding again and then accelerates responding as the *T* approaches. This fixed-interval scallop is very similar to an interval reduction strategy discussed above.

Harris and Wilkins (1982) proposed a specific model for strategic monitoring in time-based prospective memory tasks. Their Test–Wait–Test–Exit (TWTE) model, was based on the Test–Operate–Test–Exit (TOTE) framework by Miller, Galanter, and Pribram (1960), and monitoring was assumed to involve a series of test–wait cycles until a final test is made during a critical period. To test this model, Harris and Wilkins (1982) asked participants to hold up a series of cards after 3 or 9 min, while they were watching a film. For example, if the cards indicated 3 min, 9 min, 3 min, respectively, participants were to wait 3 min and hold up the first card, wait 9 min and hold up the second card, and so on. Participants monitored the time by turning to look at the clock on the wall behind them, and the experimenter recorded the number of clock checks. Harris and Wilkins found that monitoring of the clock was closely related to the latency of responding, with shorter latencies associated with a greater rate of monitoring, especially during the period immediately preceding the target time. Consistent with the TWTE model, the overall pattern of clock-checking frequency showed a J-shaped function. According to Harris and Wilkins, participants first checked the clock frequently to synchronize their internal clocks with the external clock. During the middle of the period, they could rely on their internal clocks to keep track of the time. Finally, as the response time approached, they relied frequently on the external clock to ensure they were not late in performing the prospective memory task.

Ceci and Bronfenbrenner (1985) conducted a seminal study of time-based prospective memory in school-aged children. In their study, children of ages 10 and 14 years were instructed to remove cupcakes from an oven after exactly 30 min to avoid burning them. In another condition, the children charged a battery and were instructed to turn off the charger after 30 min to prevent overcharging. During the 30-min interval, the children played a video game in a separate room (either at home or in a laboratory setting). The clock was placed behind the child, so the experimenter (sibling) could easily see when the child turned around to determine how much cooking or charging time remained. However, this checking was associated with a cost, in that the act of monitoring was a distraction from the game.

Ceci and Bronfenbrenner (1985) found that all children checked the clock frequently during the first 10 min of the waiting period and then engaged in very little clock checking until the final moments of the waiting period. Specifically, older children in both settings, and younger children in the home setting, *reduced* the frequency of monitoring actions during the middle period (from 10 to 25 min) of the task interval. When younger children were tested in the unfamiliar laboratory setting (and with an unknown experimenter), they maintained the frequency of clock checking at the same high level also during the mid-phase of the task. These findings suggest that even young school-aged children monitor deadlines strategically in that they accelerated clock checking when the deadline was approaching.

Mäntylä, Carelli, and Forman (2007) provided direct support for the notion that time monitoring is closely related to individual and developmental differences in executive control functions (see also Kerns, 2000; Mackinlay, Kliegel, & Mäntylä, 2009; Mäntylä, 2003; Mäntylä & Nilsson, 1997). In their study, children between 7 to 11 years indicated the passing of time every 5 min, while watching a film. Executive functioning had selective effects on time-based prospective memory performance (as measured by monitoring frequency and response accuracy) in that children with low performance in the updating and inhibition tasks of executive functioning checked the clock more frequently *and* made greater timing errors than did children with more efficient control functions (see also, for similar findings with older adults, Mäntylä, Del Missier, & Nilsson, in press).

In general terms, these findings are consistent with the attentional-gate model of Block and Zakay (1996; Zakay & Block, 1996; see also Block & Zakay, 2006). According to their model, prospective duration judgments depend on attention-demanding processes that occur concurrently with the processing of non-temporal information. To the extent that a person's attentional resources are limited, fewer resources can be allocated to temporal information, and fewer time signals accumulate in the cognitive counter. Duration judgments are assumed to reflect the total number of accumulated signals, and experienced durations decrease as the difficulty of the secondary task increases.

Although the attentional-gate model acknowledges the importance of attentional (executive) processes, its predictions are unspecific in that *any* task manipulation that increases attentional demands is assumed to modulate experienced durations (i.e., the amount of temporal signals that is accumulated in the counter). Thus, the attentional-gate model is neutral with respect to qualitative (rather than quantitative) differences in executive functioning: Two equally demanding tasks that reflect *different* aspects of executive functioning (e.g., task shifting and inhibition) are expected have similar effects on experienced durations. By contrast, our findings (Carelli et al., 2008; Mäntylä et al., 2007) showed selective effects in that participants with low performance in the updating and inhibition, but not in the shifting, tasks of executive functioning made greater timing errors than better performing individuals.

Representation of temporal patterns

The previous section of this chapter suggested that individual and developmental differences in frontal lobe/executive functioning are associated with difficulties in temporal information processing in goal-directed tasks such as time-based prospective memory. However, empirical support for a direct link between individual differences in executive functioning and duration judgment is weak when temporal information processing is based on psychophysical methods of time estimation and time reproduction. In other words, healthy children and adults with difficulties in executive processing have greater difficulties in coordinating time-based tasks than do individuals with more efficient control functions, but they do not seem to have problems in reproducing and estimating stimulus durations.

Although the studies summarized in the previous sections are consistent with this conclusion, a general limitation of our own work is that the criterion tasks were quite different (time-based prospective memory vs. time reproduction). An interesting possibility is that duration judgments are indeed related to individual differences in executive functioning, but that the assessment of subjective time should be based on tasks that reflect complexities of everyday cognition. In other words, traditional psychophysical methods of duration judgment might not be sufficiently sensitive for detecting the influence of individual differences in cognitive control in healthy individuals.

One limitation of past timing research is that the level of temporal complexity has been very low in most studies, including those summarized earlier. Typically, participants observe a discrete event for a few seconds, and they are instructed to make a judgment of its duration. In most cases, the observed effects (i.e., under- or overestimations) are consistent with the existing theories of timing, such as the attentional-gate model of prospective timing (Block & Zakay, 1996; Zakay & Block, 1996) and the contextual change model of retrospective timing (Block & Reed, 1978), but psychophysical methods of interval timing are not easily applied to more complex activities in everyday situations. Thus, one reason "for the lack of interaction between developments in 'mainstream' psychology and time psychology proper" (Michon, 1985, p. 6) might be that the paradigms of interval timing research are not easily translated to the complexities of everyday cognition.

However, it should be noted that not only can timing research be criticized for involving overly simplified tasks, but a similar argument holds for memory research. Most studies on episodic memory involve a list of discrete words or pictures. Typically, a list of stimulus words is assumed to simulate a real-world episode, including its temporal dynamics: "Words to the memory researcher are what fruit flies are to the geneticists: a convenient medium through which the phenomena and processes of interest can be explored and elucidated. . . . A word has well-defined boundaries, it can be presented as a single item, separately from others, or as members of a smaller or larger grouping. Its occurrence represents a discrete event that can be accurately dated in time and located in space" (Tulving, 1983, p. 146).

Although word lists are not the only stimuli in episodic memory research, one might argue that memory researchers have simplified the temporal complexities and dynamics of real-world events in their experimental simulations of these events. These simplifications are even more apparent considering that time is considered as a characteristic (or even the defining) feature of episodic memory (e.g., Tulving, 1983, 2002a, 2002b; Wheeler, Stuss, & Tulving, 1997) and that "mental time travel" is considered as a unique property of human episodic memory (Roberts, 2002; Suddendorf & Corballis, 1997, 2007; Tulving, 1983, 1999; see also Addis, Wong, & Schacter, 2007; Atance & O'Neill, 2001; Clayton & Dickinson, 1998; Hassabis, Kumaran, Vann, & Maguire, 2007).

Temporal patterns of episodic events

Most naturalistic events are temporally and structurally complex in that they comprise a number of elements and that each individual element has its temporal duration within the event. Although a stimulus word can be considered as an "episodic event", it is fair to argue that most everyday events are more complex and dynamic than word lists or a series of stimulus pictures in a recognition memory experiment. Consider, for example, a theatre play in which the actors constitute the elements of the event (along with props). A theatre play reflects different temporal levels, including the real time of the performance, which commences at a specific hour and ends a couple of hours later. Furthermore, most events are composed of sub-elements with individual temporal characteristics. For example, the actors of a play may enter and leave the scene during the course of the act (e.g., actor A entered the scene first, after which actor C appeared, then B entered, D appeared briefly and A and C left the scene together, followed by E, after which B left the scene, etc.). In other words, the play (or any other dynamic event comprising multiple elements with different onset and offset times) does not only reflect its total duration (i.e., "how long was the play?"), but the actions of individual elements constitute a temporal pattern of event information (e.g., "how long did you see B?" or "did you see A and D together?").

Furthermore, it is not only dynamic events that can be described as complex temporal patterns; a representation of static events, such as a picture of scene, may also constitute a temporal pattern of saccadic fixations (Holm & Mäntylä, 2007; see also, for an overview, Henderson & Hollingworth, 1999). Depending on the viewer's goals and perceptual properties of the scene, some of its areas are fixated in a temporal order (i.e., they "enter" and "leave" the viewer's viewpoint). However, in contrast to the theatre metaphor above, encoding of static scene attributes is serial, whereas most dynamic events are temporally complex in that the individual elements have different and partially overlapping time windows. Of course, scene perception reflects multiple levels of temporal dynamics, including the temporal pattern of the event per se (cf. the actors' script) and each observer's idiosyncratic preferences within this temporal pattern of event information.

Although most real-world events constitute complex patterns of sub-events, neither memory researchers nor timing researchers have much to say about these temporal dynamics. How is asynchronous dynamic event information encoded, stored, and retrieved? How accurately can, for example, an eyewitness report the duration of multiple parallel events with different temporal profiles? What is the role of prior expectations or schematic knowledge structures (e.g., a script of a bank robbery) in these processes?

Somewhat surprisingly, research on multiple-duration judgments is virtually non-existent. To the best of my knowledge, only two studies have examined duration judgments in the context of multiple stimulus durations (Brown & West, 1990; Vanneste & Pouthas, 1999). Both studies tested the hypothesis that prospective timing requires attentional resources and that concurrent durations impair prospective time judgments. Thus, the primary focus of their studies was on the effects of concurrent task load on single-item duration judgments, rather than examining temporal patterns of event information.

Brown and West's (1990) participants monitored the duration of one to three stimuli (letters on a computer screen) with different onset and offset times. At test, they reproduced one of the durations. As can be expected, their main finding was that the magnitude of timing error increased as the number of target stimuli increased from one to three targets. Vanneste and Pouthas (1999) reported similar findings for young and older adults. Both Brown and West (1990) and Vanneste and Pouthas (1999) interpreted their findings in terms of the attentional-gate model of prospective timing, supporting the view that cognitive timing requires attention.

Recently, we completed an unpublished study in which we used a more elaborated version of a multiple-duration task. In this study, participants observed a pantomime in which five actors appeared on the stage for varying and partly overlapping time periods. One group of participants was informed that the pantomime described a "wedding ceremony" (i.e., a schema-consistent event), whereas another group of participants was instructed that they would witness an "assault" (a schema-inconsistent event). Both groups were instructed that they should observe the play for a later memory test, but they were not informed about the exact nature of these tests. The five actors (a priest, a bride, a groom, and two witnesses) were dressed in different colours (a black, white, blue, green, and yellow shirt, respectively) and accessories. They also performed different actions (one of the actors was talking on the phone, and the other actors were checking the clock, yawning, sneezing, etc.). The actors entered and left the scene individually and at different times.

At test, the participants first completed a content recall test, followed by two duration judgment tasks. In the first timing task, referred to as the *time estimation task*, they estimated the duration of the whole play (in seconds) as well as the appearance time of each actor (i.e., how long a time each actor appeared on the stage). In the second task, referred to as the *timeline task*, they reproduced the temporal pattern of the play by drawing a "timeline" of each actor. Specifically, the participants were given a response sheet in which a line represented the duration of the pantomime. The end points of the line indicated the start and stop times of the stimulus event without providing any other numeric or temporal cues. Each actor/colour was indicated by separate "tracks," and the participants were instructed to draw a timeline within each track. For both tasks, the primary dependent measure was the absolute difference between the expected and observed times.

The results of the study were consistent with those of Brown and West (1990) and Vanneste and Pouthas (1999), in that participants made large errors in the time estimation task (the absolute mean error for the whole 3-min event was greater than 90 s!). Interestingly, the mean absolute error was nearly three times greater in the time estimation task than in the timeline task. In other words, participants had great difficulties in making absolute duration judgments of the individual actors, but when using the timeline procedure they were surprisingly good at reproducing the temporal pattern of these actors. Thus, although participants did not have an accurate temporal representation of the event in terms of seconds and minutes (as indicated by the large timing errors in the duration estimation task), the timeline task provided a procedure to construct a rather accurate temporal pattern by relating the individual timelines to each other (perhaps at an ordinal level rather than in terms of absolute durations – e.g., "C came before B but after A" etc.).

This result is also consistent with the notion that people use space to think about time. Evidence from psychophysical experiments (Casasanto & Boroditsky, 2008; Vallesi, Binns, & Shallice, 2008; see also Ornstein, 1969) and psycholinguistic studies (e.g., Boroditsky, 2000; Núñez & Sweetser, 2006; Tversky, Kugelmass, & Winter, 1991) suggest that people construct spatial representations online when processing temporal information and that this relationship is asymmetric (Boroditsky, 2000; Casasanto & Boroditsky, 2008). For example, Casasanto and Boroditsky (2008) used a temporal reproduction task, in which the duration of a line (or a dot) was varied continuously and orthogonally with its left-to-right spatial displacement. Participants had to reproduce either temporal duration or spatial displacement. Casasanto and Boroditsky (2008) found that the irrelevant spatial displacement influenced the reproduction of temporal duration and not vice versa, suggesting that mental representations of duration and spatial displacement are asymmetrically dependent on one another.

Our own and others work summarized in the previous sections of this chapter suggests that individual differences in executive control functions are only weakly related to timing performance in healthy adults and children as measured by the psychophysical tasks of time reproduction and time estimation. A reasonable hypothesis is that these tasks are not sufficiently sensitive to individual differences in executive functioning because their demands on cognitive control functions are relatively low.

In another unpublished study, we attempted to relate individual differences in executive functioning to two duration tasks that were expected to vary in cognitive demands on cognitive control. Specifically, participants completed a set of executive functioning tasks (two tasks of response inhibition and working memory updating). Subjective experience of time was assessed by means of a duration judgment task, in which participants (university students) reproduced stimulus durations varying between 4 s and 24 s. They also completed a timeline task, in which they first observed two short videos (60 s and 180 s). In both videos, four actors entered and left the scene (a room or an outdoor scene) after completing various everyday activities (e.g., reading a newspaper). Participants were informed that they should pay attention to the temporal pattern of the actors' appearances in the movie. They were also informed about the nature of the timeline procedure, including a practice phase.

The main findings of the study were that individual differences in executive functioning (the inhibition and updating data yielded a common factor in the principal component analysis) were not related to time estimation performance. This result replicated the findings of Carelli et al. (2008) and provided additional support for the notion that executive functions play only a marginal role in duration judgments, as measured by a standard task of time reproduction. In contrast, participants were again quite good at reconstructing the temporal pattern of the observed movies. Furthermore, individual differences in executive functioning were related to performance in the timeline task, so that participants with good performance in the updating and inhibition tasks of executive functioning showed better performance than participants with less efficient control functions. These findings suggest that individual differences in executive functions contribute to duration judgments, but only in conditions that involve relatively complex cognitive timing performance. That is, participants with efficient control functions were not more accurate in estimating the duration of individual actors than were participants with lower performance in the executive functioning tasks, but their superior updating and inhibition functions resulted in a more accurate reconstruction of the temporal pattern in the timeline task.

Conclusions

The aim of this chapter was to examine cognitive mechanisms of temporal information processing in children and adults. The research summarized in this chapter suggests that individual and developmental differences in executive functions are related to sense of time when temporal information processing is examined in more complex task conditions than those involved in psychophysical methods of interval timing. Studies on time-based prospective memory suggest that individual and developmental differences in executive functioning mediate both monitoring frequency and retrieval accuracy. Similarly, time keeping of patterns of temporal events appears to be closely related to individual differences in cognitive control functions.

A reasonable interpretation of these findings is that the functional role of a subjective sense of time is to initiate time keeping (e.g., monitoring actions) when more specific temporal information is needed closer to the deadline. Instead of relying on absolute duration estimates, even category-level temporal information (e.g., "not yet – soon – now") might be sufficient to minimize early clock checking and to reduce monitoring costs in time-based prospective memory tasks. Similarly, this type of lower-level temporal information can be used to reconstruct complex patterns of temporal information. This type of cognitively constructed (but functional) time might be mediated by processes related to the maintenance and updating of working memory contents. Following the notion that updating and retaining dynamic event information in working memory contributes to a sense of temporal continuity (Jonides & Smith, 1997), individuals with efficient updating functions would be able to rely on this temporal information when monitoring deadlines, reconstructing past episodic events, and thinking about the future. In contrast, an individual with difficulties in temporary maintenance and elaboration of working memory contents may experience discontinuities in the sense of time, leading to increased dependence on external time keeping.

This notion is also consistent with evidence suggesting that the dorsolateral prefrontal cortex is integral to both cognitive timing and working memory. For example, Lewis and Miall (2006) suggested that cognitively controlled timing is based on the same dorsolateral prefrontal cells that are known to be involved in working memory (see also Rammsayer, 1997, 1999). Their perspective is somewhat different from more traditional models of the scalar expectancy theory, including the attentional-gate model. Instead of merely keeping track of the progress of a separate timekeeper (i.e., an accumulator process that collects quantized ticks from a hypothetical neural pacemaker), these working memory processes might actually constitute the time-dependent process itself.

The studies summarized in this chapter suggest that most psychophysical tasks of interval timing are rather insensitive to individual and developmental differences in higher-order cognitive control functions. Although the time reproduction task is more "cognitive" than most tasks of motor timing (Lewis & Miall, 2006; Rammsayer, 1999), its demands on executive control functioning are still rather low. Considering that clinical observations suggest that individuals with frontal lobe disorders have marked difficulties in temporal information processing, a practical implication of the work summarized here is that experimental and clinical assessment of temporal dysfunctions should be based on tasks that reflect the complexities of everyday cognition.

References

Addis, D. R., Wong, A. T., & Schacter, D. L. (2007). Remembering the past and imagining the future: Common and distinct neural substrates during event construction and elaboration. *Neuropsychologia*, *45*, 1363–1377.

Atance, C. M., & O'Neill, D. K. (2001). Episodic future thinking. *Trends in Cognitive Sciences*, *5*, 533–539.

Atkin, M. S., & Cohen, P. R. (1996). Monitoring strategies for embedded agents: Experiments and analysis. *Journal of Adaptive Behavior*, *4*, 125–172.

Barkley, R. A. (1997). Behavioral inhibition, sustained attention, and executive functions: Constructing a unifying theory of ADHD. *Psychological Bulletin*, *121*, 65–94.

Barkley, R. A., Koplowitz, S., Anderson, T., & McMurray, M. B. (1997). Sense of time in children with ADHD: Effects of duration, distraction, and stimulant medication. *Journal of the International Neuropsychological Society*, *3*, 359–369.

Block, R. A., & Reed, M. A. (1978). Remembered duration: Evidence for a contextual-change hypothesis. *Journal of Experimental Psychology: Human Learning*, *4*, 656–665.

Block, R. A., & Zakay, D. (1996). Models of psychological time revisited. In H. Helfrich (Ed.), *Time and mind* (pp. 171–195). Kirkland, WA: Hogrefe & Huber.

Block, R. A., & Zakay, D. (1997). Prospective and retrospective duration judgments: A meta-analytic review. *Psychonomic Bulletin & Review*, *4*, 184–197.

Block, R. A., & Zakay, D. (2006). Prospective remembering involves time estimation and memory processes. In J. Glickson & M. Myslobodsky (Eds.), *Remembering on time: The case for a time-based prospective memory* (pp. 25–49). New York: World Scientific Publishing.

Boroditsky, L. (2000). Metaphoric structuring: Understanding time through spatial metaphors. *Cognition*, *75*, 1–28.

Brown, S. W., & West, A. N. (1990). Multiple timing and the allocation of attention. *Acta Psychologica*, *75*, 103–121.

Carelli, M. G., Foreman, H., & Mäntylä, T. (2008). Sense of time and executive functioning in children and adults. *Child Neuropsychology*, *14*, 372–386.

Casasanto, D., & Boroditsky, L. (2008). Time in the mind: Using space to think about time. *Cognition*, *106*, 579–593.

Castellanos, F. X., Sonuga-Barke, E. J. S., Milham, M. P., & Tannock, R. (2006). Characterizing cognition in ADHD: Beyond executive dysfunction. *Trends in Cognitive Science*, *10*, 117–123.

Ceci, S. J., & Bronfenbrenner, U. (1985). "Don't forget to take the cupcakes out of the oven": Prospective memory, strategic time-monitoring, and context. *Child Development*, *56*, 152–164.

Church, R. M., & Broadbent, H. (1990). Alternative representations of time and number. *Cognition*, *5*, 105–118.

Clayton, N. S., & Dickinson, A. (1998). Episodic-like memory during cache recovery by scrub jays. *Nature*, *395*, 272–278.

Cohen, P. R., Atkin. M. S., & Hansen, E. A. (1994). The interval reduction strategy for monitoring cupcake problems. *Proceedings of the Third International Conference on the Simulation of Adaptive Behavior* (pp. 82–90). Cambridge, MA: MIT Press.

Della Sala, S., Laiacona, M., Spinnler, H., & Rivelli, C. (1993). Autobiographical recollection and frontal damage. *Neuropsychologia*, *31*, 823–839.

Ferster, C. B., & Skinner, B. F. (1957). *Schedules of reinforcement*. New York: Appleton-Century-Crofts.

Fuster, J. (1993). Frontal lobes. *Current Opinion in Neurobiology*, *3*, 160–165.

Fuster, J. (2002). Physiology of executive functions: The perception–action cycle. In D. T. Stuss & R. T. Knight (Eds.), *Principles of frontal lobe function*. New York: Oxford University Press.

Harris, J. E., & Wilkins, A. J. (1982). Remembering to do things: A theoretical framework and an illustrative experiment. *Human Learning*, *1*, 123–136.

Hassabis, D., Kumaran, D., Vann, S. D., & Maguire, E. A. (2007). Patients with hippocampal amnesia cannot imagine new experiences. *Proceedings of the National Academy of Sciences USA*, *104*, 1726–1731.

Henderson, J. M., & Hollingworth, A. (1999). High-level scene perception. *Annual Review of Psychology*, *50*, 243–271.

Holm, L., & Mäntylä, T. (2007). Memory for scenes: Refixations reflect retrieval. *Memory & Cognition*, *35*, 1664–1674.

Ingvar, D. (1985). Memory of the future: An assay on the temporal organization of conscious awareness. *Human Neurobiology*, *4*, 127–136.

Janowsky, J. S., Shimamura, A. P., & Squire, L. R. (1989). Memory and metamemory: Comparisons between patients with frontal lobe lesions and amnesic patients. *Psychobiology*, *17*, 3–11.

Jonides, J., & Smith, E. E. (1997). Working memory: A view from neuroimaging. *Cognitive Psychology*, *33*, 5–42.

Kerns, K. A. (2000). The CyberCruiser: An investigation of development of prospective memory in children. *Journal of the International Neuropsychological Society*, *6*, 62–70.

Kerns, K. A., McInerney, R. J., & Wilde, N. J. (2001). Time reproduction, working memory, and behavioral inhibition in children with ADHD. *Child Neuropsychology*, *7*, 21–31.

Klein, S. B., Loftus, J., & Kihlstrom, J. F. (2002). Memory and temporal experience: The effects of episodic memory loss on an amnesic patient's ability to remember the past and imagine the future. *Social Cognition*, *20*, 353–379.

Lewis, P., & Miall, R. C. (2006). Remembering the time: A continuous clock. *Trends in Cognitive Sciences*, *10*, 401–406.

Mackinlay, R., Kliegel, M., & Mäntylä, T. (2009). Predictors of time-based prospective memory in children. *Journal of Experimental Child Psychology*, *102*, 251–264.

Mäntylä, T. (2003). Assessing absentmindedness: Prospective memory complaint and impairment in middle-aged adults. *Memory & Cognition*, *31*, 15–25.

Mäntylä, T., Carelli, M. G., & Forman, H. (2007). Time monitoring and executive functioning in children and adults. *Journal of Experimental Child Psychology*, *96*, 1–19.

Mäntylä, T., Del Missier, F., & Nilsson, L.-G. (in press). Patterns of task costs in time-based prospective memory. *Aging, Neuropsychology, and Cognition*.

Mäntylä, T., & Nilsson, L.-G. (1997). Remembering to remember in adulthood: A population-based study. *Aging, Neuropsychology, and Cognition*, *4*, 81–92.

Maté, G. (1999). *Scattered minds: A new look at the origins and healing of attention deficit disorder*. Toronto: Knopf.

Matell, M. S., & Meck, W. H. (2004). Cortico-striatal circuits and interval timing: Coincidence-detection of oscillatory processes. *Cognitive Brain Research*, *21*, 139–170.

McDermott, D. (1978). Planning and acting. *Cognitive Science*, *2*, 71–109.

Michon, J. A. (1985). Introduction: The psychology of time. In J. A. Michon & J. L. Jackson (Eds.), *Time, mind and behavior*. Berlin: Springer-Verlag.

Miller, G., Galanter, E., & Pribram K. H. (1960). *Plans and the structure of behavior*. New York: Holt, Rinehart, & Winston.

Miyake, A., Friedman, N. P., Emerson, M. J., Witzki, A. H., Howerter, A., & Wager, T. D. (2000). The unity and diversity of executive functions and their contributions to complex "frontal lobe" tasks: A latent variable analysis. *Cognitive Psychology, 41*, 49–100.

Moray, N. (1986). Monitoring behavior and supervisory control. In K. R. Boff, L. Kaufman, & J. P. Thomas (Eds.), *Handbook of perception and human performance* (Vol. 2). New York: Wiley.

Núñez, R., & Sweetser, E. (2006). Looking ahead to the past: Convergent evidence from Aymara language and gesture in the crosslinguistic comparison of spatial construals of time. *Cognitive Science, 30*, 401–450.

Ornstein, R. (1969). *On the experience of time*. Harmondsworth, UK: Penguin.

Pyke, G. H. (1984). Optimal foraging: A critical review. *Annual Review of Ecology and Systematics, 15*, 523–527.

Rammsayer, T. H. (1997). Are there dissociable roles of the mesostriatal and mesolimbocortical dopamine systems on temporal information processing in humans? *Neuropsychobiology, 35*, 36–45.

Rammsayer, T. H. (1999). Neuropharmacological evidence for different timing mechanisms in humans. *Quarterly Journal of Experimental Psychology, 52B*, 273–286.

Roberts, W. A. (2002). Are animals stuck in time? *Psychological Bulletin, 128*, 473–489.

Salthouse, T. A., Atkinson, T. M., & Berish, D. E. (2003). Executive functioning as a potential mediator of age-related cognitive decline in normal adults. *Journal of Experimental Psychology: General, 132*, 566–594.

Staddon, J. E. R., & Higa, J. J. (1996). Multiple time scales in simple habituation. *Psychological Review, 103*, 720–733.

Suddendorf, T., & Corballis M. C. (1997). Mental time travel and the evolution of the human mind. *Genetic, Social, and General Psychology Monographs, 123*, 133–167.

Suddendorf, T., & Corballis, M. C. (2007). The evolution of foresight: What is mental time travel, and is it unique to humans? *Behavioral and Brain Sciences, 30*, 299–313.

Toplak, M. E., Dockstader, C., & Tannock, R. (2006). Temporal information processing in ADHD: The findings to date and new methods. *Journal of Neuroscience Methods, 151*, 15–29.

Tulving, E. (1983). *Elements of episodic memory*. Oxford, UK: Oxford University Press.

Tulving, E. (1999). On the uniqueness of episodic memory. In L.-G. Nilsson & H. J. Markowitsch (Eds.), *Cognitive neuroscience of memory* (pp. 11–42). Seattle, WA: Hogrefe & Huber.

Tulving, E. (2002a). Episodic memory: From mind to brain. *Annual Review of Psychology, 53*, 1–25.

Tulving, E. (2002b). Chronesthesia: Conscious awareness of subjective time. In D. T. Stuss & R. T. Knight (Eds.), *Principles of frontal lobe function* (pp. 311–325). New York: Oxford University Press.

Tversky, B., Kugelmass, S., & Winter, A. (1991). Cross-cultural and developmental trends in graphic productions. *Cognitive Psychology, 23*, 515–557.

Vallesi, A., Binns, M. A., & Shallice, T. (2008). An effect of spatial–temporal association of response codes: Understanding the cognitive representations of time. *Cognition, 106*, 579–593.

Vanneste, S., & Pouthas, V. (1999). Timing in aging: The role of attention. *Experimental Aging Research, 25*, 49–67.

Wheeler, M. A., Stuss, D. T., & Tulving, E. (1997). Toward a theory of episodic memory: The frontal lobes and autonoetic consciousness. *Psychological Bulletin*, *121*, 331–354.

Zakay, D., & Block, R. A. (1996). The role of attention in time estimation processes. In M. A. Pastor & J. Artieda (Eds.), *Time, internal clocks and movement* (pp. 143–164). Amsterdam: North-Holland/Elsevier.

Zakay, D., & Block, R. A. (2004). Prospective and retrospective duration judgments: An executive-control perspective. *Acta Neurobiologiae Experimentalis*, *64*, 319–328.

6 How do brains detect novelty?

Endel Tulving

"We have to live today by what truth we can get today, and be ready tomorrow to call it falsehood."

William James

Festschrifts are among the wonderful inventions of enlightened minds. They serve many purposes. The main purpose, of course, is to honour the honouree and make him happy. Sometimes this purpose does not work because not all great scholars and scientists for whom Festschrifts are written know how to be happy. In the present case, however, the success of this part of the venture is assured because our honouree, Lars-Göran Nilsson, not only believes in happiness but also practises it wherever and whenever possible. In that sense alone, this Festschrift in his honour is especially appropriate. Festschrifts also make Festschrift organizers happy, not only because they can thereby publicly express their respect and admiration for the honouree but also because it makes for a handsome addition to their own curricula vitae. And Festschrifts make the invited contributors happy because it sometimes affords them a chance to publish something that they might not be allowed to publish under less friendly circumstances. As a contributor I am grateful to Lars-Göran Nilsson for laying the groundwork for such an opening, and to Lars Bäckman and Lars Nyberg for effecting it, thereby making it possible to tell the story that appears here.

The story is about novelty. As everyone knows, brains are very good at detecting novelty. The question is, however, how do they do it? I discuss the question and suggest an answer to it. The story has its roots in previous work that I did some time ago with colleagues in Toronto, and also at the University of California at Davis, and that was significantly extended and elaborated by Lars-Göran Nilsson and his students in Stockholm. I first summarize this work and then raise and try to answer a question that emerged from it. It is now possible to imagine that the earlier version of the story may not have been quite right. Here, then, is an opportunity to make amends.

PETting memory

The story begins back in the 1990s, in the early heady days of "PETting memory". The newly developed technique of positron emission tomography (PET) had just been adapted for studying human cognition and seemed to hold the promise of providing fascinating new insights into the mind and its relation to brain. At Toronto, too, we found ourselves learning how to play the new game with the new toy in the new sandbox. I and some colleagues constituted ourselves a "PETting memory" team and began to explore encoding and retrieval processes of episodic memory. In one of our early PET studies, we measured regional cerebral blood flow of subjects as they looked at complex coloured scenes of people and places ("travel pictures") under two conditions: when the pictures were "new", seen for the first time, and when they were "old", having already been seen on the previous day (Tulving, Markowitsch, Kapur, Habib, & Houle, 1994b). When we subtracted the PET images for the new pictures from the images for the old pictures, we found a number of brain regions in the bilateral prefrontal cortex, left retrosplenial area, right angular gyrus, as well as some other cortical regions, that "lit up", meaning that they were more active for the old than the new pictures. That was exciting, because it suggested that we were seeing the regions of the brain where "remembering happened" – a brand new facet of experimental memory research of which Ebbinghaus could not have even dreamt.

Our enthusiasm, however, was a bit dampened when we looked at the PET images made by the opposite subtraction – that is, when we subtracted the images for old (familiar, remembered) pictures from the images for new ones that the subjects had never seen before. Quite a few brain regions "lit up" in this contrast, too, especially when we decided to throw caution to the wind and used a low threshold for significance. This meant that when the owner of the brain remembered seeing the pictures that he had seen 24 hours earlier, some regions of the brain became less active. This was puzzling. What made the puzzle even more baffling was the fact that these "deactivations", as they were called then (and sometimes are called so even today), occurred in what we thought could be properly classified as the "expanded limbic region". This region included the hippocampus! (See Figure 6.1.) Thus, what we had observed was that remembering past experiences reduces the activity in the hippocampus, the "seat of memory"! This was nothing less than scandalous, although we could not say so publicly, of course. (As the informed reader can see, we were a bit more naive and innocent about the ways of memory and the brain than we are now. Among other things, we thought that all the changes in regional blood flow that one observes in a functional neuroimaging study necessarily reflect experimental manipulations!)

Early PETters of cognition did not like to see activity reductions ("deactivations") in the brain because they did not quite know what to make of them. When task-related reductions in activity were observed, they tended to be just ignored or even not reported. By 1992, however, in an early PET study of

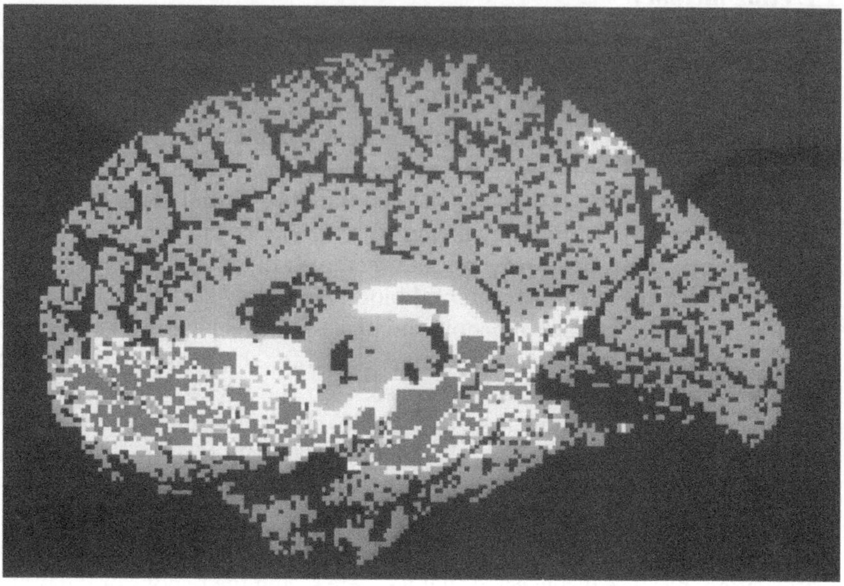

Figure 6.1 The expanded limbic region, showing greater activation by novel items than by familiar items. Data reported in Tulving et al. (1994b). (This figure is published in colour at http://www.cognitiveneurosciencearena.com/brain-scans/.)

memory retrieval (Squire et al., 1992) that showed activation near the right hippocampus, a deactivated region in the right occipital cortex was also observed and was boldly interpreted as signalling "priming", repetition-based facilitation of processing perceptual stimuli (Tulving & Schacter, 1990). Exactly how or why reduced neuronal activity should lead to improved behavioural performance was not quite spelt out – the question is still open, some 15 years later – but there was no problem with that: at the early stage of any scientific game, intuition often substitutes for logic. In our own very first PET study of what we thought was retrieval, this one with auditory sentences as the to-be-remembered material (Tulving, Kapur, Craik, Moscovitch, & Houle, 1994a), we had blithely copied the priming idea for the "deactivations" that had shown up, although we did not quite believe that all of the numerous "deactivations" signalled priming.

Novelty in the hippocampus

In the course of puzzling over the "unwanted" observation that the hippocampal formation tends to "slow down" when the subject looks at the remembered pictures, a happy, "novel" thought emerged that could be seen as "saving the phenomena" and fit reasonably into a world on which the hippocampus is central to memory. The thought was this: What if those puzzling "deactivated" brain sites did not show decreased familiarity (remembering) activation for previously studied pictures but, instead, showed relatively increased novelty of the new pictures? Thus, what we had observed was not decreased familiarity but increased novelty. Logically, of course, the two propositions are indistinguishable, being but mirror images of each other. If the brain activity for perceived familiarity, in any given region, is lower than the activity for novelty, then it must also be the case that, in that region, the activity for perceived novelty must be higher than the activity for familiarity in that region. So, perhaps the hippocampus and its adjacent structures served memory, indeed, as advertised, but perhaps they did so by detecting novelty rather than by "remembering" what had happened. We found encouragement for this thought in relatively freshly published data on single-unit recordings from monkey brains that had revealed the existence of neurons that showed more spiking activity when the monkey looked at a picture for the first time, in comparison with another picture that was shown repeatedly (Fahy, Riches, & Brown, 1993; Li, Miller, & Desimone, 1993; Wilson & Rolls, 1990.)

So, we had PET data showing "familiarity activations" that presumably had something to do with the remembering of the pictures, and we had data showing "novelty activations" that presumably also pointed to a memory-related function. But what function? How does higher brain activity for novelty fit into the larger picture? It was well known at the time, of course, that novel events are better remembered than familiar events, but the connection of that fact with our finding of "novelty activations" in the limbic system that included the hippocampus was not at all obvious.

One thought that suggested itself was that distinguishing between what is novel and what is already known is useful to the brain when it comes to deciding whether or not to store incoming information for long-term use. If brains are clever – and as products of evolution they must be – they would not clutter up their memory stores with information that is already "in there". Conversely, it is potentially advantageous to store information that is not yet "in there", novel information, because it may turn out to be relevant in the future. So, clever brains distinguish between the old and the new in order to use their memory storage capacity economically. And the hippocampus would still exercise control over declarative memory (Squire, 1992), but would do so mostly by encoding through novelty detection, a critical component of encoding.[1]

With some trepidation we published our new "discovery" of "widely distributed novelty-detection networks" (Tulving et al., 1994b) in a relatively new journal that was known for its reasonable reviewers and fast service to authors. Our message was that some brain networks are differentially involved in detecting novel stimuli, screening out the redundant information, and encoding the novel information in memory.

We specifically mentioned the hippocampus in the paper, although our "novelty activations" covered a much larger, albeit restricted, area than just the hippocampus. In those early days of PETting the mind, the hippocampus seldom showed up on the otherwise fetchingly colourful brain maps. In a review paper, Richard Frackowiak, one of the leaders of the new field, praised the overall developments, because "localizing psychological models onto distinct parts of the brain provides a much sought-after link between metaphorical description and biology", but he also pointed to the difficulties ahead, as "the hippocampus, long implicated in memory function, has been surprisingly difficult to activate" (Frackowiak, 1994, p. 111). So, lots of people were feverishly searching for the hippocampus in their PET studies of memory. Whenever a PET signal was detected anywhere near the medial temporal regions, it was warmly welcomed and eagerly labelled as "hippocampus". We were part of the crowd when we reported novelty in the expanded limbic system in the right hemisphere, a huge area that included the hippocampus.[2]

Right now this all sounds pretty weird, and certainly naive, but this realization is a sign of progress. And progress in PETting memory has been rapid. Today, with functional magnetic resonance imaging (fMRI) having largely replaced PET as the technique for neuroanatomical localization of mental activity, we know a great deal more than we did then, both about "memory in the brain" in general and about novelty/familiarity discrimination in particular. The hippocampus and its neocortical neighbours are now of equal interest to neurocognitive students of memory and are routinely observed in functional neuroimaging studies. "Back then", the idea that the phenomenal feeling of oldness and newness of an event may arise from the activity of the limbic system, perhaps among other brain regions, was purely intuitive and therefore highly speculative. Today, however, we have comforting evidence of the connection (Aggleton & Brown, 2006; Daselaar, Fleck, & Cabeza, 2006; Gonsalves, Kahn, Curran, Norman, & Wagner, 2005; Nyberg, 2005).

Novelty encoding hypothesis

"Back then", with the novelty detection networks revealed by PET (Tulving et al., 1994b), the question naturally arose as to the relation between the apparent ability of the limbic system to respond differentially to oldness/newness of stimuli and the well-known fact of superior memorability of novel stimuli. A possible answer to the question seemed to be that novel events are encoded more effectively, at the time of study, than familiar ones. The idea was formulated as the "novelty/encoding hypothesis" (Tulving & Kroll, 1995; Tulving, Markowitsch, Craik, Habib, & Houle, 1996). It postulated two sequentially organized sub-processes: novelty detection followed by "higher level" contextually determined encoding operations. The hippocampus and the limbic system would first serve to assess the novelty of the incoming information. Then, depending on the outcome of such assessment, the information would or would not be forwarded to other regions for the higher level encoding. In another one of our early PET studies (Kapur et al., 1994) we had already caught a glimpse of some such "encoding regions", including one in the left inferior prefrontal cortex. That one turned out to be a real winner, because today left inferior prefrontal cortex is acknowledged to be as important a player in the brain's memory games as the hippocampus.

At any rate, the novelty encoding hypothesis holds that when incoming information is novel, it undergoes further encoding processing and ends up successfully stored. When it is totally familiar – for instance, one and the same picture presented for the umpteenth time in a long series – it is "screened out", and its umpteenth presentation to the rememberer would not change what was already in the store before the umpteenth time. The two extremes, one of the highly novel and the other of the boringly familiar, are separated by a continuum of novelty detection and subsequent encoding, and a corresponding continuum of subsequent memory.

Now, if the novelty of an incoming item really is an important determinant of its encoding, one should be able to observe the effect even in purely behavioural tests. Furthermore, the effect should show up not just with pictorial material but with other kinds of incoming information as well. Because the behavioural data of our PET study were insufficient to test the idea – as we see below, we were missing an important control condition – I invited Neal Kroll at UC Davis to help me conduct an experiment whose design would allow a clean test of the novelty encoding hypothesis (Tulving & Kroll, 1995). We used what is known as the "3-phase recognition paradigm", or simply "3-phase paradigm". By holding constant all other variables that might affect memory performance, it allows complete control over oldness/newness of stimuli,

Here is a sketch of the 3-phase paradigm:

Phase 1	Study	A	B		
Phase 2	Study/Test	A		C	
Phase 3	Test	A	B	C	D

Each letter represents a set of individual items that subjects encounter. Thus, in Phase 1, subjects encounter items in experimental Sets A and B; in Phase 2, items in Sets A and C; and in Phase 3, items in Sets A, B, C, and D. All items "look alike" to the subjects; belongingness to different sets and subsets is known only to the experimenter.

The first two phases correspond to the classical yes/no recognition paradigm: in Phase 2, subjects are given a yes/no recognition test for items whose appearance they witnessed in Phase 1. In this test, items in Set A are the "old" targets, whereas items in Set C are the "new" lures.

In the 3-phase paradigm, Phase 1 becomes the "familiarization phase". Its purpose is to create "familiar" items for the study list presented in Phase 2, in order to compare their learning in Phase 2 and subsequent retention with "novel" (non-familiarized) items. Phase 3 provides the relevant data for this comparison. The subjects' task is to discriminate between items studied (A and C) and those not studied (B and D) in Phase 2. The experimenter's interest lies in whether the novelty/familiarity status of the test items affects such discrimination. The recognition test items in Phase 3 are A: familiar, studied; B: familiar, not studied; C: novel, studied; D: novel, not studied.

Thus, the design of the 3-phase paradigm is 2 × 2. One factor is familiarity/novelty, defined by the presence or absence of intra-experimental encounter prior to Phase 2. The second factor is study/non-study, defined by the item's appearance or non-appearance in Phase 2.

The novelty encoding hypothesis "predicts" that subjects are more accurate at recognizing C (novel) items than A (familiar) items as having occurred in Phase 2. Accuracy of recognition can be measured as the difference between hit rates and false-alarm rates. (Using other measures, such as d', does not materially change the outcome.) Thus the "prediction" of the novelty encoding hypothesis becomes one of interaction between the two factors of the 2 × 2 design. The difference between the probability of calling C items old and calling D items old should be larger than the difference between the probability of calling A items old and calling B items old – that is, (C – D) > (A – B), where each letter represents the probability of items called "old" in the corresponding subsets (i.e., as having been seen in Phase 2).

Although we tested only four subjects, the experiment produced the predicted results with a vengeance. Recognition accuracy, as defined, was .20 for familiar words and .56 for novel words. This is a large difference. The F ratio for the predicted interaction, with 1 and 3 degrees of freedom, turned out to be 280.3, which was "off the charts", although we modestly reported it as having a p value less than .01.

Physiologically oriented memory researchers took our "discovery" in stride, because it fitted snugly into the rapidly unfolding larger picture of brain and novelty. Psychologically oriented memory researchers were less keen on the study, and those few who seemed to have looked at the paper tended to be sceptical about both our findings and our thoughts about them (Chalmers & Humphreys, 1998; Dobbins, Kroll, Yonelinas, & Liu, 1998; Greene, 1999; Maddox & Estes, 1997). Among other things, doubts were expressed about the reliability and generalizability of the data. There were two earlier papers in the literature that reported the same kind of novelty effect that we had observed (Anderson & Bower, 1972, Expt. 4; Kinsbourne & George, 1974), but not too many people knew about them.

This is where Lars-Göran Nilsson led his troops into the breach (Åberg & Nilsson, 2001, 2003; Kormi-Nouri, Nilsson, & Ohta, 2005). In their experiments they adopted the general logic and design of the 3-phase paradigm and tested the effect of variables such as the format of the familiarization procedures, the nature of test materials, and the types of the activity between successive phases of the experiment. When they had finished, after several years of diligent work and spirited battles with critics, they had replicated the "novelty effect" many times. On a few occasions they had to make concessions to the referees of their papers who had their own theories as to what was going on in the 3-phase paradigm, and what the data really meant.

Thus, thanks to the effort of Lars-Göran Nilsson and his students, the "novelty effect" as captured by the 3-phase recognition paradigm was firmly established. However, a problem remained. The problem had been there from the beginning, and its existence caused the researchers in Stockholm considerable headache, because the critics of the work kept hammering away at it: Well, you may have the data, and you can claim that they are caused by novelty, but how do you explain them?

The critics were right: there was no explanation. The novelty/encoding hypothesis offered no insight into why or how novelty detection, or novelty assessment, occurs. It simply stated a generalization, derived from empirical observations, that the brain (or the long-term memory system) responds more vigorously to novel than to non-novel (recently encountered) stimuli and that this enhanced vigour is translated into more effective encoding. It was completely mute on any details of how this happens. This was not good. To invoke the concept of novelty when reporting that people can tell the old from the new, and that newness of stimuli enhances remembering, means essentially to describe the 3-phase paradigm and the findings that it yields. It does not say anything about how novelty detection "works". To attribute the effect of novelty to greater "attention" that subjects, at study, pay to novel items also amounts to the description of the experiment and its results, with an addition "epicycle" thrown in. It does not say how the subjects identify novel items in order to pay more attention to them.

So, the problem remained: What are the underlying processes or mechanisms? To put it in slightly loftier language: what are the lathomena behind the phenomena of novelty detection?[3] This issue, explaining novelty detection, will occupy us in the remainder of this chapter.

Comparator models of novelty detection

The most popular neurocognitive account of novelty detection at the present time is provided by the "comparator model", or the "match–mismatch" model (Kumaran & Maguire, 2007b). Different versions of these models have been proposed, but they share the central idea that novelty detection is based on a comparison of the incoming information with information already stored in the system. This comparison is carried out by specialized neuronal networks, usually the hippocampus, or computational mechanisms, that match incoming information against the information already in the system, or against what the system (human, animal, robot), on the basis of its previous experience, "expects" to happen. If the difference between the actual and the expected is sufficiently large there is a "mismatch", and novelty is said to have been detected. The statement in a recent paper by Kumaran and Maguire (2007a) describing relevant fMRI data neatly captures these ideas:

"the hippocampus may generate predictions about how future events will unfold, and critically detect when these expectancies are violated, even when task demands do not require it" (p. 2372). The idea of the hippocampus as a novelty comparator has a respectable history that goes back to research and thinking before PET (Gray, 1982). Our PET findings of novelty detection seemed to fit into the larger picture nicely, even if our data showed novelty activations in a wider region, beyond the hippocampus. The notion of the hippocampus as a comparator became even more respectable when other PETters also reported sightings of the medial temporal regions when they compared PET responses to old and new pictures (Stern et al., 1996). An especially striking demonstration of the central role of the hippocampus was reported by Martin and coworkers when they compared old and new coloured, totally meaningless noise patterns (Martin, Wiggs, & Weisberg, 1997). Today the literature on the medial temporal lobe and novelty detection is extensive, and the critical regions that have been shown to be implicated have extended beyond the hippocampus into adjacent parahippocampal neocortical regions, especially perirhinal cortex (Brown & Aggleton, 2001), as well as the basal forebrain and the ventral tegmental area (Lisman & Grace, 2005).

Quite apart from the issue of "where in the brain" it happens, the idea that novelty detection requires a comparison between incoming information with that previously stored has been explicitly approved or implicitly accepted by many. In the Tulving and Kroll (1995) paper, we also took it for granted. Comparison seemed inevitably necessary. How else can anyone – the human rememberer, the brain, the hippocampus – decide whether a stimulus that one is facing now has not been encountered before, or at least not encountered recently, if not by comparing it with what has been encountered before? It is this apparently inescapable involvement of past experience in novelty detection that makes novelty detection a part of memory.

Can brains actually do it? Do they have to?

There is a problem. Hippocampus as a comparator is a metaphor. Explanations of novelty detection that are based on the concepts such as mismatch or comparison are no better, nor worse, than other metaphorical explanations that Richard Frackowiak, mentioned earlier, was talking about. Even when explanations are presented in the form of highly sophisticated models of how and where in the brain the relevant computations are carried out, they are still metaphorical. Kumaran and Maguire's apt phrase that I quoted above about the hippocampus that generates predictions and detects violations of expectancies beautifully captures the spirit of this kind of explanation Kumaran & Maguire, 2007a, p. 2372). The description makes the central ideas clear, and as such it is heuristically most useful. But it need not be true.

Metaphorical explanations are among the time-honoured tools that brain/mind scientists use to fill gaps in their theories. They help us get on with the business. In many of these explanations, mind/brain processes or mechanisms are likened to events and activities in our everyday world. The domain of memory is replete with anthropomorphic processes and mechanisms, beginning with various metaphorical renderings of "memory" itself (Roediger, 1980). When we talk about "strengthening" memory, we have in mind an analogy with strengthening of the muscle with practice; when we talk about retrieval as "search", we think of the reading glasses or the car keys that we have misplaced in the house; when we talk about conscious awareness of our own experiences at times other than the present as "mental time travel", and about the "self" that has the awareness as the "traveller", we surely speak most metaphorically. In *Elements of Episodic Memory* (Tulving, 1983) I had decried the use of anthropomorphic descriptions of internal processes of memory because they created an illusion of understanding where we should have been admitting ignorance and using this ignorance as spur to further study. Among the examples of human-like activities pressed into service in encoding and retrieval that I listed were analysing, anticipating, categorizing, comparing, comprehending, computing, deciding, discriminating, estimating, filtering, generating, interpreting, locating, marking, matching, mismatching, organizing, pigeon-holing, rehearsing, rejecting, scanning, searching, sorting, supplementing, switching, transferring, and understanding (Tulving, 1983, p. 141). In those days, the brain did not play much of a role of any kind in the study of human memory, and the processes were purely "cognitive". Today, as the case of the hippocampus as the comparator shows, temptation is great to have the brain engage in these kinds of purely human activities too.

One problem with the comparator, or match–mismatch, model of novelty detection is that it leaves the fundamental problem unsolved: What is the mechanism that underlies novelty detection? To suggest that there is something like what we ordinarily mean by comparison actually going on in the brain means to stretch the credulity of many thinkers who distinguish between what the brain does, or can do, and what the whole organism, the brain's owner, can do. It is difficult to imagine the physical brain actually comparing old and new objects. Oldness/newness is not a primary quality of objects – it is not like weight or length or hardness. It is not even a secondary quality – like hue or loudness or taste – which the brain, properly outfitted with relevant sensors, could be said to be able to detect and identify, in its own way, of course. Oldness/newness is a historical quality, and histories reside in the minds of thinking people, blessed with both highly evolved brains and educated, conscious minds.

The more important reason for questioning the idea of the brain's ability to perform match–mismatch computations is that there is no need for such computations. It is not necessary to postulate any comparison mechanisms in order to account for novelty detection. There is no need to attribute to the physical brain (or the hippocampus, or its CA1 field) capabilities that they do not possess. Instead, there is a need to understand how the capabilities that they do have serve the brain's owner.

I will argue that we can explain novelty detection in the brain without invoking comparisons and matches–mismatches. The brain can record happenings within the domains of its sensors and can store the information comprising these happenings. Various resulting records (engrams, memory traces) can become a part of the brain's state at any given moment. This current state co-determines and modulates how any incoming information is processed, and it thereby shapes the consequences of that processing. In the case we are discussing here – novelty detection in the 3-phase paradigm – it is this current state that determines the differential processing of items in Sets A and C in the second phase of the 3-phase paradigm for their encoding and hence subsequent recognition. The point I am making is that it is possible to think of brain mechanisms that are involved in what the external observer of the brain calls novelty detection without attributing human-like capabilities to the human brain. One such possible mechanism is what I call "camatosis".

The concept of camatosis

Camatosis is a (hypothetical) neurophysiological process that causes specific activity-dependent reduction in the efficacy of the operation of neuronal networks that support encoding of incoming information for long-term storage. The term is derived from "kamatos", a word in classical Greek which can be translated into English as "tiredness" or "weariness".[4]

Camatosis – specific activity-dependent "weariness" of a neuronal network – is analogous to the "fatigue" that many biological systems incur as a consequence of their operations. Camatosis manifests itself in the diminution of the functional efficacy of a particular neural ensemble to do again at Time 2 what it did at an earlier time, Time 1. It applies to situations in which the presentation of an item (Event 1) occurs at time T1 and the presentation of the same, or similar, item (Event 2) occurs at a subsequent time T2. If the processing of Event 2 involves the same, or largely the same, neuronal networks that supported the processing of Event 1, and those networks are "camatotic", processing of Event 2 will suffer – it will not occur "normally", as it would in the absence of camatosis of the relevant networks. To the extent that this "processing" is responsible for encoding (conversion of a perceptual/cognitive event into a long-term memory trace), encoding of Event 2 will be impaired.[5]

The concept of camatosis was initially introduced in a theoretical treatment of the inhibiting effects of earlier "learning" on subsequent "learning", in situations where the interfering memory items were not (nominally) identical but only similar. In the very first publication on camatosis, the concept was used to account for the von-Restorff-type distinctiveness effects (Tulving & Rosenbaum, 2005). The idea was that what required explanation was not the good memory for the isolated item but, rather, the poor memory for the massed items. Camatosis was suggested as the "cause" of that poor memory. In a second paper, camatosis was proffered as an explanation, or as a factor contributing to the explanation, of a variety of primacy effects in memory (Tulving, 2007). This paper also proposed a "law of camatotic encoding": Of two events, the one whose encoding is more severely affected by camatosis is less likely to be retained. I will return to this "law" later.

The camatotic effect of Event 1 on Event 2 depends on many factors, as yet mostly unknown, although two relevant factors can be tentatively pinpointed on the basis of available evidence. One such is the similarity of Events 1 and 2: The greater this similarity, the greater the overlap between the neuronal networks processing Events 1 and 2, and the greater the camatotic effect of Event 1 on Event 2. Evidence from experiments conducted long ago and now nearly forgotten shows that in extreme cases of "massed repetition" (one and the same item presented for study twice in immediate succession), the additional opportunity for encoding afforded by the second presentation may have no effect at all (Madigan, 1969; Waugh, 1970). The other factor is the temporal interval between Events 1 and 2. Similar to the way the firing of a single spike in a single neuron is followed by a refractory period, the operation of a network is followed by a refractory period, although on a much wider timescale. A neat behavioural illustration of the refractoriness of what we now might refer to as camatosis can be found in Loess and Waugh (1967).

The camatosis hypothesis fits the 3-phase paradigm well: (nominally) identical items are repeatedly presented, and repetition impairs memory. In this paradigm, as described earlier, items familiarized in Phase 1 and presented again for study in Phase 2 (items of type A) are less likely to be identified as "old" in Phase 3, in comparison with novel items studied in Phase 2 (items of type C). What causes the difference? The answer is, camatosis. When a Set A item appears in Phase 1 of the 3-phase experiment, it is processed "normally" through the operation of a particular neuronal network whose "business" it is to register that kind of a particular input. When the same A item appears again in Phase 2, the event is again processed by very much the same network. This time, however, the processing cannot proceed quite "normally", because some of the components of the network that were engaged in registering that item in Phase 1 have not yet recovered from their earlier operations. The less-than-optimal processing of the second occurrence of Item A produces a brain signal different from that of its first occurrence, and different from that of Item C when that item occurs, for the first time, in Phase 2. The observing scientist who compares these two signals notices the difference and says "Ha, here we have it, familiarity detection", or "Ha, here we have it, novelty detection."

The camatosis hypothesis

Even more relevant to our story in this chapter is the assumption that the impaired processing of Item A, when it is encountered by the subject in Phase 2, has a deleterious effect on the process of encoding that encounter, in long-term memory. It is this camatotically handicapped treatment of Set A items that shows up in the 2 × 2 results of the 3-phase experiments (Åberg & Nilsson, 2001, 2003; Kormi-Nouri et al., 2005; Tulving & Kroll, 1995) as a difference between recognition accuracy of Set A items and Set C items. When we looked at these results "back then", we could say "Ha, novelty effect in memory", but, in the absence of an idea such as that about camatosis, we could not say anything much more about it. There was no explanation.

Now we have a possible explanation. Novelty effects in memory, revealed by the 3-phase paradigm, represent a particular instance of the general "law of camatotic encoding": Of two events, the one whose encoding is more severely affected by camatosis is less likely to be encoded and therefore less likely to be retained.

This kind of an explanation, derived from a "law", may sound anachronistic in our day and age. Scientific laws were popular in psychology in the discipline's early, formative years and decades (Teigen, 2002). Today they have all but vanished, for reasons that seem to be reasonably clear (Roediger, 2008). In this climate, to suggest a "law" seems almost heretical, especially if the temptation may be strong to glibly dismiss the proposed "law" as a definitional tautology.

The camatosis hypothesis could be illustrated graphically as shown in Figure 6.2. I have borrowed the illustration, with the authors' kind permission, from Wiggs and Martin (1998). It shows how the network of features coding a perceptual (or any cognitive) object changes, or becomes "sharpened", over its successive presentations. Wiggs and Martin created this neat diagram as an illustration of their own model of priming. Their caption was as follows:

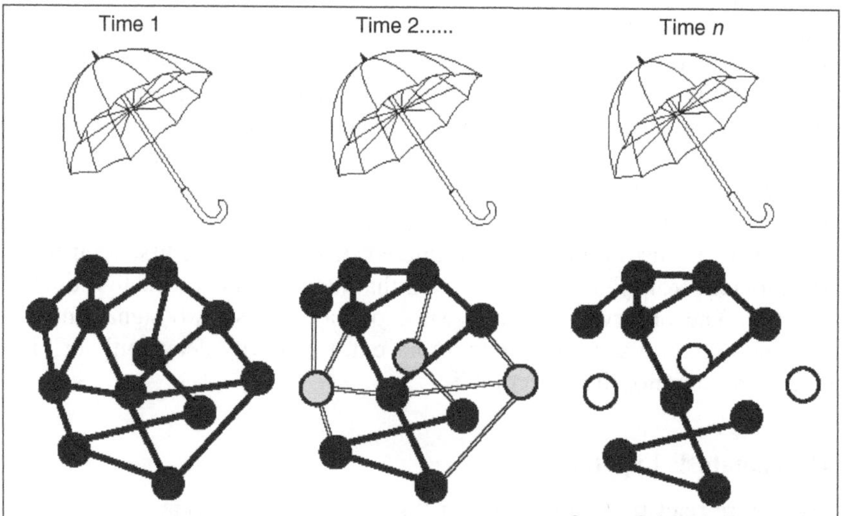

Figure 6.2 A possible schematic representation of the camatosis hypothesis. (Reproduced by permission from Wiggs & Martin, 1998.)

> Illustration of the changes in a neuronal network representing visual object features as a function of repeated experience. As an object is presented repeatedly, neurons coding features that are not essential for recognizing the object decrease their responses (from black to grey to white), thereby weakening connections with other neurons in the ensemble (from black, to open, to no lines). As a result, the network becomes sparser and more selective, yielding enhanced object recognition. (Wiggs & Martin, 1998, p. 230)

For our present purposes – namely, to illustrate camatosis – the caption might become something like this: "Illustration of the changes in a neuronal network representing features of a perceptual event as a function of its repeated occurrence. Some components involved in optimal ('normal') coding of the event become camatotic because of their previous engagement, as shown by changes from black, to open, to no lines, and the network becomes less efficient in representing the event."

The camatosis model differs from the Wiggs and Martin model in that it assumes that the initial coding of the event is always optimal. In the Wiggs and Martin model it is not, insofar as it also involves non-essential features that are shed in the subsequent "sharpening" process. It also differs in that instead of the representation becoming "sharper" over successive repetitions, it becomes impoverished. These features of the camatosis model finesse the problem of why the initial coding of a stimulus is not as sharp as it could be, and why it includes nonessential features that can be dropped. Evolved brains have been practising object identification for hundreds of millions of years, and they ought to be pretty well tuned by now when it comes to the question of what to code and what not. At any rate, and regardless of whether we can ever know how clever brains really are, the camatosis model does not have any problem with dropped features of the network. All features that are needed for optimal ("normal") processing are coded under "normal" conditions – that is, when the coding network is not camatotic by virtue of its recent engagement.

Note that according to the camatosis hypothesis there is no novelty detection in the brain, and there are no novelty detection circuits or networks. The brain does not classify the incoming information as novel, or familiar, or somewhere in between. And it does not screen out or forward to higher encoding networks information for further processing depending on its novelty/familiarity status. Our conjecture "back then" was wrong. Novelty detection exists, of course – otherwise we would not be talking about it – but it does not exist as a neural operation. It exists only as a concept, as an idea in the observing scientist's mind. All that the brain does is to process old and new stimuli differently, in keeping with its current state, including the camatosis of the networks specific to different stimuli and different combinations of stimuli. It is the external observer who describes the products of such differential processing in comparative terms. The brain is a machine; it does its thing (superbly, at least most of the time), but it cannot do things that the more powerful brain/mind system can.

The concept of camatosis is closely related to many other ideas that psychologists and other brain/mind scientists have created for the purpose of talking about what they do. There are the old perennials of habituation and adaptation that go back to the beginning of our science (Carandini, 2000; Sohal & Hasselmo, 2000). Numerous more specific terms have been used by researchers who have pursued problems in the neurophysiology of habituation and adaptation-like effects: "adaptive filtering" (Desimone, 1992), "adaptive mnemonic filtering" (Miller, Li, & Desimone, 1993), "stimulus specific adaptation" (Ringo, 1996), repetition suppression (Desimone, 1996; Henson & Rugg, 2003; Wiggs & Martin, 1998), decremental responses (Brown & Xiang, 1998), "repetition priming" or "neural priming" or just "priming" (Buckner & Koutstaal, 1998; Wagner, Koutstaal, Maril, Schacter, & Buckner, 2000), "cortical activity reduction" (Dobbins, Schnyer, Verfaellie, & Schacter, 2004), plus others. Recent developments point to the adoption of the term "repetition suppression" as a generic label of electrophysiologically and hemodynamically measured reductions of brain activity when a cognitively significant stimulus is presented repeatedly (Grill-Spector, Henson, & Martin, 2006).

Given this kind of embarrassment of riches, why yet another, new term? Why should anyone want to deliberately add to the terminological mess? There are at least two reasons. The first is relatively unimportant but worth mentioning nevertheless. Camatosis is the name of a hypothetical physiological mechanism that is introduced to explain, or help explain, particular behavioural/cognitive phenomena, such as novelty detection that leads to the novelty effect in memory. It is not a phenomenon itself; it is the hypothesized "cause" of a phenomenon. Making distinctions between causes and effects is healthy. Many terms that have cropped up even in my short essay – novelty detection, mismatch, adaptation, (repetition) priming – are ambiguous because they have been used in the sense of both observed behaviour and their underlying mechanism. It is an ancient problem in our science that persists, probably because scientists are busy people who have more important things on their minds than worrying about the cleanliness of the terms they use. Camatosis is supposed to be cleaner than many others in its circle of acquaintances, because it has a single meaning: specific activity-dependent "weariness" of a neuronal network subserving long-term memory encoding.

The second reason, a bit more substantial, has to do with camatosis not as a term but as a concept, an idea that has to do with things such as memory, repetition, and novelty detection. Like any other scientific concept, it receives its meaning and its usefulness by virtue of the role it plays in a wider theoretical context, and by virtue of its similarities to and differences from other concepts that figure in the same context (Dudai, Roediger, & Tulving, 2007). Camatosis is distinguished from other closely related concepts primarily by four ideas: (a) The insistence on the centrality of the fact that novelty is a relational concept and must be dealt with as such, as one end of a continuum between the novelty and non-novelty; (b) The idea that novelty is "normal" and reflects what the brain can do, and does, when its operations are not being hampered by nuisances such as camatosis, whereas non-novelty reflects the workings of the brain handicapped by camatosis; (c) The idea that there probably are no "novelty detection" mechanisms, circuits, or neuronal networks in the brain; (d) The idea that there is no need to endow brains with human-like powers, such as the ability to make decisions on the basis of comparisons. It is this combination of features encompassed by the concept of camatosis that makes it unique and worth thinking and talking out.

Summary

So, how do brains detect novelty? Strictly speaking, as I have suggested, they do not. Physical brains deal with the physical universe, and in the physical universe there is no such thing as novelty. This is why brains cannot "detect" novelty. Brains respond differentially to inputs, depending on their current state, which includes traces of past experiences. Intelligent observers can interpret some of the differences as reflecting novelty, but that is a propositionally expressed human judgment, not a brain decision.

In this chapter I have dealt with the problem of how to explain the observer-identified novelty detection as a necessary component of novelty effect in memory, the well-known phenomenon that novel events are remembered better than non-novel events. I limited the discussion to a special case of the novelty effect demonstrated in the 3-phase recognition paradigm, but it seems reasonable to expect that the same reasoning applies more generally to novelty effects of memory in other situations as well.

I noted that the popular comparator, or match–mismatch, models of novelty detection are unnecessarily complicated and attribute capacities to the brain as a physical/physiological "machine" that the brain probably does not possess. I also noted that "novelty" is a relational concept. To explain it means to explain the difference between the novel and the non-novel.

I described and discussed a recently introduced new concept, "camatosis" – the idea that the efficacy of neural networks involved in the process of encoding incoming information for long-term memory is reduced as a consequence of their own operations. Camatosis produced by earlier events deleteriously affects the encoding of subsequent events, depending on the extent to which the events in question are similar and are therefore subserved by correspondingly similar neural networks.

The concept of camatosis helps us understand the novelty effect observed in the 3-phase recognition paradigm – that items previously encountered in the experimental situation are less well recognized than items not previously encountered in the situation, or, in other words, that novel items are better remembered than familiar items. Camatosis leads to reduced efficacy of encoding of familiar items and thereby to their impaired retention in relation to the non-familiar (novel) items. When an external observer, contemplating the difference, focuses on the novel items, their higher memorability is seen as the "novelty effect". I suggested that this novelty effect can be viewed as a particular instance of a general law of camatotic encoding: Of two events, the one whose encoding is more severely affected by camatosis is less likely to be retained.

The idea of camatosis as a co-determinant of encoding processes provides only a broad and rough guide to exploring phenomena of the kind that led to the novelty encoding hypothesis. Its practical merits are unknown and remain to be determined by research. It claims the existence of physiological mechanisms that, automatically, inevitably come to restrain "normal" processes that are involved in converting a perceptual object or event into a long-term memory trace. The neurophysiological specifics of these mechanisms are not specified and remain to be identified. This will happen in the future. The important point is that even in its broad form the concept of camatosis allows us to systematically relate phenomena of novelty and familiarity to other interference phenomena of memory. When testing the camatosis hypothesis, in real life or in laboratory experiments, however, it is imperative to mind the *ceteris paribus* clause. It can be easily overlooked, yet it applies to the case of camatosis as it does to all other cases of explanatory abstractions.

Acknowledgements

My research is supported by an endowment by Anne and Max Tanenbaum in support of research in cognitive neuroscience.

Notes

1 The idea was not terribly original, as other thinkers had already discussed it (Kohonen, Oja, & Lehtiö, 1989, Metcalfe, 1993), but that did not matter, because very few ideas ever are. Although there was no experimental data directly relevant to it, one thing that made it attractive was the fact that an obvious alternative possibility that the brains store everything that happens and, every now and then, somehow or other clears out the redundant or otherwise unneeded stuff – perhaps at night, when the owner sleeps – sounded unnecessarily complicated, too much like Rube Goldberg. An early selection mechanism seemed preferable, a bit more worthy of the evolved brain.

2 In the context of Lars-Göran Nilsson's Festschrift, an interesting detail of our "travel pictures" PET study may be worth noting. The Talairach and Tournoux (1988) coordinates of one of the "peaks" of novelty activation in the right medial temporal region in that study were xyz = 26 –32 –8 (Tulving et al., 1994b, Table 1). In an fMRI study, co-authored by the celebree of this Festschrift and its two editors (Lind et al., 2006), the same hippocampal region (xyz = 30 –30 –8, MNI [Montreal Neurological Institute] coordinates) was identified as one in which a similar novelty activation (novel > familiar) for words was observed for one of two groups of APOE carriers (ε3/3), while the other group (ε4) showed activation in the reverse direction (familiar > novel). APOE ε4 carriers are known to be at high risk for Alzheimer's disease and impairment of episodic memory, hence the potential

significance of the observation. But regardless of that implication, the close match between the "novelty activations" in the two studies, widely separated geographically and historically, is "cool".

3 As noted earlier, one can write things in a Festschrift that diligent censors would cross out elsewhere. "Lathomena" (plural of "lathomenon") is a real word that one can find in a real book (Tulving, 1983, pp. 123, 349), as well as in Simple English Wikipedia on the Internet, if you look up "phenomenon" there, although it is not in any dictionary, yet.

4 I am grateful to Jaan Puhvel for creating the term for its intended purpose.

5 As brains are permanently active, in one way or another, they are also permanently camatotic, in one way or another. What I refer to as "normal" processing of given input refers to processing under the conditions where there has been no recent brain activity involving components of the specific functionally relevant networks underlying the processing of that particular input.

References

Åberg, C. S., & Nilsson, L.-G. (2001). Facilitation of source discrimination in the novelty effect. *Scandinavian Journal of Psychology*, *42*, 349–357.

Åberg, C. S., & Nilsson, L.-G. (2003). A strict response criterion yields a mirror effect in the novelty paradigm. *Scandinavian Journal of Psychology*, *44*, 425–432.

Aggleton, J. P., & Brown, M. W. (2006). Interleaving brain systems for episodic and recognition memory. *Trends in Cognitive Sciences*, *10*, 455–463.

Anderson, J. R., & Bower, G. H. (1972). Recognition and retrieval processes in free recall. *Psychological Review*, *79*, 97–123.

Brown, M. W., & Aggleton, J. P. (2001). Recognition memory: What are the roles of the perirhinal cortex and hippocampus? *Nature Reviews Neuroscience*, *2*(1), 51–61.

Brown, M. W., & Xiang, J. Z. (1998). Recognition memory: Neuronal substrates of the judgment of prior occurrence. *Progress in Neurobiology*, *55*, 184–189.

Buckner, R. L., & Koutstaal, W. (1998). Functional neuroimaging studies of encoding, priming, and explicit memory retrieval. *Proceedings of the National Academy of Sciences USA*, *95*(3), 891–898.

Carandini, M. (2000). Visual cortex: Fatigue and adaptation. *Current Biology*, *10*, R605–R607.

Chalmers, K. A., & Humphreys, M. S. (1998). Role of generalized and episode specific memories in the word frequency effect in recognition. *Journal of Experimental Psychology: Learning, Memory, and Cognition*, *24*(3), 610–632.

Daselaar, S. M., Fleck, M. S., & Cabeza, R. (2006). Triple dissociation in the medial temporal lobes: Recollection, familiarity, and novelty. *Journal of Neurophysiology*, *96*(4), 1902–1911.

Desimone, R. (1992). The physiology of memory: Recordings of things past. *Science*, *258*, 245–246.

Desimone, R. (1996). Neural mechanisms for visual memory and their role in attention. *Proceedings of the National Academy of Sciences, USA*, *93*, 13494–13499.

Dobbins, I. G., Kroll, N. E. A., Yonelinas, A. P., & Liu, Q. (1998). Distinctiveness in recognition and free recall: The role of recollection in the rejection of the familiar. *Journal of Memory and Language*, *38*(4), 381–400.

Dobbins, I. G., Schnyer, D. M., Verfaellie, M., & Schacter, D. L. (2004). Cortical activity reductions during repetition priming can result from rapid response learning. *Nature*, *428*(6980), 316–319.

Dudai, Y., Roediger, H. L. III, & Tulving, E. (2007). Memory concepts. In H. L. Roediger III, Y. Dudai, & S. M. Fitzpatrick (Eds.), *Science of memory: Concepts* (pp. 1–9). New York: Oxford University Press.

Fahy, F. L., Riches, I. P., & Brown, M. W. (1993). Neuronal activity related to visual recognition memory: Long-term memory and the encoding of recency and familiarity information in the primate anterior and medial inferior temporal and rhinal cortex. *Experimental Brain Research, 96*(3), 457–472.

Frackowiak, R. S. J. (1994). Functional mapping of verbal memory and language. *Trends in Neurosciences, 17*(3), 109–115.

Gonsalves, B. D., Kahn, I., Curran, T., Norman, K. A., & Wagner, A. D. (2005). Memory strength and repetition suppression: Multimodal imaging of medial temporal cortical contributions to recognition. *Neuron, 47*(5), 751–761.

Gray, J. A. (1982). The neuropsychology of anxiety: An enquiry into the functions of the septo-hippocampal system. Oxford, UK: Oxford University Press.

Greene, R. L. (1999). The role of familiarity in recognition. *Psychonomic Bulletin & Review, 6*, 309–312.

Grill-Spector, K., Henson, R., & Martin, A. (2006). Repetition and the brain: Neural models of stimulus-specific effects. *Trends in Cognitive Sciences, 10*(1), 14–23.

Henson, R. N. A., & Rugg, M. D. (2003). Neural response suppression, haemodynamic repetition effects, and behavioural priming. *Neuropsychologia, 41*(3), 263–270.

Kapur, S., Craik, F. I. M., Tulving, E., Wilson, A. A., Houle, S., & Brown, G. M. (1994). Neuroanatomical correlates of encoding in episodic memory: Levels of processing effect. *Proceedings of the National Academy of Sciences USA, 91*(6), 2008–2011.

Kinsbourne, M., & George, J. 1974). The mechanism of the word-frequency effect on recognition memory. *Journal of Verbal Learning and Verbal Behavior, 13*, 63–69.

Kohonen, T., Oja, E., & Lehtiö, P. (1989). Storage and processing of information in distributed associative memory systems. In G. E. Hinton & J. A. Anderson (Eds.), *Parallel models of associative memory* (pp. 129–167). Hillsdale, NJ: Lawrence Erlbaum Associates, Inc.

Kormi-Nouri, R., Nilsson, L. G., & Ohta, N. (2005). The novelty effect: Support for the Novelty-Encoding Hypothesis. *Scandinavian Journal of Psychology, 46*(2), 133–143.

Kumaran, D., & Maguire, E. A. (2007a). An unexpected sequence of events: Mismatch detection in the human hippocampus. *PLoS Biology, 4*, 2372–2382.

Kumaran, D., & Maguire, E. A. (2007b). Match-mismatch processes underlie human hippocampal responses to associative novelty. *Journal of Neuroscience, 27*(32), 8517–8524.

Li, L., Miller, E. K., & Desimone, R. (1993). The presentation of stimulus-familiarity in anterior inferior temporal cortex. *Journal of Neurophysiology, 69*(6), 1918–1929.

Lind, A., Persson, J., Ingvar, M., Larsson, A., Cruts, M., Van Broeckhoven, C., et al. (2006). Reduced functional brain activity response in cognitively intact apolipoprotein E €4 carriers. *Brain, 129*, 1240–1248.

Lisman, J. E., & Grace, A. A. (2005). The hippocampal–VTA loop: Controlling the entry of information into long-term memory. *Neuron, 46*(5), 703–713.

Loess, H., & Waugh, N. C. (1967). Short-term memory and inter-trial interval. *Journal of Verbal Learning and Verbal Behavior, 6*, 455–460.

Maddox, W. T., & Estes, W. K. (1997). Direct and indirect stimulus-frequency effects in recognition. *Journal of Experimental Psychology: Learning, Memory, and Cognition, 23*(3), 539–559.

Madigan, S. A. (1969). Intraserial repetition and coding processes in free recall. *Journal of Verbal Learning and Verbal Behavior, 8*, 828–835.

Martin, A., Wiggs, C. L., & Weisberg, J. (1997). Modulation of human medial temporal lobe activity by form, meaning, and experience. *Hippocampus, 7*(6), 587–593.

Metcalfe, J. (1993). Novelty monitoring, metacognition, and control in a composite holographic associative recall model: Implications for Korsakoff amnesia. *Psychological Review, 100*, 3–22.

Miller, E. K., Li, L., & Desimone, R. (1993). Activity of neurons in anterior inferior temporal cortex during a short-term memory task. *Journal of Neuroscience, 13*, 1460–1478.

Nyberg, L. (2005). Any novelty in hippocampal formation and memory? *Current Opinion in Neurology, 18*(4), 424–428.

Ringo, J. L. (1996). Stimulus specific adaptation in inferior temporal and medial temporal cortex of the monkey. *Behavioural Brain Research, 76*(1–2), 191–197.

Roediger, H. L., III. (1980). Memory metaphors in cognitive psychology. *Memory & Cognition, 8*, 231–246.

Roediger, H. L., III. (2008). Relativity of remembering: Why the laws of memory vanished. *Annual Review of Psychology, 59*, 225–254.

Sohal, V. S., & Hasselmo, M. E. (2000). A model for experience-dependent changes in the responses of inferotemporal neurons. *Network: Computation in Neural Systems, 11*(3), 169–190.

Squire, L.R. (1992). Memory and the hippocampus: A synthesis from findings with rats, monkeys, and humans. *Psychological Review, 99*, 195–231.

Squire, L. R., Ojemann, J. G., Miezin, F. M, Petersen, S. E., Videen, T. O., & Raichle, M. E. (1992). Activation of the hippocampus in normal humans: A functional anatomical study of memory. *Proceedings of the National Academy of Sciences, USA, 89*, 1837–1841.

Stern, C. E., Corkin, S., Gonzalez, R. G., Guimaraes, A. R., Baker, J. R., Jennings, P. A., et al. (1996). The hippocampal formation participates in novel picture encoding: Evidence from functional magnetic resonance imaging. *Proceedings of the National Academy of Sciences, USA, 93*, 8660–8665.

Talairach, J., & Tournoux, P. (1988). *Co-planar stereotaxic atlas of the human brain*. New York: Thieme.

Teigen, K. H. (2002). One hundred years of laws in psychology. *American Journal of Psychology, 115*, 103–118.

Tulving, E. (1983). *Elements of episodic memory*. Oxford, UK: Clarendon Press.

Tulving, E. (2007). On the law of primacy. In M. A. Gluck, J. R. Anderson, & S. M. Kosslyn (Eds.), *Memory and mind: A festschrift for Gordon H. Bower* (pp. 31–48). Hillsdale, NJ: Lawrence Erlbaum Associates, Inc.

Tulving, E., Kapur, S., Craik, F. I. M., Moscovitch, M., & Houle, S. (1994a). Hemispheric encoding/retrieval asymmetry in episodic memory: Positron emission tomography findings. *Proceedings of the National Academy of Sciences, USA, 91*(6), 2016–2020.

Tulving, E., & Kroll, N. (1995). Novelty assessment in the brain and long-term-memory encoding. *Psychonomic Bulletin & Review, 2*(3), 387–390.

Tulving, E., Markowitsch, H. J., Craik, F. I. M., Habib, R., & Houle, S. (1996).

Novelty and familiarity activations in PET studies of memory encoding and retrieval. *Cerebral Cortex*, *6*, 71–79.

Tulving, E., Markowitsch, H. J., Kapur, S., Habib, R., & Houle, S. (1994b). Novelty encoding networks in the human brain: Positron emission tomography data. *NeuroReport*, *5*(18), 2525–2528.

Tulving, E., & Rosenbaum, R. S. (2005). What do explanations of the distinctiveness effect need to explain? In R. R. Hunt & J. B. Worthen (Eds.), *Distinctiveness and memory* (pp. 407–422). New York: Oxford University Press.

Tulving, E., & Schacter, D. L. (1990). Priming and human memory systems. *Science*, *247*, 301–306.

Wagner, A. D., Koutstaal, W., Maril, A., Schacter, D. L., & Buckner, R. L. (2000). Task-specific repetition priming in left inferior prefrontal cortex. *Cerebral Cortex*, *10*(12), 1176–1184.

Waugh, N. C. (1970) On the effective duration of a repeated word. *Journal of Verbal Learning and Verbal Behavior*, *9*, 587–595.

Wiggs., C. L., & Martin, A. (1998). Properties and mechanisms of perceptual priming. *Current Opinion in Neurobiology*, *8*, 227–233.

Wilson, F. A. W., & Rolls, E. T. (1990). Neuronal responses related to the novelty and familiarity of visual stimuli in the substantia innominata, diagonal band of Broca and periventricular region of the primate basal forebrain. *Experimental Brain Research*, *80*, 104–120.

Part II

Aging

7 Bilingualism and aging

Costs and benefits

Fergus I. M. Craik and Ellen Bialystok

In previous papers we have suggested that many aspects of cognitive development and cognitive aging can be described in terms of the interplay between knowledge representations and cognitive control (Craik & Bialystok, 2006, 2008). One obvious difference between the cognitive changes observed in childhood and during aging is that in childhood both representational knowledge and control of that knowledge are growing in efficiency and complexity, whereas in aging control declines but knowledge remains relatively intact (Craik & Bialystok, 2008; Light, 1992). Although knowledge representations remain "available" in old age, in the sense that they still exist in the older person's brain, access to that knowledge is typically impaired unless the information is retrieved and used on a regular basis. Everyday examples include difficulties experienced in recollecting names of people and details of events that the older adult has not thought of for some time. In the laboratory, such age-related problems of accessibility may be illustrated by slower recognition latencies, lower word fluency and category generation scores, and the relatively greater deficit in recall relative to recognition (Craik & Jennings, 1992; Light, 1992). With regard to the age-related decline in control processes, many studies have shown that working memory abilities fall off with increasing age (e.g., Park et al., 2002), as does inhibitory control (Hasher, Zacks, & May, 1999), task-switching performance (Meiran & Gotler, 2001), and other aspects of executive control (Daniels, Toth, & Jacoby, 2006).

On the positive side of the ledger, there is growing evidence that various factors can attenuate these negative effects of aging. The idea that remaining active intellectually, socially, and physically has beneficial effects on cognitive performance has been popular for some time, although initially it was not well supported scientifically. However, the concept of "cognitive reserve" (Stern, 2002) is now widely accepted, and the relevant evidence is plentiful and convincing (Fratiglioni, Paillard-Borg, & Winblad, 2004; Kramer, Bherer, Colcombe, Dong, & Greenough, 2004; Staff, Murray, Deary, & Whalley, 2004; Valenzuela & Sachdev, 2006). The increased willingness to accept the idea that a good level of cognitive functioning can be maintained by pursuing an active lifestyle is partly attributable to other recent demonstrations of experience-based cognitive change. Some of these demonstrations have been at the behavioural level – for example, findings that video-game players have enhanced visual selective attention (Green & Bavelier, 2003) and that such skills can be increased by extensive video-game training (Feng, Spence, & Pratt, 2007). Other demonstrations have shown direct effects of specific experience on brain mechanisms and processes – for example, the finding that London taxi drivers (who have extensive route-finding abilities) have enlarged hippocampi (Maguire et al., 2000); also the finding that musicians who play stringed instruments such as guitars or violins have increased cortical representation of the fingers of the left hand (Elbert, Pantev, Wienbruch, Rockstroh, & Taub, 1995).

The studies described in the present chapter were carried out to explore the possibility that bilingualism may be a further condition associated with a range of cognitive changes. There is good evidence that the representations of both languages in a bilingual are always active to some extent (Dijkstra, Grainger, & van Heuven, 1999; Marian, Spivey, & Hirsch, 2003; Sumiya & Healey, 2004), so an inhibitory mechanism is needed to select the wanted language (Green, 1998). Bialystok (2001) suggested that the conflict created by the joint activation of two languages creates a problem in selection and inhibition of the unwanted language for bilinguals and that the constant exercise of this inhibitory control over many years might result in enhanced cognitive control over other cognitive processes. If there is evidence for a generalized cognitive control advantage in bilinguals, a further question concerns its interactions with aging – does bilingualism act to slow age-related cognitive decline?

Not all aspects of bilingualism are positive, however. Studies of children have consistently shown that bilingual children have smaller vocabularies (in each of their two languages) than their monolingual counterparts (Bialystok, 2001). Also, work by Gollan and colleagues has found that bilinguals are slower to name pictures of objects, produce fewer words in a word generation task, and have more tip-of-the-tongue experiences (Michael & Gollan, 2005). It is clear that bilinguals have a verbal access problem, and an interesting question is whether this difficulty also stems from the overlap between two language systems. That is, when a concept is activated and its name sought, is there interference between the two sets of representations that results in a slowing or failure of production? Bialystok (2001) has suggested that there is a link between the enhanced cognitive control and impaired lexical access associated with bilingualism – that competition between the two sets of representations results in both difficulty of access and more effective cognitive control. This suggestion will be reviewed again after surveying some recent evidence. Finally, what are the effects of aging on these opposite aspects of bilingualism? Again, this question will be reviewed in light of the results of recent experiments from our laboratories.

Bilingualism and cognitive control

One problem of control unique to bilingual individuals is the need to switch between their two language systems whenever appropriate (Hernandez, Dapretto, Mazziotta, & Bookheimer, 2001; Price, Green, & von Studnitz, 1999), and it is possible that the constant exercising of this function leads to a generalized improvement in cognitive control. A somewhat different idea arises from the well-substantiated claim that both language systems are always active in the bilingual brain (Gollan & Kroll, 2001) and that a mechanism is therefore needed to inhibit one language system while the other is being used. Such an inhibitory control mechanism is needed to prevent intrusions from the non-used language (Green, 1998).

The possibility that bilinguals have a general advantage in cognitive control has been investigated by Bialystok and colleagues and also by Costa and colleagues in recent years (Bialystok, Craik, Klein, & Viswanathan, 2004; Costa, Hernández, & Sebastián-Gallés, 2008). In one study (Bialystok et al., 2004, Study 2), younger and older adult bilinguals performed various versions of the Simon task (reviewed by Lu & Proctor, 1995). Participants are shown either a red square or a green square on a computer screen, and the task is simply to press a key on the left to one colour (e.g. green) and a key on the right to the other colour (red). In one condition, the squares appear in the centre of the screen, and the task thus measures 2-choice reaction time; no response conflict is involved. In a second condition, the squares appear either on the left or right of the screen, in a position that is either congruent or incongruent spatially with the appropriate response key. Participants typically respond faster in congruent cases given that the incongruent case requires some resolution of the conflicting cues carried by spatial position and task instructions. The Simon effect is the additional time needed to resolve the conflict in the incongruent trials relative to the time to respond to the congruent trials, with smaller Simon effects signalling greater levels of attentional control, given that such participants are better able to counteract the distracting effects of the misleading position information in the incongruent condition.

The results are shown in Figure 7.1. Performance levels on the control condition are seen in Figure 7.1a; mean reaction times (RTs) increase in the later age groups, but there is clearly no effect of bilingualism. Figure 7.1b shows values of the Simon effect, and the graph makes it clear that the increase with age is much greater for monolinguals – bilingualism apparently acts to increase inhibitory control, and this beneficial effect is stronger in older adults.

We have also conducted a second experiment on another variant of the Simon task (Bialystok, Craik, & Luk, 2008). In this version, participants were shown an arrow pointing either left or right on a computer screen, and the task was to press the corresponding (left or right) response key as rapidly as possible. In one condition the arrow was located centrally, and in the Simon

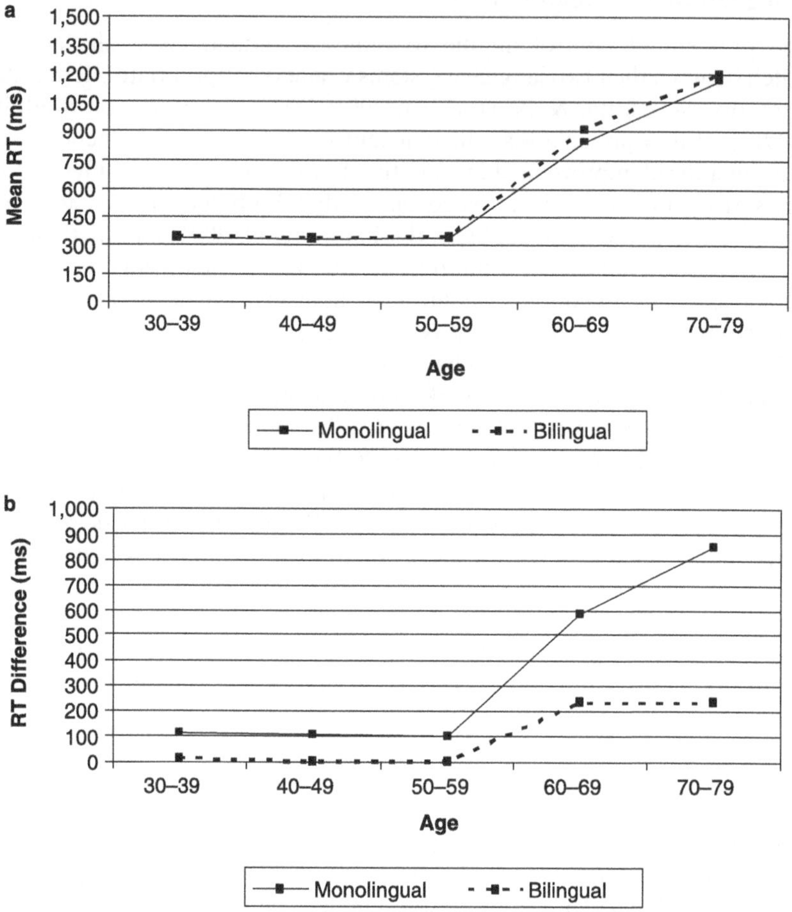

Figure 7.1 Mean reaction time (RT) by decade for monolinguals and bilinguals. (a): Mean RT for control condition. (b): Mean RT cost as the difference between congruent and incongruent trials (Simon effect).

condition the arrow appeared on one side or other of the screen, with its direction of pointing either congruent or incongruent with spatial position. The study involved 96 participants, made up of 24 individuals in each of four groups – young and older adult monolinguals and bilinguals. The younger adults' mean age was 20.2 years, and the older adults' mean age was 67.8 years. The non-English languages of the bilingual participants included a wide range of languages, of which French, Polish, Cantonese, and Spanish were the most common. All bilinguals reported using both English and their other language on a daily basis. In the control condition (centre arrow), the mean RTs for younger and older adults were 395 ms and 490 ms respectively, with no effect of bilingualism in either case. For the Simon conditions, the mean RTs were 510 ms and 720 ms for the younger and older adults, respectively, but now there were also effects of language group. The Simon effects (incongruent minus congruent RTs) were 8 ms for young monolinguals, 22 ms for young bilinguals, 61 ms for older monolinguals, and only 0.2 ms for older bilinguals. This pattern resulted in a significant 3-way interaction of age, language, and congruence, showing that the difference between congruent and incongruent trials was not significant for older bilinguals, as it was for participants in the other three groups. That is, a bilingual advantage in control was found in the older adults but, in this case, was not found in the younger group.

The Stroop effect is the gold standard for the measurement of inhibitory control, and this test was also presented to the same group of 96 participants. In two control conditions, participants either named a colour word (printed in black) as rapidly as possible, or named the colour in which a row of Xs was printed. In other conditions, they named the ink colour of a colour word (e.g., GREEN, BLUE) when the ink colour was either the same as (congruent) or different from (incongruent) the colour word itself. In the control conditions, older adults were slightly slower than their younger counterparts, but there was no effect of language group and no interactions between age and language. The results from the Stroop conditions are shown in Figure 7.2 in terms of facilitation and cost scores. Facilitation refers to the speed advantage in RT between (for example) saying "red" to ink colour when the word RED is printed in red and when the row of Xs is printed in red; in this case the lexical information is compatible with the colour information and so confers an advantage over naming the colour of the Xs. Cost refers to the slowing typically observed when naming the ink colour of a *different* colour word relative to naming that colour for Xs. Figure 7.2 shows that facilitation scores were largest for older bilinguals but also that bilinguals showed less cost than monolinguals, especially for the older group. This pattern yielded a

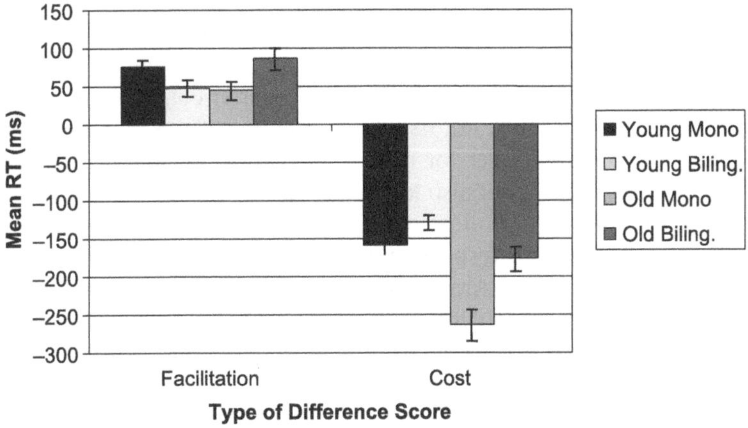

Figure 7.2 Mean RT and standard error for facilitation and cost scores in the Stroop task (see text for details).

significant 3-way interaction of age, language, and contrast (facilitation/cost), $F(1, 92) = 9.49$, $p < .002$, reflecting the fact that older bilinguals showed more facilitation and less cost than their monolingual peers and that these markers of a bilingual advantage in control were larger in the older groups than in the younger groups.

This analysis thus confirms the findings on the Simon task reported by Bialystok et al. (2004) – that bilingualism confers an advantage that increases throughout the lifespan. Put another way, many cognitive abilities decline during the course of aging, and inhibitory control appears to be one such ability (Hasher et al., 1999). Bilingualism may be one condition that acts to slow this normal age-related decline. However, the data do not always support the conclusion that the bilingual advantage increases with age. In the Stroop data reported previously, the differences between congruent and incongruent word stimuli (the Stroop effect) were significantly larger for older participants and for monolinguals, but there was no age × language interaction. The bilingual advantage was actually slightly larger for the younger participants in this instance. At this stage of data collection, the finding of a bilingual advantage in cognitive control seems reasonably well established, but the changes with age in that advantage remain to be confirmed. One last point about the data shown in Figure 7.2 is that whereas cognitive control is usually taken to mean ability to resist misleading information, good control can also be manifested as the ability to capitalize on a positive circumstance. This is what apparently happened in the facilitation part of the experiment; older bilinguals were able to gain more from the positive aspects as well as being better able to resist interference in the incongruent trials. Control can work in both directions (Hay & Jacoby, 1999).

The finding that bilingualism is associated with a benefit in attentional control has also been reported by other investigators. Zied and colleagues (2004) speculated that this might be the case on the basis of their results from a bilingual Stroop task. In the relevant conditions, French–Arabic bilinguals read incongruent colour words (that is, colour words printed in a different colour) and named the ink colour *either* in the same language as the word itself or in the participant's other language; the latter condition reflects inter-lingual interference, in the authors' terms. The size of this between-language interference effect was larger for older adult participants than for younger adults (not surprisingly) but also larger for unbalanced bilinguals when they had to respond in their non-dominant language. Balanced bilinguals of both age groups were faster to respond in all Stroop conditions than were either the French-dominant or Arabic-dominant bilinguals; on this basis, the authors suggest that manipulating and mastering two languages may enhance the efficiency of inhibitory mechanisms.

More direct evidence on the point comes from a recent study by Costa et al. (2008). They tested groups of 100 young adult (mean age = 22 years) Catalan–Spanish bilinguals and Spanish monolinguals on the attentional network task (ANT), which is a variant of the flanker task using arrows. In addition to the main measure of conflict resolution – the difference in response times between congruent and incongruent trials – the task provides measures of overall speed of responding, the benefit provided by an alerting cue, and switch costs – the slower response times on switch than on non-switch trials (where switch trials are those cases in which participants must perform congruent and incongruent trials in succession and so must switch their mindset). The results were that the bilinguals responded faster overall and also showed a smaller conflict effect, a greater benefit from the alerting cue, and smaller switch costs. That is, in confirmation of the results of Bialystok et al. (2004), bilingualism aids conflict resolution. Two other interesting results from the study are, first, that the bilingual advantage on the conflict effect decreased across blocks during the experiment so that it was no longer significant in the third and final block. Second, the bilingual participants did benefit more from an alerting stimulus but not from a further manipulation in which the alerting cue signalled the future spatial position of the arrow display on the screen. The significance of these further effects awaits replication and further experiments, but the main point of the work by Costa and colleagues is that the bilingual advantage in attentional control now seems well established and occurs throughout the lifespan.

Bilingual advantages have been reported in other domains also, and it is worth mentioning in the present context that work in Lars-Göran Nilsson's laboratory has found such advantages in both episodic and semantic memory tests in bilingual children ranging in age from 8 to 13 years (Kormi-Nouri, Moniri, & Nilsson, 2003). We have also found a bilingual advantage in certain aspects of episodic memory, although the effects were slight (Fernandes, Craik, Bialystok, & Kreuger, 2007).

Bilingualism and working memory

Working memory (WM) tasks typically involve a strong attentional control component, given that participants must hold some material in mind while carrying out further operations on the material or on new incoming stimuli. Support for this statement comes from a variety of sources – for example, Kane et al. (2004) found that WM measured by complex span tasks correlated substantially with measures of fluid intelligence, generally taken to be reflective of executive control. Neuroimaging evidence also points to a correspondence between WM and executive control, given that both sets of functions are associated with activations of the dorsolateral prefrontal cortex (Schacter, Wagner, & Buckner, 2000). And indeed, an article by Engle, Tuholski, Laughlin, and Conway (1999) explicitly provides evidence for links among WM, fluid intelligence, controlled attention, and functions of the prefrontal cortex. For these reasons we confidently expected to find strong positive relations between bilingualism and WM performance, but in fact the evidence to date has been mixed.

In the study by Bialystok et al. (2004), two control conditions in the Simon task involved coloured squares appearing in the centre of the screen. In the Center-2 condition, the squares were either brown or blue; each colour mapped to a specific response key. In the Center-4 condition, the stimulus was one of four colours (pink, yellow, red or green), two of which were mapped to one response key and two to the other. Thus in Center-2, participants had to hold a relatively simple mapping rule in mind, whereas the rule was more complex and more demanding on WM capacity in the Center-4 condition. Reaction times were predictably longer in the Center-4 condition, and we argued that the difference in RT between Center-2 and Center-4 reflected "WM Costs". Table 7.1A shows these costs for younger and older adults who were either monolinguals or bilinguals. The data show that older adults had substantially greater costs than younger adults, and that monolinguals had larger costs than bilinguals. Furthermore, the interaction between age and language was highly significant; as in the Simon task itself, bilingualism acted to mitigate the large age-related increase in WM costs. So in this first demonstration we obtained the predicted beneficial effect of bilingualism and also the Age × Bilingualism interaction.

Two further tasks studied by Bialystok et al. (2008) yielded results that were less compelling, however. One task was the self-ordered pointing task (Petrides & Milner, 1982) in which participants viewed a 12-page booklet, each page containing 12 abstract drawings. The same 12 drawings appeared on each page, but in a different random order, and the participant's task was to point to a different drawing on each page. WM ability was indexed by the number of repetitions (errors) made by the individual, with the best possible performance being no errors and the worst performance being 11 errors. The results for four groups of participants (younger/older adults, monolingual/bilingual) are shown in Table 7.1B. Statistical analysis revealed a strong effect of age (older adults were less successful) but no effect of language or of the Age × Language interaction. The second task used with the same participants was the Corsi blocks test (Milner, 1971), in which 10 wooden blocks are spread out in a random array. The experimenter touches a sequence of

Table 7.1 Scores on working memory tasks as a function of age and language

		Monolingual	*Bilingual*
A. Simon task (ms)	Young	246	113
	Old	704	210
B. SOPT (errors)	Young	5.0	5.4
	Old	8.4	8.5
C. Corsi span forward	Young	3.3	3.8
	Old	3.5	3.5
D. Corsi span backward	Young	2.8	3.5
	Old	2.5	2.3

blocks, and the participant's task is to reproduce the sequence. Performance is measured by the longest series that the participant can reproduce correctly. The results for the forward-span (repeat the sequence in the same order) and backward-span procedures (repeat the sequence in reverse order) are shown in Tables 7.1C and 7.1D. The forward-span data showed no effects of either age or language, but the more difficult backward-span task was performed significantly better by younger adults. Additionally, there was a significant bilingual advantage in the backward-span task, but only in the younger adults.

Feng (2008) has also reported results on a nonverbal WM task similar to Corsi blocks. In the adult version of this Matrix Task, participants viewed a 5 × 5 matrix that was initially blank. They were then presented with a sequence of red squares at 1-s intervals; each square filled one cell in the matrix, was then replaced by the next square, and so on until (say) 5 squares had been presented. The participant's task was to point to the cells that had been filled, but in *matrix order*, not presentation order; matrix order involves starting at the top left square, proceeding left to right along the first row, then right to left along the second row, left to right along the third, and so on. Participants must therefore hold the presentation positions in mind, but also re-order them during the response sequence. Feng found a significant bilingual advantage in a group of young adults (mean age = 20 years) on this task, and also a bilingual advantage in a group of 7-year-old children on a simpler version of the task. Older adults have not been tested so far on this test. Other related studies from Bialystok's lab have explored adult age and bilingual differences in versions of number span and alpha span. In alpha span (Craik, 1986), participants are presented with a short list of words and must repeat them back in correct alphabetical order; number span follows the same basic principle, but with 2-digit numbers as material. The results (on over 500 participants) showed age differences in performance (young adults were better than older adults) and a very slight (but nonsignificant) bilingual *disadvantage* on both tasks.

The reasons for these different results are not clear. Both self-ordered pointing (SOPT) and Corsi blocks are supposedly measures of WM, yet there was no trace of a bilingual advantage in the SOPT and an advantage for bilinguals in the Corsi blocks task, but only for younger adults. There was also no trace of a bilingual advantage on the number span and alpha span task. The answer to this puzzle probably depends on understanding that "working memory" is not one mechanism or structure and is not even the stable tripartite construct advocated by Baddeley and Hitch (1974). We suggest instead that the term "working memory" should refer to a class of tasks, where the tasks all involve some degree of short-term memory maintenance, as well as some degree of processing of the material held or processing of other material. However, given that the component processes and the types of material maintained and manipulated vary considerably from one WM task to another, the effects of bilingualism and other individual-difference variables may depend on the specific processes and materials involved in a particular WM task rather than on the simple fact that the task taps "working memory".

The same line of argument was put forward by Craik and Rabinowitz (1984) in an attempt to understand adult age differences in "short-term memory". They proposed that,

> in our view it is misleading to think of PM (primary memory), SM (secondary memory), and WM as structures or mechanisms that are or are not impaired by the aging process. Rather, the terms may be thought of as describing related processes; age decrements will occur as a function of the complexity and novelty of the specific processes required by any particular task . . . primary memory and working memory may be regarded as lying on a complex continuum as opposed to being truly dichotomous types of memory. (Craik & Rabinowitz, 1984, p. 481).

More recently, Unsworth and Engle (2007) have proposed similar arguments concerning the similarities and differences between short-term and working memory.

So what kinds of WM processes do bilinguals perform particularly well, and are there language-related differences in the ability to deal with different types of material? We suggest that bilingual children and adults exhibit an advantage when the task is *nonverbal* and involves attentional control. Bilinguals may show a disadvantage when dealing with verbal materials, however, as described in the next section.

Bilingualism and verbal access

Given that balanced bilingual speakers use each language approximately half as often as their monolingual counterparts, it would not be surprising to find that bilinguals have a less extensive vocabulary in each language. This possibility is borne out by recent research. For example, Oller and Eilers (2002) reported vocabulary deficits in fluently bilingual children, and Bialystok and Feng (in press) reported an analysis based on almost 1,000 children ranging in age from 5 to 9 years in which there was also a consistent disadvantage in vocabulary scores for the bilinguals. Access to lexical information is also impaired in bilinguals. In a series of studies, Gollan and her colleagues have found longer picture-naming times for bilingual adults, reduced scores on letter and category fluency tests, and increased frequency in adults' tip-of-the-tongue states (Gollan, Montoya, Fennema-Notestine, & Morris, 2005; Gollan, Montoya, & Werner, 2002; Gollan & Silverberg, 2001). Other researchers have also demonstrated poorer scores on fluency tests for bilinguals (Rosselli et al., 2000), more errors in picture naming (Roberts, Garcia, Desrochers, & Hernandez, 2002), and poorer word identification through noise (Rogers, Lister, Febo, Besing, & Abrams, 2006). The naming difficulties for bilinguals apparently persist into older age, although the magnitude of the effect does not change from young to older adulthood (Gollan, Fennema-Notestine, Montoya, & Jernigan, 2007).

We have conducted further exploratory studies on the effects of bilingualism and aging on lexical access using the same 96 participants who were tested on measures of cognitive control (Bialystok et al., 2008). As described previously, the sample consisted of four groups of 24 participants: younger and older adults who were monolingual or bilingual. All participants were given an English vocabulary test (PPVT-III), a version of the Boston naming test, and two tests of verbal fluency. The PPVT-III is a standardized test of receptive vocabulary in which the participant is shown four pictures and must indicate which of the four corresponds to a name spoken by the experimenter. Similar 4-choice trials of progressively greater difficulty continue until the participant makes 8 errors in a block of 12 trials. Raw scores are converted to standard scores on the basis of the person's age. In the Boston naming task (Kaplan, Goodglass, & Weintraub, 1983) participants are asked to name a series of line drawings of objects. In our version we substituted verbal definitions for half of the drawings on the speculative assumption that accessing relatively uncommon words would be more difficult (and perhaps relatively *more* difficult for bilinguals) from abstract definitions as opposed to relatively concrete drawings. That is, drawings might provide more contextual support and might thus be of particular benefit to older adults (Craik, 1983) and perhaps also to bilinguals. Finally, in the fluency tests, participants had to say as many words as possible within one minute starting with a given letter. Following standard procedure, the letters were F, A, and S. Again following standard practice, participants were also asked to name as many animals as they could within a minute (category fluency).

The results are shown in Table 7.2. Confirming previous findings, the vocabulary scores were substantially higher in the monolingual groups, $F(1, 92) = 40.1$, $MSE = 128$, $p < .0001$, with no interaction of age and language. The PPVT scores are standardized for age, so the data show no effect of aging; but when raw scores were analysed, there was a strong (and typical) advantage for older adults, an advantage for monolinguals, but

Table 7.2 Mean score (and standard deviation) by age and language group for the PPVT-III vocabulary test, Boston naming, and category fluency tasks from the verbal task battery

		Boston naming		*Fluency*	
Group	*PPVT-III*	*Picture*	*Definition*	*Letter*	*Category*
Young monolinguals	122.3 (9.3)	26.9 (2.2)	25.5 (3.2)	49.8 (7.4)	23.3 (5.4)
Young bilinguals	109.2 (10.3)	24.0 (4.6)	20.4 (4.3)	42.4 (11.1)	21.3 (3.8)
Older monolinguals	119.5 (10.2)	27.1 (2.3)	26.5 (2.9)	45.4 (7.7)	20.1 (3.9)
Older bilinguals	103.3 (14.9)	23.0 (3.0)	22.5 (3.3)	34.9 (13.9)	15.7 (5.4)

no Age × Language interaction. In the Boston naming task, monolinguals again outperformed bilinguals in both the picture and definition version (both *p*s $< .0001$). There was also an effect of aging; older participants outperformed younger ones, but only in the definition condition. Finally, monolingual advantages were also found in the fluency tests, both for letter and for category conditions. In this case, younger participants generated more items than older participants, again for both letter and category tests. There was no interaction between age and language in either task. In summary, strong and consistent negative effects of bilingualism were found in all three measures of verbal ability, despite the fact that strong bilingual *advantages* were found when the same participants performed the cognitive control tasks described in the previous section.

It is thus clear from our own results and from those reported by other researchers that bilingualism carries the cost of a smaller vocabulary and less efficient access to lexical knowledge – even in perfectly fluent bilingual speakers who use English on a daily basis. It is important to note that the linguistic deficit for bilinguals appears to be confined to the rapid access of lexical items and does not extend to the retrieval of semantic/conceptual information. For example, Gollan et al. (2005) found that whereas bilinguals were slower at naming pictures than were their monolingual peers, the two language groups were equivalent in their ability to classify the pictures rapidly as natural or human-made. A final major question concerns the relations (if any) between the bilingual advantage in cognitive control and the bilingual *disadvantage* in lexical access. Are these two phenomena independent, or are they somehow related? This question is taken up in the final section.

Bilingualism, access, and control

Research results to date thus show a clear disadvantage to bilinguals of all ages in vocabulary level and lexical access, a bilingual *advantage* in at least some aspects of cognitive control, and a possible advantage in nonverbal WM tasks. These strengths and weaknesses may reflect independent processes; it is quite possible, for example, that the bilingual disadvantage in verbal processing is simply a function of reduced frequency of use. On the other hand, it is attractive to consider the possibility that the positive and negative effects reflect some common underlying cause. If the bilingual advantage in cognitive control stems from years of practice in selecting the wanted language system while inhibiting the second language, the advantage may be attributed to excellent "interference suppression" – one aspect of cognitive control described by Bunge, Dudukovic, Thomason, Vaidya, and Gabrieli (2002). In turn we assume that this superior ability in interference suppression is also seen in tasks such as Stroop and Simon, where misleading information must again be suppressed.

Bunge et al. (2002) describe another form of cognitive control that they term “response inhibition”, in which a habitual response must be replaced by no response or by a non-salient response. Go/no-go tasks fall into this category, as does the reverse Simon condition, in which participants must always respond in the opposite direction to that indicated by the arrow. We see no reason for bilinguals to excel in this type of cognitive control; so this analysis provides a reason for why the bilingual advantage is found in some but not all executive control tasks. As one example, Carlson and Meltzoff (2008) found that 6-year-old bilingual children outperformed their monolingual peers on tasks that measured conflict, but that the groups were equivalent on tasks involving delay, whose primary feature was the need to refrain from responding. A second example is provided by an experiment (Bialystok, Craik, & Ryan, 2006) in which young adult bilinguals and monolinguals performed equivalently on a task in which they were required to press a key on the side opposite to stimulus presentation. In a second condition, participants had to ignore misleading information, and in this case a bilingual advantage was found.

The bilingual difficulty with tasks requiring rapid lexical access may stem from this same necessity to resolve conflict between competing lexical items. Thus, paradoxically, the disadvantage in lexical access may reflect the same feature of bilingualism that results in the advantage in cognitive control (Bialystok, 2001; Green, 1998). It might be expected that those bilingual individuals who show greatest cognitive control in the Stroop and Simon tasks would also show least problems in lexical access, given their more effective control mechanisms. That is, performance on cognitive control tasks and lexical access tasks may be negatively correlated. Such correlations were not found in the data collected by Bialystok et al. (2008), however; values ranged from –0.26 to +0.03 in young bilinguals and from –0.59 to +0.23 in the old bilinguals. The search for an adequate account continues.

With regard to aging, the results on vocabulary level and lexical access seem clear – the bilingual disadvantage remains stable across the lifespan. For cognitive control the results are less clear-cut. In the Bialystok et al. (2004) study, we found that control declined with increasing age in adults, but that bilingualism reduced the rate of decline. This result was found again on the Simon task experiment reported by Bialystok et al. (2008) and also in the facilitation and cost analysis of Stroop data (Figure 7.2). We have also reported preliminary evidence pointing to the possibility that bilingualism delays the onset of dementia (Bialystok, Craik, & Freedman, 2007). There is thus some reasonable evidence in favour of the notion that the bilingual advantage in cognitive control is enhanced in older adults, although more data are required to make this conclusion definitive.

As a final word, this programme of experiments speaks to the larger issue of the interrelations between representations and control and to how these relations change across the lifespan (Craik & Bialystok, 2006, 2008). The development of two language systems creates a degree of representational complexity that in turn promotes enhanced control to manage the complexity.

The positive result appears to be a general advantage in cognitive control that increases, if anything, from childhood to old age.

In summary, the emerging pattern of results from our laboratory shows that bilingual adults demonstrate an advantage in cognitive control over their monolingual counterparts, but that monolinguals outperform bilinguals on tests of vocabulary and verbal access. Some studies have shown that the bilingual advantage in control increases with age; however, that result has not always been found. On the other hand, the monolingual advantage in verbal access appears to remain constant across the adult lifespan. It is tempting to believe that the control advantage and the access disadvantage reflect the same underlying cognitive mechanism, but the evidence for this position is still incomplete. Nonetheless, the clear interactions among measures of language, attention, decision-making, and memory underline the point that cognitive processes do not exist in isolation.

This chapter was prepared to honour the accomplishments of Lars-Göran Nilsson as he finishes a long and distinguished career in departmental and scientific administration in order to devote more time to research. Lars-Göran is fluently bilingual and has been for many years. We have not detected any marked signs of word-finding difficulties at this point, but (if he believes our results) he can draw comfort from the knowledge that his ability to suppress distracting thoughts and stimuli will increase, if anything, in the coming years!

References

Baddeley, A. D., & Hitch, G. J. (1974). Working memory. In G. H. Bower (Ed.), *Recent advances in learning and motivation* (Vol. 8, pp. 47–90). New York: Academic Press.

Bialystok, E. (2001). *Bilingualism in development: Language, literacy, and cognition.* New York: Cambridge University Press.

Bialystok, E., Craik, F. I. M., & Freedman, M. (2007). Bilingualism as a protection against the onset of symptoms of dementia. *Neuropsychologia, 45*, 459–464.

Bialystok, E., Craik, F. I. M., Klein, R., & Viswanathan, M. (2004). Bilingualism, aging, and cognitive control: Evidence from the Simon task. *Psychology and Aging, 19*, 290–303.

Bialystok, E., Craik, F. I. M., & Luk, G. (2008). Cognitive control and lexical access in younger and older bilinguals. *Journal of Experimental Psychology: Learning, Memory, and Cognition, 34*, 859–873.

Bialystok, E., Craik, F. I. M., & Ryan, J. (2006). Executive control in a modified anti-saccade task: Effects of aging and bilingualism. *Journal of Experimental Psychology: Learning, Memory, and Cognition, 32*, 1341–1354.

Bialystok, E., & Feng, X. (in press). Language proficiency and its implications for monolingual and bilingual children. In A. Durgunoglu (Ed.), *Challenges for language learners in language and literacy development*. New York: Guilford Press.

Bunge, S. A., Dudukovic, N. M., Thomason, M. E., Vaidya, C. J., & Gabrieli, J. D. E. (2002). Immature frontal lobe contributions to cognitive control in children: Evidence from fMRI. *Neuron, 33*, 301–311.

Carlson, S. M., & Meltzoff, A. N. (2008). Bilingual experience and executive functioning in young children. *Developmental Science, 11*, 282–298.

Costa, A., Hernández, M., & Sebastián-Gallés, N. (2008). Bilingualism aids conflict resolution: Evidence from the ANT task. *Cognition, 106*, 59–86.

Craik, F. I. M. (1983). On the transfer of information from temporary to permanent memory. *Philosophical Transactions of the Royal Society of London, Series B, 302*, 341–359.

Craik, F. I. M. (1986). A functional account of age differences in memory. In F. Klix & H. Hagendorf (Eds.), *Human memory and cognitive capabilities, mechanisms, and performances* (pp. 409–422). Amsterdam: Elsevier.

Craik, F. I. M., & Bialystok, E. (2006). Cognition through the lifespan: Mechanisms of change. *Trends in Cognitive Sciences, 10*, 131–138.

Craik, F. I. M., & Bialystok, E. (2008). Lifespan cognitive development: The roles of representation and control. In F. I. M. Craik & T. A. Salthouse (Eds.), *The handbook of aging and cognition* (3rd ed., pp. 557–601). New York: Psychology Press.

Craik, F. I. M., & Jennings, J. M. (1992). Human memory. In F. I. M. Craik & T. A. Salthouse (Eds.), *The handbook of aging and cognition* (pp. 51–110). Hillsdale, NJ: Lawrence Erlbaum Associates, Inc.

Craik, F. I. M., & Rabinowitz, J. C. (1984). Age differences in the acquisition and use of verbal information: A tutorial review. In H. Bouma & D. G. Bouwhuis (Eds.), *Attention and Performance X* (pp. 471–499). Hillsdale, NJ: Lawrence Erlbaum Associates, Inc.

Daniels, K., Toth, J., & Jacoby, L. (2006). The aging of executive functions. In E. Bialystok & F. I. M. Craik (Eds.), *Lifespan cognition: Mechanisms of change* (pp. 96–111). New York: Oxford University Press.

Dijkstra, T., Grainger, J., & van Heuven, W. J. B. (1999). Recognition of cognates and interlingual homographs: The neglected role of phonology. *Journal of Memory and Language, 41*, 496–518.

Elbert, T., Pantev, C., Wienbruch, C., Rockstroh, B., & Taub, E. (1995). Increased cortical representation of the fingers of the left hand in string players. *Science, 270*, 305–307.

Engle, R. W., Tuholski, S. W., Laughlin, J. E., & Conway, A. R. A. (1999). Working memory, short-term memory, and general fluid intelligence: A latent-variable approach. *Journal of Experimental Psychology: General, 128*, 309–331.

Feng, J., Spence, I., & Pratt, J. (2007). Playing an action game reduces gender differences in spatial cognition. *Psychological Science, 18*, 850–855.

Feng, X. (2008). *Working memory and bilingualism: An investigation of executive control and processing speed.* Unpublished doctoral dissertation, York University, Toronto, Canada.

Fernandes, M. A., Craik, F. I. M., Bialystok, E., & Kreuger, S. (2007). Effects of bilingualism, aging, and semantic relatedness on memory under divided attention. *Canadian Journal of Experimental Psychology, 61*, 128–141.

Fratiglioni, L., Paillard-Borg, S., & Winblad, B. (2004). An active and socially-integrated lifestyle in late life might protect against dementia. *Lancet Neurology, 3*, 343–353.

Gollan, T. H., Fennema-Notestine, C., Montoya, R. I., & Jernigan, T. L. (2007). The bilingual effect on Boston Naming Test performance. *Journal of the International Neuropsychological Society, 13*, 197–208.

Gollan, T. H., & Kroll, J. F. (2001). The cognitive neuropsychology of bilingualism.

In B. Rapp (Ed.), *What deficits reveal about the human mind/brain: A handbook of cognitive neuropsychology* (pp. 321–345). Philadelphia, PA: Psychology Press.

Gollan, T. H., Montoya, R. I., Fennema-Notestine, C., & Morris, S. K. (2005). Bilingualism affects picture naming but not picture classification. *Memory & Cognition, 33*, 1220–1234.

Gollan, T. H., Montoya, R. I., & Werner, G. (2002). Semantic and letter fluency in Spanish–English bilinguals. *Neuropsychology, 16*, 562–576.

Gollan, T. H., & Silverberg, N. B. (2001). Tip-of-the-tongue states in Hebrew–English bilinguals. *Bilingualism: Language and Cognition, 4*, 63–83.

Green, C. S., & Bavelier, D. (2003). Action video game modifies visual selective attention. *Nature, 423*, 534–537.

Green, D. W. (1998). Mental control of the bilingual lexico-semantic system. *Bilingualism: Language and Cognition, 1*, 67–81.

Hasher, L., Zacks, R. T., & May, C. P. (1999). Inhibitory control, circadian arousal, and age. In D. Gopher & A. Koriat (Eds.), *Attention and performance XVII* (pp. 653–675). Cambridge, MA: MIT Press.

Hay, J. F., & Jacoby, L. L. (1999). Separating habit and recollection in young and older adults: Effects of elaborative processing and distinctiveness. *Psychology and Aging, 14*, 122–134.

Hernandez, A. E., Dapretto, M., Mazziotta, J., & Bookheimer, S. (2001). Language switching and language representation in Spanish–English bilinguals: An fMRI study. *NeuroImage, 14*, 510–520.

Kane, M. J., Hambrick, D. Z., Tuholski, S. W., Wilhelm, O., Payne, T. W., & Engle, R. W. (2004). The generality of working-memory capacity: A latent variable approach to verbal and visuo-spatial memory span and reasoning. *Journal of Experimental Psychology: General, 133*, 189–217.

Kaplan, E. F., Goodglass, H., & Weintraub, S. (1983). *Boston naming test*. Philadelphia, PA: Lea & Febiger.

Kormi-Nouri, R., Moniri, S., & Nilsson, L.-G. (2003). Episodic and semantic memory in bilingual and monolingual children. *Scandinavian Journal of Psychology, 44*, 47–54.

Kramer, A. F., Bherer, L., Colcombe, S. J., Dong, W., & Greenough, W. T. (2004). Environmental influences on cognitive and brain plasticity during aging. *Journals of Gerontology. Series A, Biological Sciences and Medical Sciences, 59*, 940–957.

Light, L. L. (1992). The organization of memory in old age. In F. I. M. Craik & T. A. Salthouse (Eds.), *The handbook of aging and cognition* (pp. 111–165). Hillsdale, NJ: Lawrence Erlbaum Associates, Inc.

Lu, C.-H., & Proctor, R. W. (1995). The influence of irrelevant location information on performance: A review of the Simon and spatial Stroop effects. *Psychonomic Bulletin & Review, 2*, 174–207.

Maguire, E. A., Gadian, D. G., Johnsrude, I. S., Good, C. D., Ashburner, J., Frackowiak, R. S., et al. (2000). Navigation-related structural changes in the hippocampi of taxi drivers. *Proceedings of the National Academy of Sciences USA, 97*, 4398–4403.

Marian, V., Spivey, M., & Hirsch, J. (2003). Shared and separate systems in bilingual language processing: Converging evidence from eyetracking and brain imaging. *Brain and Language, 86*, 70–82.

Meiran, N., & Gotler, A. (2001). Modelling cognitive control in task switching and ageing. *European Journal of Cognitive Psychology, 13*, 165–186.

Michael, E. B., & Gollan, T. H. (2005). Being and becoming bilingual: Individual differences and consequences for language production. In J. F. Kroll & A. M. B. de Groot (Eds.), *Handbook of bilingualism: Psycholinguistic approaches* (pp. 389–407). New York: Oxford University Press.

Milner, B. (1971). Interhemispheric differences in the localization of psychological processes in man. *British Medical Bulletin*, *27*, 272–277.

Oller, D. K., & Eilers, R. E. (Eds.). (2002). *Language and literacy in bilingual children*. Clevedon, UK: Multilingual Matters.

Park, D. C., Lautenschlager, G., Hedden, T., Davidson, N. S., Smith, A. D., & Smith, P. K. (2002). Models of visuospatial and verbal memory across the adult lifespan. *Psychology and Aging*, *17*, 299–320.

Petrides, M., & Milner, B. (1982). Deficits on subject-ordered tasks after frontal- and temporal-lobe lesions in man. *Neuropsychologia*, *20*, 249–262.

Price, C. J., Green, D. W., & von Studnitz, R. (1999). A functional imaging study of translation and language switching. *Brain*, *122*, 2221–2235.

Roberts, P. M., Garcia, L. J., Desrochers, A., & Hernandez, D. (2002). English performance of proficient bilingual adults on the Boston Naming Test. *Aphasiology*, *16*, 635–645.

Rogers, C. L., Lister, J. J., Febo, D. M., Besing, J. M., & Abrams, H. B. (2006). Effects of bilingualism, noise, and reverberation on speech perception by listeners with normal hearing. *Applied Psycholinguistics*, *27*, 465–485.

Rosselli, M., Ardila, A., Araujo, K., Weekes, V. A., Caracciolo, V., Padilla, M., et al. (2000). Verbal fluency and repetition skills in healthy older Spanish–English bilinguals. *Applied Neuropsychology*, *7*, 1–24.

Schacter, D. L., Wagner, A. D., & Buckner, R. L. (2000). Memory systems of 1999. In E. Tulving & F. I. M. Craik (Eds.), *The Oxford handbook of memory* (pp. 627–643). New York: Oxford University Press.

Staff, R. T., Murray, A. D., Deary, I. J., & Whalley, L. J. (2004). What provides cerebral reserve? *Brain*, *27*, 1191–1199.

Stern, Y. (2002). What is cognitive reserve? Theory and research application of the reserve concept. *Journal of the International Neuropsychological Society*, *8*, 448–460.

Sumiya, H., & Healy, A. F. (2004). Phonology in the bilingual Stroop effect. *Memory and Cognition*, *32*, 752–758.

Unsworth, N., & Engle, R. W. (2007). On the division of short-term and working memory: An examination of simple and complex span and their relation to higher order abilities. *Psychological Bulletin*, *133*, 1038–1066.

Valenzuela, M. J., & Sachdev, P. (2006). Brain reserve and dementia: A systematic review. *Psychological Medicine*, *36*, 441–454.

Zied, K. M., Phillipe, A., Karine, P., Valerie, H.-T., Ghislaine, A., Arnaud, R., et al. (2004). Bilingualism and adult differences in inhibitory mechanisms: Evidence from a bilingual Stroop task. *Brain and Cognition*, *54*, 254–256.

8 Sex differences in episodic memory

The where but not the why

Agneta Herlitz, Johanna Lovén, Petra Thilers, and Jenny Rehnman

Lars-Göran Nilsson's genuine and deep interest in sex (variations) is well known by his friends and colleagues. Luckily, Lars-Göran has successfully been able to transfer his interest to this academic child and these grandchildren, which is why we in this chapter present an overview of sex differences in episodic memory. Our main messages are that women perform at a substantially higher level than men on verbal episodic memory and face recognition tasks, whereas there are no sex differences on tasks assessing episodic memory for nonverbal information. Men, on the other hand, outperform women on tasks requiring us to remember visuospatial episodic information. Although attempts have been made to explain these differences in terms of sex-specific influences from steroid hormones, we conclude that there is not enough evidence to support this claim at present. Much of the data presented here stem from the longitudinal population-based Betula project on memory, health, and aging, initiated and generously shared by Lars-Göran Nilsson (e.g., Nilsson et al., 1997, 2004).

Verbal episodic memory tasks

Although sex is the most basic individual-difference variable, its potential effects on episodic memory functions have been largely neglected. Nonetheless, there are a number of studies, not specifically investigating sex differences in episodic memory, reporting that women perform at a higher level than do men on episodic memory tasks. For example, sex differences in favour of women are found in word recall (Kramer, Delis, Kaplan, O'Donnell, & Prifitera, 1997), word recognition (Hill et al., 1995), story recall (Hultsch, Masson, & Small, 1991), name recognition (Larrabee & Crook, 1993), and recognition of concrete pictures and objects (Herlitz, Airaksinen, & Nordström, 1999). Confirming this pattern of data in a large population-based study of 1,000 adults, ranging in age between 35 and 80 years, we found sex differences on episodic memory tasks in which the participants were told to remember lists of words, objects, and activities (Herlitz, Nilsson, & Bäckman, 1997). The difference between men and women on a word recall task was $d = 0.25$ ($d = M_W - M_M/SD$; Cohen, 1977), indicating a moderate female advantage.

Most research on episodic memory has used verbal material or material in which it is possible to verbalize the material. As noted above, women have repeatedly outperformed men on such tasks. Women also surpass men on verbal production tasks, such as rapid word retrieval (i.e., verbal fluency; Hyde & Linn, 1988). Therefore, it could be hypothesized that women's higher performance on episodic memory tasks with a verbal component is a result of a general female advantage in verbal abilities. However, in a study specifically testing this hypothesis, we found that controlling statistically for verbal ability did not eliminate, and only marginally decreased, the sex difference in episodic memory. This finding indicates that verbal ability cannot fully explain the female advantage in verbal episodic memory tasks (Herlitz et al., 1999).

Visuospatial episodic memory tasks

As men typically perform at a higher level than do women on visuospatial tasks – for instance, understanding what an irregular figure looks like when it is rotated in space ($d = 0.56$; Voyer, Voyer, & Bryden, 1995) – men can be expected to perform at a higher level than women on episodic memory tasks requiring visuospatial processing. Although relatively few studies have examined sex differences in visuospatial episodic memory tasks, it is clear that the pattern of sex differences is different from that seen in verbal episodic memory tasks (Lewin, Wolgers, & Herlitz, 2001). Interestingly, the magnitude of the male advantage seems to vary as a function of the extent to which the task relies on visuospatial processing versus the extent to which verbal processing can be utilized. A task requiring participants to remember the route walked in a maze with little or no external information results in large sex differences favouring men (e.g., Astur, Ortiz, & Sutherland, 1998), whereas smaller sex differences are found in environments in which external verbal information can support memory performance (e.g., Crook, Youngjohn, & Larrabee, 1993).

Nonverbal, non-visuospatial episodic memory tasks

Also of interest is whether there are sex differences on episodic memory tasks requiring both verbal and visuospatial processing. Notably, women outperform men on tasks in which an object's position is to be remembered, such as when playing the game Memory, or when trying to remember where you last saw your glasses (Voyer, Postma, Brake, & Imperato-McGinley, 2007). Even though such tasks require visuospatial processing, women may utilize their verbal advantage in order to remember the objects' position. Whether there are sex differences on episodic memory tasks requiring a minimum of either verbal or visuospatial processing – such as when remembering unfamiliar odours or an unfamiliar piece of music – is yet an open question. This issue is of interest, as the presence of sex differences on such tasks would suggest that there is a sex difference in basic episodic memory capacity, irrespective of the type of material to be remembered. Although there are findings suggesting that women have a slight advantage over men on such tasks (Öberg, Larsson, & Bäckman, 2002), more studies are clearly needed.

Face recognition

Many studies have shown that women outperform men on face recognition tasks (e.g., Lewin & Herlitz, 2002; Lewin et al., 2001). Although face recognition cannot readily be assumed to rely on verbal processing, we hypothesized that women could utilize their greater verbal abilities to encode faces, by verbalizing the face: "a dark, blue-eyed handsome man". We investigated this hypothesis by showing faces, in rapid succession, prohibiting the participants from verbalizing the faces (Lewin & Herlitz, 2002). Nonetheless, women recognized more faces than men did, irrespective of whether or not verbal encoding was suppressed, thus providing no support for the hypothesis that women use their greater verbal abilities to encode faces. The results also revealed that the female recognition advantage was magnified for female faces. The tendency for females to remember more faces of their own sex than faces of the opposite sex (i.e., "own-sex effect") is found across age. Both young girls and adult women remember more female faces, irrespective of the age of the faces (e.g., faces of young girls or adult women), and across ethnicity (e.g., ethnically familiar or unfamiliar faces). In contrast, men tend to remember male and female faces equally well (e.g., Rehnman & Herlitz, 2006, 2007). Why might this be the case?

To address this question, we created a set of androgynous faces and showed them to three groups of participants (unpublished data). The three groups received different instructions – that they would be presented with a series of faces, either (a) female faces, (b) male faces, or (c) faces – and their task was to remember the faces for a later recognition task. Interestingly, women in the group of participants who were told to remember "women" remembered more faces than did women in the groups of participants who were told to remember "male faces", or just "faces", despite all participants having seen the same androgynous faces. By contrast, the men in the three groups performed at similar levels across instructional conditions. Furthermore, in the group of participants instructed to remember just "faces", women remembered more androgynous faces than did the men.

Based on these findings, we suggest that women allocate more attention to female than to male faces. A study on infants has shown that infant girls devote more attention to faces than infant boys do (Connellan, Baron-Cohen, Wheelwright, Batki, & Ahluwalia, 2000). Speculatively, the attention that infant girls devote to faces may form the basis of women's superior face recognition ability. Moreover, developmentally, categorization of female faces precedes that of male faces for both sexes, possibly as a result of greater early exposure to female than to male faces (Ramsey-Rennels & Langlois, 2006). With increasing age, girls may develop their interest in other females, which also might be strengthened through reciprocal interactions with other women. By contrast, developing boys may orient themselves towards other males, resulting in a loss of their early advantage for categorization of female faces and, as a consequence, an absence of an own-sex bias.

Explanations: The environment

What are the possible explanations for sex differences in episodic memory tasks? We know that expectations from society play a role in shaping the magnitude of sex differences. For example, the size of the difference can be increased or decreased by altering the instructions given to the participants, although the direction of the sex difference cannot be reversed (O'Brien & Crandall, 2003). The importance of education and culture is illustrated in a study in which we compared the magnitude and pattern of cognitive sex differences in literate and illiterate older adults from Bangladesh and Sweden (Herlitz & Kabir, 2006). The participants were tested on the Mini-Mental State Examination (MMSE; Folstein, Folstein, & McHugh, 1975). Although the MMSE is not intended to be divided into subtasks, we analysed the tasks assessing verbal episodic memory (a 3-word word list) and spatial visualization (drawing or forming, with sticks, a geometrical form) separately. In general, men performed at a higher level than did women on the spatial visualization task, whereas women performed at a higher level than did men on the episodic memory task. Among the illiterate Bangladeshis, there were large differences favouring men – also on tasks where no differences were expected, such as orientation in time and space. In fact, the only task in which these men did not outperform the women was the episodic memory task. Illiterate Bangladeshi women, in contrast to Bangladeshi men, have little or no access to the world outside the immediate home and family. Therefore, we interpreted the results as indicating that the pattern of cognitive sex differences is similar irrespective of nationality and literacy, but that the magnitude of the differences is related to both education and sociocultural factors. Importantly, the low performance of the illiterate women demonstrates the penalizing effect restrictions in public exposure might have on cognitive performance, thereby underscoring the importance of environmental factors.

Explanation: Hormones

In the search for biological influences on cognitive sex performance, steroid hormones have received considerable interest during the last 20 years. Indeed, the notion that estrogen and testosterone influence cognitive performance is considered an undisputable fact and is stated as such in articles, often without providing reference to the statement. However, a review of the area demonstrates that the results are inconsistent, suggesting that the evidence for an association between hormones, sex differences, and cognition is far from unequivocal.

Testosterone

The notion that testosterone influences human behaviour comes from experimental research on other mammals. A number of studies show that testosterone plays an important role in the neural and behavioural sexual differentiation in rodents and non-human primates (i.e., Goy & McEwen, 1980). Whether testosterone has the same influence on humans is, however, less clear.

The organizational (i.e., permanent) effect of androgens has been studied in girls with congenital adrenal hyperplasia (CAH). CAH is a rare disorder in which a genetic mutation on the short arm of chromosome 6 results in a deficient enzyme in the adrenal cortex. This deficiency results in unusually high levels of androgens during gestation among CAH girls. Thus, the prenatal effect of testosterone on behaviour can be studied in CAH girls. A number of studies have shown that prenatal testosterone influences later childhood play behaviour, so that girls with CAH show an increased preference for toys that are typically chosen by boys, such as vehicles and weapons, and for rough-and tumble play (i.e., Hines, 2006; Nordenström, Servin, Bohlin, Larsson, & Wedell, 2002; Servin, Nordenström, Larsson, & Bohlin, 2003). However, research attempting to establish a link between prenatal testosterone levels and visuospatial abilities has been less conclusive. Although there are studies reporting higher visuospatial performance in CAH girls than in controls (Berenbaum, 2001; Hampson, Rovet, & Altmann, 1998), a larger number of studies indicate no differences (Hines et al., 2003; McGuire, Ryan, & Omenn, 1975), or even lower performance in CAH girls (Helleday, Bartfai, Ritzén, & Forsman, 1994).

Other studies have investigated the activational effect that testosterone may have on cognitive abilities, the argument being that testosterone receptors can be found in brain areas implicated in cognition, such as the hypothalamus (Krithivas et al., 1999) and the hippocampus (Janowsky, 2006). Therefore, men with higher levels of endogenous testosterone are expected to perform at a higher level on visuospatial tasks than men with lower levels of endogenous testosterone. In line with this reasoning, there are studies showing positive associations between testosterone and visuospatial performance in both young and old men (Christiansen & Knussmann, 1987; Gordon & Lee, 1986; Hogervorst, De Jager, Budge, & Smith, 2004; Hooven, Chabris, Ellison, & Kosslyn, 2004; Moffat et al., 2002; Silverman, Kastuk, Choi, & Phillips, 1999; Thilers, MacDonald, & Herlitz, 2006), but there are also studies reporting nonsignificant associations throughout the adult lifespan (Fonda, Bertrand, O'Donnell, Longcope, & McKinlay, 2005; Gouchie & Kimura, 1991; Hassler, Gupta, & Wollmann, 1992; Wolf & Kirschbaum, 2002). Complicating the pattern, negative associations between testosterone and visuospatial performance have also been reported throughout the adult lifespan (Moffat & Hampson, 1996; Yonker et al., 2006). Although the discrepancies in the literature could be a consequence of diverse hormone sampling, time-of-day, and different age groups being investigated, it is at present not possible to conclude that there is positive association between testosterone and visuospatial abilities in men.

Estrogen

As with testosterone, estrogen receptors can be found in a variety of brain areas – for example, the cerebral cortex, the hypothalamus, the amygdala, and the hippocampus (Bixo, Bäckström, Winblad, & Andersson, 1995; McEwen, 2002) – suggesting that estrogen may influence cognitive performance.

One line of research investigating this issue has focused on the influence of estrogen in pre-menopausal women. Here, cognitive performance is studied in relation to the normal fluctuations in endogenous estrogen levels associated with the menstrual cycle. A number of studies have found that cognitive performance varies as a function of menstrual-cycle phase (Hampson, 1990; Hampson & Kimura, 1988; Hausmann, Slabbekoorn, Van Goozen, Cohen-Kettenis, & Güntürkün 2000; Philips & Silverman, 1997; Saucier & Kimura, 1998). These studies suggest that estrogen has an inhibitory influence on the right hemisphere, resulting in decreased performance on visuospatial tasks. In contrast, estrogen is thought to have a facilitating effect on tasks in which women typically excel, such as articulation, manual speed, and coordination. Therefore, women have been hypothesized to perform at a higher level on these tasks in the mid-luteal phase of the menstrual cycle, when estrogen levels are high. Although some studies have reported this pattern of data, the effects are often not found (Epting & Overman, 1998; Gordon & Lee, 1993; Maki, Rich, & Rosenbaum, 2002; Postma, Winkel, Tuiten, & van Honk, 1999).

A second line of research has investigated the effects that hormone therapy (HT) around menopause may have on cognitive performance. Although results from observational epidemiological and cohort investigations have largely demonstrated beneficial effects of HT, findings from randomized controlled clinical trials show a more diverse pattern of results. As observational studies typically have problems with subject selection, often with a "healthy user bias", clinical trials provide more unbiased evidence. By now, there are a number of well-conducted clinical trials reporting no, or even negative, effects of HT on cognition (e.g., Almeida et al., 2006; Dunkin et al., 2005; Espeland et al., 2004; Polo-Kantola et al., 1998; Resnick et al., 2006; Yaffe et al., 2006). The negative effects of HT on cognitive performance found by Women's Health Initiative (Rapp et al., 2003) have invoked uncertainty and fear against HT. However, most studies indicate that relatively healthy women can use HT without notable concern about cognitive consequences.

A third line of research has investigated whether the drop in endogenous estrogen levels around menopause is accompanied by a similar drop in cognitive performance. A cross-sectional study reported that the menopausal transition was associated with cognitive decline. However, when the influences of age and education were controlled, the menopausal effect disappeared (Fuh, Wang, Lu, Juang, & Lee, 2003; Herlitz, Thilers, & Habib, 2007). Longitudinal investigations have replicated these results and failed to find the expected negative effects of the menopausal transition on cognitive performance (Fuh, Wang, Lee, Lu, & Juang, 2006; Meyer et al., 2003).

Taken together, the findings in the extant literature make it difficult to conclude that estrogen has a positive effect on cognitive performance in women, thereby contributing to cognitive sex differences. Instead, the available evidence suggests that if estrogen positively affects cognition in women, its effects are marginal.

Summary

Women consistently outperform men on episodic memory tasks that require remembering items that are verbal in nature or can be verbally labelled. However, women also excel on tasks requiring little or no verbal processing, such as in recognition of unfamiliar odours or faces. In contrast, there is a male advantage on episodic memory tasks requiring visuospatial processing. These findings suggest that women's episodic memory advantage can increase or be reversed, depending on the nature of the material to be remembered. Although the environment can influence the magnitude of these sex differences, it does not seem to be able to change their direction, suggesting that the explanation for these differences should be sought elsewhere. The potential effects of steroid hormones on cognitive functions have been investigated thoroughly. However, no definite conclusions regarding hormonal effects can be drawn, although it seems fair to state that estrogen and testosterone have, at best, relatively small effects on cognition. A more fruitful avenue for future research may be to examine the potential relationship between structural and functional sex differences reported in cerebral cortex and cognitive performance (e.g., Goldstein et al., 2001; Maller et al., 2007; Nyberg, Habib, & Herlitz, 2000). Also, the role of sex chromosome genes and the effect they may have on sex dimorphic cognitive performance is a relatively unexplored area of research, which deserves attention in the future (Skuse, 2005).

References

Almeida, O. P., Lautenschlager, N. T., Vasikaran, S., Leedman, P., Gelavis, A., & Flicker, L. (2006). 20-week randomized controlled trial of estradiol replacement therapy for women aged 70 years and older: Effect on mood, cognition and quality of life. *Neurobiology of Aging*, *27*, 141–149.

Astur, R. S., Ortiz, M. L., & Sutherland, R. J. (1998). A characterization of performance by men and women in a virtual Morris water task: A large and reliable sex difference. *Behavioural Brain Research*, *93*, 185–190.

Berenbaum, S. A. (2001). Cognitive function in congenital adrenal hyperplasia. *Endocrinology and Metabolism Clinics of North America, 30*, 173–192.

Bixo, M., Bäckström, T., Winblad, B., & Andersson, A. (1995). Estradiol and testosterone in specific regions of the human female brain in different endocrine states. *Journal of Steroid Biochemistry & Molecular Biology, 55*, 297–303.

Christiansen, K., & Knussmann, R. (1987). Sex hormones and cognitive functioning in men. *Neuropsychobiology, 18*, 27–36.

Cohen, J. (1977). *Statistical power analysis for the behavioral sciences*. Hillsdale, NJ: Lawrence Erlbaum Associates, Inc.

Connellan, J., Baron-Cohen, S., Wheelwright, S., Batki, A., & Ahluwalia, J. (2000). Sex differences in human neonatal social perception. *Infant Behavior & Development, 23*, 113–118.

Crook, T. H., Youngjohn, J. R., & Larrabee, G. J. (1993). The influence of age, gender, and cues on computer-simulated topographic memory. *Developmental Neuropsychology, 9*, 41–53.

Dunkin, J., Rasgon, N., Wagner-Steh, K., David, S., Altshuler, L., & Rapkin, A. (2005). Reproductive events modify the effects of estrogen replacement therapy on cognition in healthy postmenopausal women. *Psychoneuroendocrinology, 30*, 284–296.

Epting, L. K., & Overman, W. H. (1998). Sex-sensitive tasks in men and women: A search of performance fluctuations across the menstrual cycle. *Behavioral Neuroscience, 112*, 1304–1317.

Espeland, M. A., Rapp, S. R., Shumaker, S. A., Brunner, R., Manson, J. E., Sherwin, B. B., et al. (2004). Conjugated equine estrogens and global cognitive function in postmenopausal women: Women's Health Initiative memory study. *Journal of the American Medical Association, 291*, 2959–2968.

Folstein, M. F., Folstein, S. E., & McHugh, P. R. (1975). "Mini-mental state:" A practical method for grading the cognitive state of patients for the clinician. *Journal of Psychiatric Research, 12*, 189–198.

Fonda, S. J., Bertrand, R., O'Donnell, A., Longcope, C., & McKinlay, J. B. (2005). Age, hormones, and cognitive functioning among middle-aged and elderly men: Cross-sectional evidence from the Massachusetts male aging study. *Journals of Gerontology. Series A, Biological Sciences and Medical Sciences, 60A*, 385–390.

Fuh, J. L., Wang, S. J., Lee, S. J., Lu, S. R., & Juang, K. D. (2006). A longitudinal study of cognition change during early menopausal transition in a rural community. *Maturitas, 53*, 447–453.

Fuh, J. L., Wang, S. J., Lu, S. R., Juang, K. D., & Lee, S. J. (2003). Alterations in cognitive function during the menopausal transition. *Journal of the American Geriatric Society, 51*, 431–442.

Goldstein, J. M., Seidman, L. J., Horton, N. J., Makris, N., Kennedy, D. N., Caviness, V. S., et al. (2001). Normal sexual dimorphism of the adult human brain assessed by in vivo magnetic resonance imaging. *Cerebral Cortex, 11*, 490–497.

Gordon, H. W., & Lee, P. A. (1986). A relationship between gonadotropins and visuospatial function. *Neuropsychologia, 24*, 563–576.

Gordon, H. W., & Lee, P. A. (1993). No difference in cognitive performance between phases of the menstrual cycle. *Psychoneuroendocrinology, 18*, 521–531.

Gouchie, C., & Kimura, D. (1991). The relationship between testosterone levels and cognitive ability patterns. *Psychoneuroendocrinology, 16*, 323–334.

Goy, R. W., & McEwen, B. S. (1980). *Sexual differentiation of the brain*. Cambridge, MA: MIT Press.

Hampson, E. (1990). Variations in sex-related cognitive abilities across the menstrual cycle. *Brain & Cognition*, *14*, 26–43.

Hampson, E., & Kimura, D. (1988). Reciprocal effects of hormonal fluctuations on human motor and perceptual-spatial skills. *Behavioral Neuroscience*, *102*, 456–459.

Hampson, E., Rovet, J. F., & Altmann, D. (1998). Spatial reasoning in children with congenital adrenal hyperplasia due to 21-hydroxylase deficiency. *Developmental Neuropsychology*, *14*, 299–320.

Hassler, M., Gupta, D., & Wollmann, H. (1992). Testosterone, estradiol, ACTH and musical, spatial and verbal performance. *International Journal of Neuroscience*, *65*, 45–60.

Hausmann, M., Slabbekoorn, D., Van Goozen, S. H. M., Cohen-Kettenis, P. T., & Güntürkün, O. (2000). Sex hormones affect spatial abilities during the menstrual cycle. *Behavioral Neuroscience*, *114*, 1245–1250.

Helleday, J., Bartfai, A., Ritzén, E. M., & Forsman, M. (1994). General intelligence and cognitive profile in women with congenital adrenal hyperplasia (CAH). *Psychoneuroendocrinology*, *19*, 343–356.

Herlitz, A., Airaksinen, E., & Nordström, E. (1999). Sex differences in episodic memory: The impact of verbal and visuospatial ability. *Neuropsychology*, *13*, 590–597.

Herlitz, A., & Kabir, Z. N. (2006). Sex differences in cognition among illiterate Bangladeshis: A comparison with literate Bangladeshis and Swedes. *Scandinavian Journal of Psychology*, *47*, 441–447.

Herlitz, A., Nilsson, L.-G., & Bäckman, L. (1997). Gender differences in episodic memory. *Memory & Cognition*, *25*, 801–811.

Herlitz, A., Thilers, P., & Habib, R. (2007). Endogenous estrogen is not associated with cognitive performance before, during, and following menopause. *Menopause*, *14*, 425–431.

Hill, R. D., Grut, M., Wahlin, Å., Herlitz, A., Winblad, B., & Bäckman, L. (1995). Predicting memory performance in optimally healthy very old adults. *Journal of Mental Health & Aging*, *1*, 57–67.

Hines, M. (2006). Prenatal testosterone and gender-related behavior. *European Journal of Endocrinology*, *155*, S115–S121.

Hines, M., Fane, B. A., Pasterski, V. L., Mathews, G. A., Conway, G. S., & Brook, C. (2003). Spatial abilities following prenatal androgen abnormality: Targeting and mental rotations performance in individuals with congenital adrenal hyperplasia. *Psychoneuroendocrinology*, *28*, 1010–1026.

Hogervorst, E., De Jager, C., Budge, M., & Smith, A. D. (2004). Serum levels of estradiol and testosterone and performance in different cognitive domains in healthy elderly men and women. *Psychoneuroendocrinology*, *29*, 405–421.

Hooven, C. K., Chabris, C. F., Ellison, P. T., & Kosslyn, S. M. (2004). The relationship of male testosterone to components of mental rotation. *Neuropsychologia*, *42*, 782–790.

Hultsch, D. F., Masson, M. E., & Small, B. J. (1991). Adult age differences in direct and indirect tests of memory. *Journal of Gerontology*, *46*, 22–30.

Hyde, J. S., & Linn, M. C. (1988). Gender differences in verbal ability: A meta-analysis. *Psychological Bulletin*, *104*, 53–69.

Janowsky, J. S. (2006). Thinking with your gonads: Testosterone and cognition. *Trends in Cognitive Sciences*, *10*, 77–82.

Kramer, J. H., Delis, D. C., Kaplan, E., O'Donnell, L., & Prifitera, A. (1997). Developmental sex differences in verbal learning. *Neuropsychology*, *11*, 577–584.

Krithivas, K., Yurgalevitch, S. M., Mohr, B. A., Wilcox, C. J., Batter, S. J., Brown, M. et al. (1999). Evidence that the CAG repeat in the androgen receptor gene is associated with the age-related decline in serum androgen levels in men. *Journal of Endocrinology, 162*, 137–142.

Larrabee, G. J., & Crook, T. H., III. (1993). Do men show more rapid age-associated decline in simulated everyday verbal memory than do women? *Psychology and Aging, 8*, 68–71.

Lewin, C., & Herlitz, A. (2002). Sex differences in face recognition: Women's faces make the difference. *Brain & Cognition, 50*, 121–128.

Lewin, C., Wolgers, G., & Herlitz, A. (2001). Sex differences favoring women in verbal but not in visuospatial episodic memory. *Neuropsychology, 15*, 165–173.

Maki, P. M., Rich, J. B., & Rosenbaum, R. S. (2002). Implicit memory varies across the menstrual cycle: Estrogen effects in young women. *Neuropsychologia, 40*, 518–529.

Maller, J. J., Anstey, K. J., Réglade-Meslin, C., Christensen, H., Wen, W., & Sachdev, P. (2007). Hippocampus and amygdala volumes in a random community-based sample of 60–64 year olds and their relationship to cognition. *Psychiatry Research: Neuroimaging, 156*, 185–197.

McEwen, B. S. (2002). Estrogen actions throughout the brain. *Recent Progression in Hormone Research, 57*, 357–384.

McGuire, L. S., Ryan, K. O., & Omenn, G. S. (1975). Congenital adrenal hyperplasia. II. Cognitive and behavioral studies. *Behavior Genetics, 5*, 175–188.

Meyer, P. M., Powell, L. H., Wilson, R. S., Everson-Rose, S. A., Kravitz, H. M., Luborsky, J. L., et al. (2003). A population-based longitudinal study of cognitive functioning in the menopausal transition. *Neurology, 61*, 801–806.

Moffat, S. D., & Hampson, E. (1996). A curvilinear relationship between testosterone and spatial cognition in humans: Possible influence of hand preference. *Psychoneuroendocrinology, 21*, 323–337.

Moffat, S. D., Zonderman, A. B., Metter, E. J., Blackman, M. R., Harman, S. M., & Resnick, S. M. (2002). Longitudinal assessment of serum free testosterone concentration predicts memory performance and cognitive status in elderly men. *Journal of Clinical Endocrinology and Metabolism, 87*, 5001–5007.

Nilsson, L.-G., Adolfsson, R., Bäckman, L., de Frias, C. M., Molander, B., & Nyberg, L. (2004). Betula: A prospective cohort study on memory, health and aging. *Aging, Neuropsychology, and Cognition, 11*, 134–148.

Nilsson, L.-G., Bäckman, L., Erngrund, K., Nyberg, L., Adolfsson, R., Bucht, G., et al. (1997). Betula prospective cohort study: Memory, health and aging. *Aging, Neuropsychology, and Cognition, 4*, 1–32.

Nordenström, A., Servin, A., Bohlin, G., Larsson, A., & Wedell, A. (2002). Sex-typed toy-play behavior correlates with the degree of prenatal androgen exposure assessed by CYP21 genotype in girls with congenital adrenal hyperplasia. *Journal of Clinical Endocrinology & Metabolism, 87*, 5119–5124.

Nyberg, L., Habib, R., & Herlitz, A. (2000). Brain activation during episodic memory retrieval: Sex differences. *Acta Psychologica, 105*, 181–194.

Öberg, C., Larsson, M., & Bäckman, L. (2002). Differential sex effects in olfactory functioning: The role of verbal processing. *Journal of the International Neuropsychological Society, 8*, 691–698.

O'Brien, L. T., & Crandall, C. S. (2003). Stereotype threat and arousal: Effects on women's math performance. *Personality and Social Psychology Bulletin, 29*, 782–789.

Phillips, K., & Silverman, I. (1997). Differences in the relationship of menstrual cycle phase to spatial performance on two- and three-dimensional tasks. *Hormones and Behavior*, *32*, 167–175.

Polo-Kantola, P., Portin, R., Polo, O., Helenius, H., Irjala, K., & Erkkola, R. (1998). The effect of short-term estrogen replacement therapy on cognition: A randomised, double-blind, cross-over trial in postmenopausal women. *Obstetrics and Gynecology*, *91*, 459–466.

Postma, A., Winkel, J., Tuiten, A., & van Honk, J. (1999). Sex differences and menstrual cycle effects in human spatial memory. *Psychoneuroendocrinology*, *24*, 175–192.

Ramsey-Rennels, J. L., & Langlois, J. H. (2006). Infants' differential processing of female and male faces. *Current Directions in Psychological Science*, *15*, 59–62.

Rapp, S. R., Espeland, M. A., Shumaker, S. A., Henderson, V. W., Brunner, R. L., Manson, J. E., et al. (2003). Effect of estrogen plus progestin on global cognitive function in postmenopausal women. The Women's Health Initiative Study: A randomized controlled trial. *Journal of the American Medical Association*, *289*, 2663–2672.

Rehnman, J., & Herlitz, A. (2006). Higher face recognition in girls: Magnified by own-sex and own-ethnicity bias. *Memory*, *14*, 289–296.

Rehnman, J., & Herlitz, A. (2007). Women recognize more faces than men do. *Acta Psychologica*, *124*, 344–355.

Resnick, S. M., Maki, P. M., Rapp, S. R., Espeland, M. A., Brunner, R., Coker, L. H., et al. (2006). Effects of combination estrogen plus progestin hormone treatment on cognition and affect. *Journal of Clinical Endocrinology and Metabolism*, *91*, 1802–1810.

Saucier, D. M., & Kimura, D. (1998). Intrapersonal motor but not extrapersonal targeting skill is enhanced during the midluteal phase of the menstrual. *Developmental Neuropsychology*, *14*, 385–398.

Servin, A., Nordenström, A., Larsson, A., & Bohlin, G. (2003). Prenatal androgens and gender-typed behavior: A study of girls with mild and severe forms of congenital adrenal hyperplasia. *Journal of Developmental Psychology*, *39*, 440–450.

Silverman, I., Kastuk, D., Choi, J., & Phillips, K. (1999). Testosterone levels and spatial ability in men. *Psychoneuroendocrinology*, *24*, 813–822.

Skuse, D. H. (2005). X-linked genes and mental functioning. *Human Molecular Genetics*, *14*, R27–R32.

Thilers, P., MacDonald, S., & Herlitz, A. (2006). The association between endogenous free testosterone and cognitive performance: A population-based study in 35 to 90 year-old men and women. *Psychoneuroendocrinology*, *31*, 565–756.

Voyer, D., Postma, A., Brake, B., & Imperato-McGinley, J. (2007). Gender differences in object location memory: A meta-analysis. *Psychonomic Bulletin & Review*, *14*, 23–38.

Voyer, D., Voyer, S., & Bryden, M. P. (1995). Magnitude of sex differences in spatial abilities: A meta-analysis and consideration of critical variables. *Psychological Bulletin*, *117*, 250–270.

Wolf, O. T., & Kirschbaum, C. (2002). Endogenous estradiol and testosterone levels are associated with cognitive performance in older women and men. *Hormones and Behavior*, *41*, 259–266.

Yaffe, K., Vittinghoff, E., Ensrud, K. E., Johnson, K. C., Diem, S., Hanes, V., & Grady, D. (2006). Effects of ultra-low-dose transdermal estradiol on cognition and health-related quality of life. *Archives of Neurology*, *63*, 945–950.

Yonker, J. E., Adolfsson, R., Eriksson, E., Hellstrand, M., Nilsson, L.-G., & Herlitz, A. (2006). Verified hormone therapy improves episodic memory performance in healthy postmenopausal women. *Aging, Neuropsychology, and Cognition*, *13*, 291–307.

9 An epidemiological approach to cognitive health in aging

Roger A. Dixon

The purpose of this chapter is to explore the foundations and implications of an epidemiological approach to understanding the multiple change trajectories and outcome patterns in the field of cognitive aging. Whereas it is reasonably apparent that there are multiple trajectories of cognitive changes with aging (ranging, in principle, from gains to losses), there is a correspondingly large range of functional outcomes of these trajectories (ranging, colloquially, from successful to normal to pathological cognitive aging). Well known, as well, is the fact that these trajectories and outcomes are often multiply-determined, with influential precursors, moderators, and mediators originating in levels of analyses from the neurobiological to the cognitive and to the sociocultural (Cabeza, Nyberg, & Park, 2004; Dixon, Bäckman, & Nilsson, 2004; Hess & Blanchard-Fields, 1999; Park, Nisbett, & Hedden, 1999). The present goal is to explore the development of a framework for considering multiple precursors, profiles, and patterns of cognitive health in aging. The framework is broadly epidemiological and includes both theoretical and methodological implications, but this is not primarily a theoretical or a methodological chapter. Rather, the focus is on exploring and illustrating the concept of cognitive health and how it can be approached in an epidemiological framework.

I am pleased to acknowledge that this chapter is inspired by the opportunity to honour the influential research career and seminal ideas of Lars-Göran Nilsson. Although broadly active in a variety of fields in the cognitive and health sciences, Nilsson's large body of research on cognitive aging and cognitive neuroscience is pivotal for this chapter. Specifically, in his role as director of the Betula project (BP), one of the most internationally prominent epidemiological studies of cognitive aging, Nilsson has sponsored research that has covered the gamut of the field (see Nilsson et al., 1997, 2004). The BP has produced momentous publications charting many descriptive characteristics of cognitive aging, neurobiological underpinnings, health moderators, and genomic precursors of individual differences in cognitive decline. Notably for the present chapter, Nilsson and BP colleagues have also generated novel perspectives on the possibility of healthy or stable cognitive changes with aging. For example, Nilsson's multidisciplinary BP group has examined cognitive, noncognitive, biohealth (e.g., teeth), and neurobiological influences on altered or preserved cognitive functioning in older adults (e.g., Bergdahl, Habib, Bergdahl, Nyberg, & Nilsson, 2007; Habib, Nyberg, & Nilsson, 2006; Persson et al., 2006). In addition, in the context of a five-year programme of collaborative research between the Swedish BP and the Canadian Victoria Longitudinal Study (VLS), Nilsson was instrumental in sponsoring and leading conferences (e.g., Dixon et al., 2004) and publications (e.g., Dixon & Nilsson, 2004; Nyberg et al., 2003; Wahlin, MacDonald, de Frias, Nilsson, & Dixon, 2006) bearing on the epidemiological approach to selective cognitive decline (or preservation). The goal of the present chapter is to sketch a model that could promote additional and more systematic research on cognitive health in the context of ongoing epidemiological studies of cognitive decline and illness. The chapter is presented in four parts, tracing the logical progression from conceptual overview (e.g., what is cognitive health?), to select theoretical and methodological issues (e.g., multivariate epidemiological approaches to cognitive health), to evolving research questions and directions.

Considering cognitive health and aging in an epidemiological context

Of central concern to older adults themselves, and to public health observers, are the twin possibilities of (a) preserving or maintaining cognitive health into late life and (b) preventing or compensating for some of the cognitive decline or illness that inevitably occurs. How do we discover the confluence of factors, crossing multiple levels of analysis, that may lead to healthier cognitive aging or to gentler patterns of cognitive decline? At a global level, much theoretical work in cognitive aging appears to draw such precursor factors from the biological, psychological, or sociocultural realms (see collections edited by Cabeza et al., 2004; Craik & Salthouse, 2007; Dixon et al., 2004; Hess & Blanchard-Fields, 1999; Stern, 2006). That these factors might interact across realms or levels of analysis is at least implicit. Popular in the current vernacular are terms such as "biocultural" and "biopsychosocial" context (Baltes & Smith, 2004). Indeed, lifespan development is frequently portrayed as intrinsically unfolding in the generous context of various aspects of interior and exterior "biopsychosocial" worlds (e.g., Baltes, Staudinger, & Lindenberger, 1999). The unfolding or temporal idea, however, points to another important factor – namely, that of time: Arguably, time, change, or aging may be considered a fourth horseman of this enveloping and evolving context. If the epidemiological context involves multiple broad factors, and if they function interactively as risk or protective factors, relevant cognitive outcomes could be wide ranging indeed. Figure 9.1 models this approach.

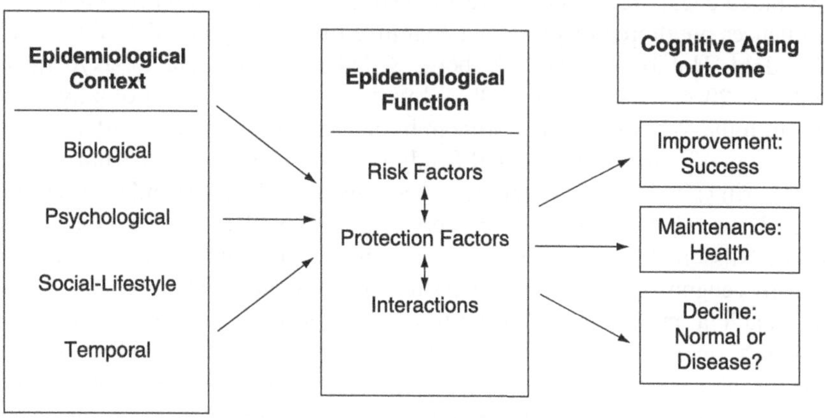

Figure 9.1 Framing the epidemiological influence of interactive contexts on the outcome of cognitive health in aging.

Biopsychosocial (+ temporal) factors

Considering Figure 9.1, it is useful to unpack briefly each of the elements of these integrated but generic factors associated with cognitive aging. First, the "bio" aspect of the lifespan refers to the underlying and tangible reality that we "age" as biological organisms. Not incidentally, this axiom includes the corresponding facts that (a) lifespan biological development follows, except for the first 25% of the life course, a narrative of differential but gradually declining vitality, and (b) throughout adulthood many dimensions of biological functioning, from those central to cognition (i.e., neurological) to those peripheral to cognition (i.e., cardiovascular, sensory), can affect cognitive performance in aging (e.g., Baltes et al., 1999; Raz, 2004; Waldstein, 2000). Unsurprisingly, changes in basic biological vitality or health are prominent sources of risk factors for late-life cognitive decline (e.g., MacDonald, Dixon, Cohen, & Hazlitt, 2004; Wahlin, 2004).

Second, the "psycho" aspect refers to the well-documented notion that virtually all psychological or behavioural processes – including systems of memory, affect and emotion, appraisal and beliefs, attention and cognition, awareness and executive functioning, personality and mental health, reserve and resilience, motor and sensory functioning, wisdom and creativity – change throughout adulthood (see recent reviews in Birren & Schaie, 2006; Craik & Salthouse, 2007). Mattering little for the present chapter is the otherwise weighty theoretical question of whether the changes within processes specific to each of these domains are differential, variable, universal, gradual, or directional. Instead, of more immediate pertinence are the following key considerations: (a) relatively few reviewers of (or theories pertaining to) these psychological processes feature or even identify robust "gains" with aging (see below), and (b) decremental changes in each of these processes could very well have an influence on the attainment and maintenance of cognitive health in late life. Clearly, for cognitive aging, the "psycho" factors are by far the most comprehensively examined. Although many basic cognitive resources and factors are associated with robust aging-related losses, some exceptions and perhaps even protective, rehabilitative, or compensatory functions or practices may emerge (Dixon, Garrett, & Bäckman, 2008; Einstein & McDaniel, 2004; McDaniel, Einstein, & Jacoby, 2007; Reuter-Lorenz & Lustig, 2005; Stern, 2006).

Third, the "social" aspect refers to multiple facets of the relatively "external" worlds of aging individuals. If pushed to oversimplify, one might locate most influential features in conceptual and geographical space exterior to that typically associated with the individual-biological and individual-psychological. These contexts are external in the sense of being (a) conceptually non-overlapping with the relatively internal (i.e., residing interior to the individual) biological contexts of individual cognitive development and (b) only moderately overlapping with the relatively more internal (i.e., individual in social and cultural worlds) psychological context of cognitive aging. As can be seen in the recent handbook edited by Binstock and George (2006), the social context of aging includes cultural issues, demographic characteristics, economic conditions, ethnicity and racial issues, familial and friendship circles and roles, geographical distribution and movement, historical and generational era, interactive situations, role transitions, social influences in health and health care, social institutions, and work and retirement roles. From the present perspective, the "social" factor may also refer to a collection of lifestyle (cognitive, social, physical) activities and other aspects of social engagement that can influence patterns and directions of cognitive aging. Some aspects of social engagement may serve as protection factors for cognitive health and even occurrence of dementia (e.g., Ghisletta, Bickel, & Lövdén, 2006; Scarmeas, 2006; Small, Hughes, Hultsch, & Dixon, 2006; Wang, Karp, Winblad, & Fratiglioni, 2002).

Fourth, the "temporal" factor refers to the simple fact that each element of each factor changes over time. As elements or units they may interact (couple or decouple, lead or lag) in novel ways within and across factors over time. Moreover, these complex and temporal interactions may be modelled quantitatively (e.g., McArdle et al., 2004; Ram & Nesselroade, 2007). Naturally, time (aging) per se is more an index than a source or cause of cognitive changes with aging, but its unavoidable dynamic characteristic and function do carry the implication that epidemiological research could involve time-structured research designs (e.g., longitudinal; see Hofer & Sliwinski, 2006; Hultsch, 2004). Therefore, the temporal factor is neither a risk nor protection factor for cognitive aging, except in the sense that it is associated with increases in the opportunities for (and prevalence of) cognitive decline.

This unpacking of the new (and even more awkward) term "biopsychosocialtemporal" factors into equal (and interacting) parts is temporary and tentative. Temporary, because unpacking the term jeopardizes the richness of the concept. For example, it risks reifying a "geographic" error – that is, in locating essential and influential contexts of aging in different geographical and disciplinary spaces. A possible and incorrect implication is that they do not or cannot interact (Little, Bouvaird, & Card, 2007). Tentative, in that we quickly return to the elaborated notion of "biopsychosocialtemporal" factors and explore further the potential application to cognitive health in aging. In sum, the implication is that there are temporally interactive (whether crossed, coupling, decoupling, leading, or lagging) systems of influences on the production and maintenance of cognitive health with aging. Such factors, although changing themselves, can be identified as risking or promoting cognitive health in aging. The use of such complex neologisms can (and should) be avoided, but endorsing the concept commits researchers to considering factors across a wide range of "levels of analysis" as indicated by the nature of the target cognitive process, despite the fact that these levels or factors may be commonly associated with neighbouring (or even disparate) disciplines or research traditions.

Preliminary to an epidemiology of cognitive health

Cognitively healthy adults, like their contexts, change – and they change in a variety of ways. Various trajectories of changes can be expected in all manner of observable performances, as well as indirect indicators of reserves or resources, and in a variety of underlying biological (e.g., neurochemical, neuroanatomical, physical health) and coordinating psychological (e.g., compensation, selection, resilience) mechanisms that control, exacerbate, or modify cognitive health. In sum, both the developmental and the epidemiological approaches to understanding current phenomena could involve an investigation of temporally preceding (or concurrent) factors from the bio, psycho, or social trends of the individual or population. The full range of contexts of cognitive health in late life includes aspects drawn from the bio, psycho, and social contexts, as rendered and applied through the changing prism of time (e.g., Little et al., 2007).

A goal of epidemiological approaches to health and illness is to identify the causes, distributions, risk factors, and protection factors associated with a given disease. This goal could apply equally to understanding the factors contributing to continuing health, recovery or rehabilitation, or avoidance of disease. Just as epidemiological approaches are suitably applied to cognitive diseases (e.g., such neurodegenerative diseases as Alzheimer's disease, AD), they could apply to the study of continuing cognitive health, cognitive rehabilitation or recovery, maintenance of cognitive health into very late life, and avoidance or postponement of cognitive diseases such as impairment or AD. Such an application would be enhanced if a demonstrably valid healthy outcome, parallel to the diagnosis of (say) AD, could be identified, measured, and tracked over time. Therefore, a goal of the epidemiological study of phenomena of cognitive health in late life would also focus on risk factors (which hinder maintenance or accelerate decline) or protection factors (which promote maintenance or buffer decline). Some theoretical guidance is required, including attention to the simple question of what constitutes cognitive health in late life – that is, what pertinent outcomes might be identified. Some methodological guidance is also required, including attention to how cognitive health is measured and what methods might best establish its presence, absence, operations, implications, or fluctuations.

By convention, epidemiological research includes the study of factors that both hinder or promote the maintenance of physical or mental health. In order to appreciate the protection factors that promote or spare cognitive health in aging, it is crucial to understand the risk factors that are associated with less propitious outcomes. Thus, the idea of considering cognitive health in the contexts of space (social, biological) and time (social, biological, and chronological) is germane. Perhaps two assumptions are required: (a) that considering factors involved in the development of healthy or unhealthy cognition involves essentially similar operations; (b) that these operations are fundamentally the same as those for detecting precursors to physical diseases. In the next sections we sketch sequentially some of the most pertinent definitional, theoretical, and methodological considerations.

Towards a model of cognitive health and aging

What is cognitive health?

What is meant by "cognitive health" and how does it map on to extant concepts in cognitive aging research? The adjective "healthy" has, of course, numerous definitions, including a variety of synonyms, from the superordinate (e.g., wholesome and fit) to the subordinate (e.g., flourishing, hale, hardy, unimpaired, disease-free, and useful). Somewhat more qualified and lenient (but still propitious) definitions include the notion that good health can result from processes that balance or adjust losses with gains. Terms loosely synonymous with this concept include compensatory, corrective, consistent, resilient, normal, and restored. Obvious antonyms of "healthy" include the counter-indicators of delicate, feeble, infirm, sick, diseased, and weak. Regarding older adults, cognitive health is, in this respect, like physical health. If applied to older adults, an uncontaminated and unqualified definition of physical health might secure but a few real-world exemplars. How many older adults are truly as healthy and biologically vital as they were in their peak years (e.g., their 20s)? Instead, healthy and normal aging may be defined not as the closeness to perfectly wholesome, disease-free, and fit – the young adult template – but, rather, as a cluster of characteristics that reflect the fact that time (aging) is associated with decline in the biological-health context (Siegler, Bosworth, & Poon, 2003; Wahlin, 2004) and subsequently with more challenging conditions in the very late years (e.g., Baltes & Smith, 2004).

For aging adults, the status of being healthy should not be defined exclusively by invoking pure criteria such as robust and disease-free. This anchor of the continuum, while entirely accurate and important, would produce a population in which older adults are decidedly under-sampled and unique. Nevertheless, the criteria should be explicit, for they provide the purest standard of selection. Therefore, an operational definition of cognitive health in older adults would include observed levels of performance on a given cognitive indicator that might be interpreted as (a) high with respect to the cohort today, (b) high with respect to other cognitive skills or abilities, (c) high with respect to the individual's recent past (i.e., stabilized or improving over time), (d) maintained level of performance into late life (intra-individually) in contrast to cohort-normative trajectories, and (e) consistent within the individual (across trials or opportunities) in the same window of observation. Each of these profiles would reflect the fit, flourishing, and unimpaired version of the definition of healthy. Taken literally and in combination, they set a lofty standard indeed. Taken leniently and separately, however, they provide a selective but attainable criterion that could be applied to the concept of cognitive health.

This perspective is similar to that for the study of cognitive "gains" with aging (Dixon, 2000; Ebner, Freund, & Baltes, 2006). Notably, it may be advantageous and practical to operationally define healthy cognition in more relative, generous, and encompassing terms. Accordingly, cognitive health, in the context of old age, may also be observed under the following conditions: suboptimal or lower than expected performance on any of the above five items could accurately reflect sustained losses or variability, disease, injury, or other adversities and imperfections. But if the level and trajectory of cognitive performance can be interpreted as managing lower or declining performance (despite disease, adversity, injury, or health restrictions), or as adapting to decline and inconsistency, then relative cognitive health for older adults may be a viable concept (Dixon, 2000). Healthy cognition, therefore, is not only characterized as high in performance (which is the most robust way to define it) but also as performance that is reasonably good despite the decremental temporal-related effects of the aging biopsychosocial context. Specifically, healthy cognition may be indicated by good performance despite the confluence of neurobiological decline, psychological constraints and impediments, and the absence of support social structures and functions. In this case, the level of performance of a cognitively healthy older adult is still of interest, but if the inference of cognitive health is to be viable despite suboptimal performance, it must be supported by information pertaining to qualifying mechanisms (e.g., compensation, plasticity). The methodological challenge is that identifying healthy cognition in later life may require not only raw performance information, but also a rich appreciation of qualitative characteristics of performance, mechanisms of execution, adaptivity of the effort and result, and pertinent elements of the context. As noted in a later section, such challenges can be met in part through creative assembly of data from ongoing longitudinal epidemiological studies (Nilsson et al., 2004).

Naturally, at the anchor point opposite that of cognitive health is the exemplar of unhealthy cognition. As derived from the larger concept of physical ill-health, some of the parallel terms include feeble, infirm, impaired, diseased, or progressively degenerating. Accordingly, diagnostic of cognitive ill-health in older adults are indications of (a) neurodegenerative diseases, (b) abrupt or collapsing neurocognitive resources or cognitive reserve, (c) dramatically lower than expected performance in a select or specialized domain (e.g., an area of personal expertise), (d) absence or diminished evidence for resilience or adaptation (including lack of compensation, reduced strategic or goal-adjusted behaviours, or depressed range of plasticity), and (e) significant or increasing intra-individual variability (inconsistency). Typically, distinguishing healthy normal aging from mildly impaired or unhealthy cognitive aging requires a cluster of observations. Optimally, the observations would include dynamic multivariate distributions derived with time-structured data from more than one factor of the context (e.g., Little et al., 2007; McArdle et al., 2004). Ideally, such dynamic diagnostic data could include concurrent and intra-individual patterns that would be available to either indicate (confirm) or counter-indicate (disconfirm) diagnostic status.

From related concepts to a provisional model

Although we are lacking a general unifying conceptual model for understanding the development and maintenance of cognitive health, theoretical guidance is available from several sources. These include the following literatures, briefly recognized: (a) lifespan approaches to general developmental-aging phenomena and conceptual models of successful aging (e.g., Baltes et al., 1999; Bengtson & Schaie, 1999; Perlmutter, 1990; Rowe & Kahn, 1999; Vaillant, 2002), (b) research on presumably healthy cognition phenomena such as wisdom and creativity in late life (Baltes & Staudinger, 2000; Habib et al., 2006; Simonton, 1990; Sternberg & Lubart, 2001), (c) social- or emotional-cognitive aspects of engagement, resilience, self-efficacy, and personal optimization (e.g., Berry, 1999; Blanchard-Fields, 2005; Brandtstädter, 1999; Carstensen, Mikels, & Mather, 2006; Small et al., 2006; Staudinger, 1999), (d) research on plasticity and the health benefits of cognitive training, practice, and physical exercise on neurobiological and cognitive levels (e.g., Ball et al., 2002; Kramer, Colcombe, McAuley, Scalf, & Erickson, 2005), and (e) a cluster of theories accounting for aging-related cognitive decline as a function of the declining operations or volume of underlying biological or neurological processes or cognitive resources (e.g., Cabeza et al., 2004; Raz, 2004; Reuter-Lorenz & Lustig, 2005; Salthouse, 1991).

Derived from these and other sources, Figure 9.2 presents a conceptual model for linking temporally the factors potentially influencing (favourably and unfavourably) the concurrent state and longitudinal trajectory of

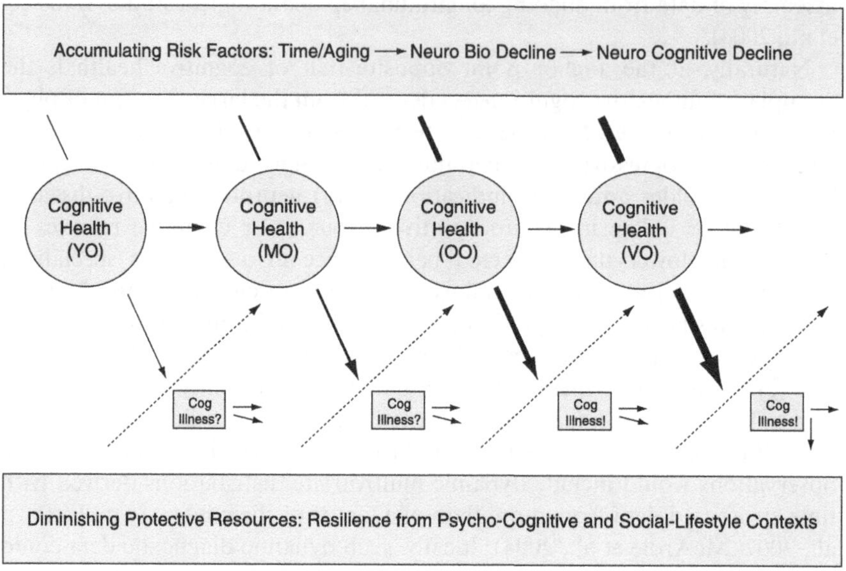

Figure 9.2 Modelling accumulating risk factors and diminishing protective resources for maintaining cognitive health in late life. (YO: young-old; MO: mid-old; OO: old-old; VO: very old.)

cognitive health in aging. As can be seen in the middle panel of the figure, cognitive health is portrayed from the input (arbitrary starting point in late midlife), through transition phases, and to the output (aging-related goal of successful cognitive health). This stability model reflects the typical case that the actual aging-related goal is maintenance (rather than continually escalating or initial achievement) of cognitive health through late life. Therefore, Figure 9.2 presents cognitive health at both the input (left margin; young-old adults, 50s and 60s) and output (right margin, very old adults, 80s and 90s) linked by a sequence of stability arrows. In brief, the most likely goal is "maintenance" of cognitive health throughout a reasonably extended period of late life. To some extent, cognitive and physical health may be essentially givens (at the population level) among young adults, but the prevalence rates (and the meanings) of "health" are very different in the population of older adults (Wahlin, 2004). In epidemiological terms, the ratio of protective to risk factors (vis-à-vis cognitive health) is likely more favourable for younger than for older adults and, as the model postulates, even for young-old versus old-old adults.

In order to understand how this goal-related scenario may be either imperilled and compromised or promoted and enhanced, one might consult the expected effects of the pertinent biopsychosocial factors of cognitive changes with aging. These are represented in the model by the panels above and below the target (maintenance) process. Together, they represent categories of the epidemiological factors – both risk and protection factors – of healthy cognitive aging. First, the passage of time in adulthood inevitably leads to decline in cognitive performance with aging. Age per se is a prominent risk factor for cognitive decline or, put differently, for the development of cognitive "illnesses" such as Alzheimer's disease. Therefore, time is symbolically portrayed by the overall flow of Figure 9.2. Although the goal (of the middle panel) is maintenance of cognitive health, much robust research supports the proposition that normal cognitive aging declines in a variety of processes across late life (e.g., Craik & Salthouse, 2007). Crucial, intrinsic, and inevitable aging-related forces are operating over time in a manner antagonistic to its attainment and detrimental to its long-term maintenance. These dynamic forces are represented in the top panel of the figure.

Put simply, the top panel represents decline in biological, neurobiological, and neurocognitive integrity and functioning (Hedden & Gabrieli, 2004; Raz, 2004). If the passage of time is a risk factor of decremental trajectories of cognitive health, it is arguably related to its underlying association with normal biological aging. Essentially, it is simply the old idea that normal neurodegeneration, pathogenic neurodegeneration, and decrements in biological and sensory health can lead, exacerbate, interfere, and delimit cognitive performance at any point in time. Eventually, over a succession of late-life time points, ineluctable cognitive decline is established. In contrast, what effects could sustained or recovered biological vitality, preserved or improved biological health and physical condition, or neurobiologically related compensatory functions have on overall late-life cognitive health (Dixon et al., 2008; Persson & Nyberg, 2006; Reuter-Lorenz & Lustig, 2005)? If biological illness (or suboptimal health) acts as a risk factor for cognitive decline, then stabilized or favourable biological health or vitality may act as a protective factor. In a sense, the dynamic relationship between the top and middle panels of the figure portrays cognitive health in the context of biological health. It implies that they are mutually implicative, with persuasive arguments that changes in the latter may often lead or be a precursor to changes in the former (Wahlin, 2004; Wahlin et al., 2006). For example, individual differences in aging-related changes in biological health may be associated with differential mean-level trajectories and intra-individual variability in cognitive health (MacDonald, Nyberg, & Bäckman, 2006).

In the third and lower panel of Figure 9.2, the inevitable decline in biological health (and potentially cognitive health) is linked with factors drawn from a broad psycho-sociocultural realm. Some of these factors may restrict or imperil cognitive health, whereas others may provide the nexus from which particular rehabilitative, compensatory, optimizing, selective, restorative, or supportive actions and programmes may derive. Conceivably, through the operation of elements in this context, cognitive health may be maintained despite the fact that it would normally decline with aging as a function of the factors in the top panel. Strategies for maintenance of cognitive health in late life may reside at the individual psychological level (e.g., mnemonic or compensatory techniques), social interactive or situative level (e.g., recruitment and using cognitively intact human aids), social structural level (e.g., adjusting demand conditions for older adults in given situations, providing health and activity support for older adults), or perhaps even the cultural level (e.g., systems of expectations and rewards for aging generations) (e.g., Baltes & Smith, 2004; Park et al., 1999).

Finally, note also that Figure 9.2 contains three sets of internal arrows, two of which have not been discussed. One set originates in the top – accumulating risk factor – panel. The arrows follow an unrelenting 45°-angle downward direction, with increasing thicknesses with aging. These characteristics are intended to symbolize that the hazardous effects of biological decline on cognitive health increase in intensity with aging (Bäckman, Small, & Wahlin, 2001). A second set of arrows originate in the lower – diminishing protective resources – panel. The dotted depiction and more limited extension (only to the middle panel, cognitive health) are intended to indicate the notion that these resources may serve to interrupt the steady push from biological decline to cognitive illness, but that they are unlikely to mitigate the opposing effect from the accumulating risk factors in the top panel.

Given the incidental geography of Figure 9.2, a "gravity" principle of cognitive health may appear to apply: The "downward" push of neurobiological decline may be cumulatively stronger than the available supportive or "upward" pushes from the protective resources. Overall, the epidemiological model is intended to provide a provisional framework for considering the problem with which we are faced: Can (and if so how may) cognitive health be maintained given the robust (and often sobering) realities of cognitive and biological aging, along with the intriguing qualifications or opportunities potentially available but certainly not always realized in the bio-, psycho-, and socio-worlds of aging adults?

Selected methodological considerations for an epidemiology of cognitive health

Given the model (Figure 9.2), what are some of the key methodological considerations to consider in formulating a developmental epidemiology of cognitive health in aging? In brief, the themes seem to be "selectivity" and "multiples". Just as in epidemiological research on cognitive aging disease, helpful characteristics include having a multidimensional pool (e.g., multi-level data archives) available from which researchers may select specific indicators, represent relevant levels of analyses, identify appropriate measurement occasions, recruit expert collaborators, and even share or compare data and results. The ideal is rarely reached and not always necessary; as always, much depends on the target processes, purposes of a study, and theories of influences. The multiple levels (etc.) are merely hypothetical (if not ambiguous) unless included in actual research projects, and then not only included but integrated and analysed interactively (McArdle et al., 2004;

Ram & Nesselroade, 2007). Such projects could include many of the features highlighted in Figure 9.3. To the extent they do, they may constitute large-scale longitudinal studies (LSLS), of which Nilsson's Betula project is a prominent example. Among the other international projects with a sampling of such characteristics are the Australian Longitudinal Study of Ageing, Berlin Aging Study, Kungsholmen Project, Seattle Longitudinal Study, and the Victoria Longitudinal Study (see also Hultsch, 2004).

Although new studies could be launched, extant large-scale longitudinal studies represent a favourable alternative for new research on the factors influencing cognitive health in aging. Most of the active LSLS represent the methodological expansion and theoretical growth of both differential and experimental research traditions, as they have been applied to cognitive aging. Given the range and complexity of potential influences on cognitive decline with aging, it is natural and possible that many of these LSLS may therefore contain a pool of indicators from which particular researchers could harvest data pertaining to cognitive health and aging. Unsurprisingly, for several decades, the notion that some phenomena of human cognitive aging may involve multiple levels of analysis has been a fixture among theoreticians, methodologists, and LSLS (e.g., Baltes & Smith, 2004; Dixon et al., 2004; Hofer & Sliwinski, 2006; Park et al., 1999; Ram & Nesselroade, 2007).

To their advantage in conducting epidemiological studies of cognitive aging, LSLS frequently recruit multiple expert collaborators, include research measures, and evaluate novel research questions – often imported from neighbouring disciplines such as neuroscience, genetics, pharmacology, sociology, and psychology. By design, LSLS may include large samples, multiple occasions of observation, and a host of potential predictors drawn from a

Designs for Developmental-Epidemiological Research on Cognitive Health

- Research Designs Could Include Indicators of:
  - Time: Change in Levels of Performance
  - Observation: Gains, Losses, Maintenance
  - Interpretation: Level, Resilience, Adaptation, Compensation
  - Inputs: From Bio, Psycho, Social Levels
  - Output: Multiple Indicators of Cognitive Health/Disease
  - Crossing: Interactions Within/Across Levels
  - Risk Factors: Precursors to Loss
  - Protective Factors: Promoting Maintenance or Managed Loss
- LSLS have some of these features:
  - ALSA, BASE, Betula, Kungsholmen, SLS, VLS

Figure 9.3 Key methodological issues in epidemiological aging research. (ALSA: Australian Longitudinal Study of Ageing; BASE: Berlin Aging Study; SLS: Seattle Longitudinal Study; VLS: Victoria Longitudinal Study.)

wide range of disciplines. Many of the active longitudinal studies reviewed by Schaie and Hofer (2001), or those featured in lengthier formats in a special issue of *Aging, Neuropsychology, and Cognition* (Hultsch, 2004), essentially fit these generous criteria. Together, they have produced voluminous results pertaining to cognitive aging, using combinations of differential, experimental, cross-sectional, simple longitudinal, and epidemiological techniques. To be sure, the foci of each of the LSLS are broad, different, and balanced. For example, whereas the Kungsholmen Project has made enormous contributions to understanding the epidemiological factors in the emergence of Alzheimer's disease and other dementias (e.g., Fratiglioni et al., 1991), the Berlin Aging Study (e.g., Baltes et al., 1999) has contributed uniquely to our understanding of differential courses and characteristics of aging, and the Seattle Longitudinal Study (e.g., Schaie, 1996) has produced prodigious information pertaining to normal intellectual development across decades of historical time. Nevertheless, despite the non-redundancy, there is also considerable methodological overlap among the studies, a characteristic that offers many opportunities for cross-national (if not yet cross-cultural) comparisons. Among many other examples internationally, Nilsson's Betula project (Nilsson et al., 1997, 2004) and the Victoria Longitudinal Study (Dixon & de Frias, 2004; Hultsch, Hertzog, Dixon, & Small, 1998) have collaborated on several such integrative projects (e.g., Dixon et al., 2004; Nyberg et al., 2003; Wahlin et al., 2006).

One advantage of LSLS is that data pertaining to differentiating processes of normal aging from probable neurodegenerative (or decline-based) or from probable cognitively healthy can be assembled. Whether it is the data, the researchers, the tools and techniques, or the levels of analyses, assembling information across studies and domains can produce templates approaching the comprehensive. On a large scale, some researchers are pursuing this agenda aggressively indeed, linking longitudinal data sets focused on selected methods, problems, and issues in cognitive aging (e.g., Hofer & Sliwinski, 2006). On a more limited scale of a single LSLS, Figure 9.4 shows how assembled archival data, organized by outcome condition, could yield a template upon which differential patterns of change could be depicted. Moreover, not only descriptive analyses (e.g., incidence and prevalence) would be available, but so too would more explanatory studies of associated risk and protection factors and, as occasions of measurement accumulate, lead and lag relationships. Notably, such studies are limited only by start date as to the available window of time for examining various lagged, interactive, and coupling effects, perhaps even deep into the history and background of emerging target cases and groups. In brief, underlying processes from relevant levels of analyses could be linked with the various patterns of transitions, trajectories, correlates, and outcome conditions (McArdle et al., 2004).

Using Figure 9.4 and the VLS as a model, the vertical rectangle on the left margin represents the archives of a panel followed in a longitudinal study. The key point is that, as the aging panel is followed over time, identifiable

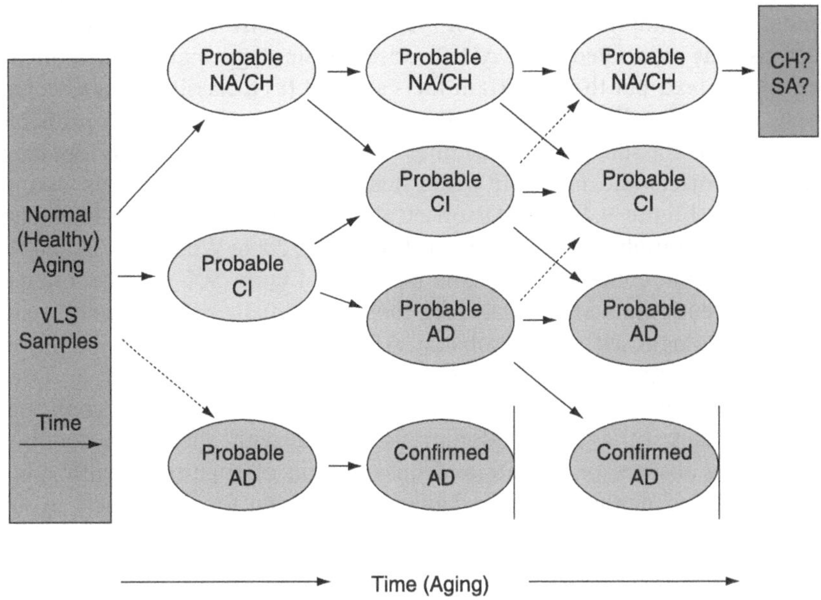

Figure 9.4 Differentiating cognitively healthy from neurodegenerative trajectories in longitudinal studies of aging. (AD: Alzheimer's disease; CH: cognitive health; CI: cognitive impairment; NA: normal aging; SA: successful aging.)

clusters of diagnostically separable groups emerge. In the case of the VLS, little time is required for even initially healthy 55–85-year-old participants to begin to show signs of three clusters of tentatively separable outcomes. One cluster of longitudinal participants are differentiated quickly (or eventually) into classic cognitive illnesses, such as that represented by a diagnosis of probable AD. At some point, as shown in the lower portion of Figure 9.4, these diagnoses can be confirmed using traditional clinical procedures. Another cluster of participants are evident from inspection of intra-individual patterns of change, depicted in the upper portion of Figure 9.4. Their performance meets several of the above-noted criteria for cognitive health, such as relatively (a) high performance with respect to the cohort, (b) sustained levels of intra-individual performance over time, and (c) consistent (low intra-individual variability in) performance across observations. Because there is no known and validated outcome measure of normal aging (NA in Figure 9.4), cognitive health (CH), or successful aging (SA), the Figure (a) emphasizes the tentative nature of the cluster by referring to the "diagnosis" as probable CH and (b) includes explicit question marks in the final-outcome box (upper-right corner). Figure 9.4 also represents a middle-range collection of older adults, those possibly at risk for impaired or accelerated decline. Although presently imprecise conceptually and diagnostically (see Tuokko &

Hultsch, 2006), this group is increasingly referred to as bearing signs of a mild cognitive impairment but not (yet or at all) converted into a dementia such as that associated with AD. Precise terminology matters little in the present context, but the important facts are that (a) a classification as cognitively impaired (CI in Figure 9.4) is prospectively tentative or probable, because (b) classification procedures vary dramatically across epidemiological projects and most are associated with instability in status, as represented in Figure 9.4 (e.g., Dixon et al., 2007; Palmer, Wang, Bäckman, Winblad, & Fratiglioni, 2002; Tuokko & Hultsch, 2006; Winblad et al., 2004).

Two general conclusions emanating from Figure 9.4 can be offered. First, firm endpoints are available for those individuals who are quickly and accurately diagnosed with probable AD, and the same firm but more extended endpoints occur for those individuals who transition more slowly from normal aging to cognitive impairment to probable and then confirmed AD. The lack of a firm endpoint associated with successful cognitive aging – the absence of definite and final criteria of cognitive health – is a theoretical and methodological challenge remaining for researchers in this field. Second, although data are not shown in Figure 9.4, the template reflects trends actually observed in some longitudinal studies (including the VLS) that include large samples of initially physically and cognitively healthy older adults. Understandably, much of the focus is on tracking, detecting, and analysing patterns and factors associated with individuals and groups that resolve their participation in a condition of unhealthy cognition. Equally interesting – if not equally frequent – are those individuals and groups that appear to maintain relatively, if not absolutely, high and successful cognitive health through late life. Epidemiological approaches can be fruitfully applied, with some assumptions, to cognitive health and aging.

The VLS and cognitive health: Tapping data archives for novel questions

The VLS is a project similar to Nilsson's Betula project (Dixon & de Frias, 2004; Nilsson et al., 2004). Both began in the late 1980s, featured large samples followed at regular intervals, with measures from multiple domains at multiple levels (memory, cognition, biohealth, demographic, neuropsychological, psychosocial, and others). The general purpose of the BP was to examine memory change in adulthood, with some focus on identifying risk factors and preclinical signs of dementia. The general purpose of the VLS was to examine differential memory change in adulthood, with some focus on identifying risk factors and preclinical signs of accelerated memory decline and dementia. Nevertheless, as long-term intra-individual longitudinal data poured into these studies, notable individual differences in change patterns occurred in rate and relative direction of decline with aging. In addition, however, surprisingly vivid portraits of long-term patterns consistent with inferences of sustained cognitive health were also observed. In the VLS, several recent initiatives have begun to explore selected aspects of probable cognitively healthy aging. We have used selected subsamples (e.g., highly engaged, cognitively intact), a variety of methods (e.g., longitudinal analyses such as growth curve and multilevel modelling, as well as matched group comparative designs), and new indicators of potential cognitive health (cognitive consistency, compensatory behaviour) to begin our studies of the phenomenon. This buffet-style or opportunistic sampling of potential cognitive health phenomena is perhaps similar to that of the BP (e.g., Habib et al., 2006), for the likely common reason that both studies were set up with cognitive decline and illness in mind and were not focused on more favourable outcomes. Fortunately, in the large-scale collection of longitudinal data, many opportunities to address unanticipated questions can emerge.

In the remainder of the chapter, three brief sketches of recent VLS research on the initially unforeseen but fortuitously available topics are sketched. In the interest of continuity, the examples are linked to our earlier discussion of the foundations and opportunities for research in cognitive health. Other epidemiological aspects of cognitive health were planned at the outset of the VLS (e.g., the role of lifestyle engagement) and will not be further discussed (Small et al., 2006). Notably, the research examples summarized are not unique to the VLS; many other projects could engage in each of these lines of inquiry (e.g., as in Ghisletta et al., 2006). To emphasize the emerging and unfinished nature of them, they are presented as provocative research questions.

Does neurocognitive consistency signal cognitive health?

If neurocognitive inconsistency at the "bio" level is an indicator of impairment or disease (MacDonald et al., 2006), could relative consistency in older adults' performance signal sustained cognitive health? Like many other epidemiological projects, the VLS has been interested in identifying early markers of impending transition to cognitive impairment or dementia. In one recent project, we observed that inconsistency in performance on speeded tasks was a powerful predictor of cognitive impairment status (Dixon et al., 2007). As can be seen in Figure 9.5, the cognitively healthy older adults performed across trials in various speeded tasks considerably more consistently than did the mild cognitively impaired group (mCI Mild) and especially the more impaired moderate group (mCI Moderate). This leads to new research questions requiring valid outcome indicators of cognitive health, which are not yet developed. Supporting the idea, however, are other studies along this line that show, for example, that consistency in neurocognitive performance is even related to the most significant aspect of health – lower rates of impending death (MacDonald, Hultsch, & Dixon, 2008).

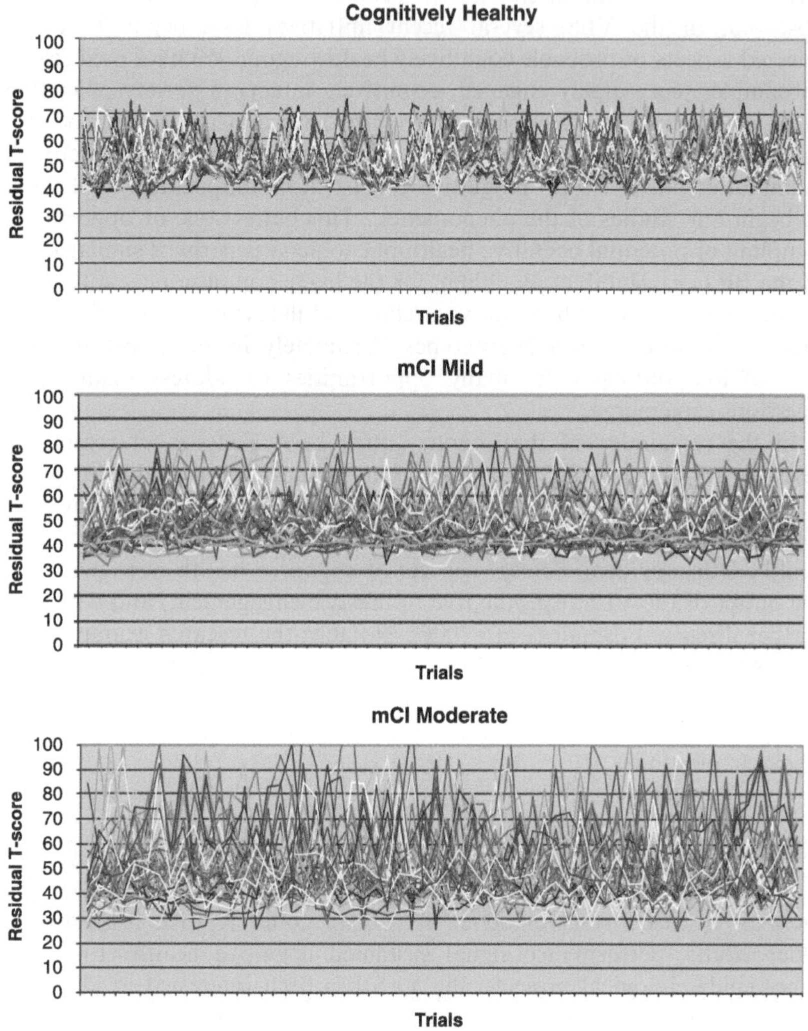

Figure 9.5 Displaying intra-individual inconsistency in multi-trial (horizontal axis) speeded performance, with older groups varying in cognitive health: less inconsistency for those classified as cognitively healthy, more inconsistency for those classified as mild cognitively impaired (mCI Mild), and most inconsistency for those classified as moderately impaired (mCI Moderate). (Adapted from Dixon et al., 2007; prepared by D. Garrett and S. MacDonald.)

Is cognitive health indicated by compensatory recruitment?

The concept of *recruitment* refers to the notion that cognitive health may be supported by effort or success in engaging (whether deliberately or automatically) resources that are not commonly applied to cognitive adaptivity, in general, or cognitive performance on a given task, in particular. At the "bio" level, recruitment may be observed in the form of compensatory brain activation (Cabeza, Anderson, Locantore, & McIntosh, 2002; Dixon et al., 2008; Persson & Nyberg, 2006; Reuter-Lorenz & Lustig, 2005). Recent VLS research has addressed whether recruitment may also occur from the "social" (interactional) to the "psycho" (cognitive) levels. Arguably as a function of cognitive losses, some adults may consult or collaborate on everyday cognitive problems – a process of recruiting other brains that is conceptually homologous with recruiting other regions of the same brain. The other brains recruited may be colleagues, spouses, or caregivers in the immediate social world of the cognitively impaired older adult. New experimental observations consistent with this general hypothesis have been observed for normal cognitive aging, in which married couples perform complex cognitive tasks through relatively unique mechanisms and at levels consistent with the recruitment idea (e.g., Gagnon & Dixon, 2008). Using VLS archives, other recent work has reported the propensity of memory-impaired older adults to use changing memory compensatory techniques in apparent efforts to maintain cognitive adaptation in everyday life (Dixon & de Frias, 2007). In addition, using Kungsholmen Project archival data, a collaborative team also observed that AD patients increased their use of cognitively intact spouses to help in managing everyday cognitive problems (Dixon, Hopp, Cohen, de Frias, & Bäckman, 2003). Compensatory recruitment may be an indicator of relative cognitive health, and one that spans more than one level of analysis.

Is younger biological "age" related to better cognitive health?

Researchers in the VLS explored the potential for biological vitality (and an associated construct of biological age or "bioage") to account for long-term changes in memory and other cognitive functions. A common observation is that chronological age is often a poor indicator of relative health, with some 70-year-olds seeming frail and others seeming vital and much younger (Liang et al., 2003). Do individual differences in biological health map onto individual differences in cognitive health? MacDonald et al. (2004) found that a bioage construct (a composite of several physiological indicators) accounted for 12-year cognitive change at a level that was at least as powerful as the more common chronological age construct. Moreover, when considered from one perspective, a younger (lower) bioage was associated with less 12-year cognitive decline. Cognitive health was at least in part associated with biological vitality, even when no constituent biomarker represented directly neurological functioning. Maintaining biological vitality, biological health, and perhaps even beliefs in health vitality may be associated with cognitive health (Wahlin, 2004; Wahlin et al., 2006). Many LSLS will have physiological indicators and could also construct markers of biological health and age.

Conclusion

The purpose of this chapter was to explore conceptual, methodological, and empirical perspectives on the nature, influences, and possible maintenance of cognitive health through late life. By linking standard epidemiological perspectives with multivariate dynamic models and cognitive aging theories, effective methodological tools may be available for conducting research on novel research questions pertaining to cognitive health in aging. In particular, many LSLS may have data archives that could be mined for evidence pertaining to cognitive health, at least supplemental to the overarching tasks of charting the patterns and precursors of cognitive disease. The concept of cognitive health in aging is an intriguing one in a field in which robust evidence of decline often (and understandably) dominates the empirical and theoretical scenery. The concept does not imply that this scenery is in any way flawed, but it does reveal novel (and interactive) aspects of the landscape that may be otherwise hidden or overlooked.

Acknowledgements

Research in the Victoria Longitudinal Study is supported by a grant (R37 AG008235) from the National Institute on Aging (NIA) to Roger Dixon, who also acknowledges support from the Canada Research Chairs program.

References

Bäckman, L., Small, B. J., & Wahlin, Å. (2001). Aging and memory: Cognitive and biological perspectives. In J. E. Birren & K. W. Schaie (Eds.), *Handbook of the psychology of aging* (5th ed., pp. 349–377). San Diego: Academic Press.

Ball, K., Berch, D. B., Helmers, K. F., Jobe, J. B., Leveck, M. D., Marsiske, M., et al. (2002). Effects of cognitive training interventions with older adults: A randomized control trial. *Journal of the American Medical Association, 288*, 2271–2281.

Baltes, P. B., & Smith, J. (2004). Lifespan psychology: From developmental contextualism to developmental biocultural co-constructionism. *Research in Human Development, 1*, 123–144.

Baltes, P. B., & Staudinger, U. M. (2000). Wisdom: A metaheuristic (pragmatic) to orchestrate mind and virtue toward excellence. *American Psychologist, 55*, 122–136.

Baltes, P. B., Staudinger, U. M., & Lindenberger, U. (1999). Lifespan psychology: Theory and application to intellectual functioning. *Annual Review of Psychology, 50*, 471–507.

Bengtson, V. L., & Schaie, K. W. (Eds.). (1999). *Handbook of theories of aging*. New York: Springer.

Bergdahl, M., Habib, R., Bergdahl, J., Nyberg, L., & Nilsson, L.-G. (2007). Natural teeth and preserved cognitive functions in humans. *Scandinavian Journal of Psychology, 48*, 557–565.

Berry, J. M. (1999). Memory self-efficacy in its social cognitive context. In T. M. Hess & F. Blanchard-Fields (Eds.), *Social cognition and aging* (pp. 69–96). San Diego: Academic Press.

Binstock, R. H., & George, L. K. (Eds.). (2006). *Handbook of aging and the social sciences*. Amsterdam: Elsevier.

Birren, J. E., & Schaie, K. W. (Eds.). (2006). *Handbook of the psychology of aging* (6th ed.). San Diego: Academic Press.

Blanchard-Fields, F. (2005). Introduction to the special section on emotion–cognition interactions and the aging mind. *Psychology and Aging*, *20*, 539–541.

Brandtstädter, J. (1999). Sources of resilience in the aging self: Toward integrating perspectives. In T. M. Hess & F. Blanchard-Fields (Eds.), *Social cognition and aging* (pp. 123–141). San Diego: Academic Press.

Cabeza, R., Anderson, N. D., Locantore, J. K., & McIntosh, A. R. (2002). Aging gracefully: Compensatory brain activity in high-performing older adults. *NeuroImage*, *17*, 1394–1402.

Cabeza, R., Nyberg, L., & Park, D. C. (Eds.). (2004). *Linking cognitive and cerebral aging*. Oxford, UK: Oxford University Press.

Carstensen, L. L., Mikels, J. A., & Mather, M. (2006). Aging and the intersection of cognition, motivation, and emotion. In J. E. Birren & K. W. Schaie (Eds.), *Handbook of the psychology of aging* (6th ed., pp. 343–362). San Diego: Academic Press.

Craik, F. I. M., & Salthouse, T. A. (Eds.). (2007). *Handbook of aging and cognition* (3rd ed.). New York: Psychology Press.

Dixon, R. A. (2000). The concept of gains in cognitive aging. In D. C. Park & N. Schwarz (Eds.), *Cognitive aging: A primer*. Philadelphia, PA: Psychology Press.

Dixon, R. A., Bäckman, L., & Nilsson, L.-G. (Eds.). (2004). *New frontiers in cognitive aging*. Oxford, UK: Oxford University Press.

Dixon, R. A., & de Frias, C. M. (2004). The Victoria Longitudinal Study: From characterizing cognitive aging to illustrating changes in memory compensation. *Aging, Neuropsychology, and Cognition*, *11*, 346–376.

Dixon, R. A., & de Frias, C. M. (2007). Mild memory deficits differentially affect six-year changes in compensatory strategy use. *Psychology and Aging*, *22*, 632–638.

Dixon, R. A., Garrett, D. D., & Bäckman, L. (2008). Principles of compensation in cognitive neuroscience and neurorehabilitation. In D. T. Stuss, G. Winocur, & I. H. Robertson (Eds.), *Cognitive neurorehabilitation* (2nd ed., pp. 22–38). Cambridge, UK: Cambridge University Press.

Dixon, R. A., Garrett, D. D., Lentz, T., MacDonald, S. W. S., Strauss, E., & Hultsch, D. F. (2007). Neurocognitive markers of cognitive impairment: Exploring the roles of speed and inconsistency. *Neuropsychology*, *21*, 381–399.

Dixon, R. A., Hopp, G. A., Cohen, A.-L., de Frias, C. M., & Bäckman, L. (2003). Self-reported memory compensation: Similar patterns in Alzheimer's disease and very old adult samples. *Journal of Clinical and Experimental Neuropsychology*, *25*, 382–390.

Dixon, R. A., & Nilsson, L.-G. (2004). Don't fence us in: Probing the frontiers of cognitive aging. In R. A. Dixon, L. Bäckman, & L.-G. Nilsson (Eds.), *New frontiers in cognitive aging* (pp. 3–15). Oxford, UK: Oxford University Press.

Ebner, N. C., Freund, A. M., & Baltes, P. B. (2006). Developmental changes in personal goal orientation from young to late adulthood: From striving for gains to maintenance and prevention of loss. *Psychology and Aging*, *21*, 664–678.

Einstein, G. O., & McDaniel, M. A. (2004). *Memory fitness: A guide for successful aging*. New Haven, CT: Yale University Press.

Fratiglioni, L., Grut, M., Forsell, Y., Viitanen, M., Grafström, M., Holmen, K., et al.

(1991). Prevalence of Alzheimer's disease and other dementias in an elderly urban population. *Neurology, 41*, 1886–1892.

Gagnon, L. M., & Dixon, R. A. (2008). Remembering and retelling stories in individual and collaborative contexts. *Applied Cognitive Psychology, 22*, 1275–1297.

Ghisletta, P., Bickel, J.-F., & Lövdén, M. (2006). Does activity engagement protect against cognitive decline in old age? Methodological and analytical considerations. *Journal of Gerontology: Psychological Sciences, 61B*, P253–P261.

Habib, R., Nyberg, L., & Nilsson, L.-G. (2006). Cognitive and non-cognitive factors contributing to the longitudinal identification of successful older adults in the Betula study. *Aging, Neuropsychology, and Cognition, 14*, 257–273.

Hedden, T., & Gabrieli, J. D. E. (2004). Insights into the aging mind: A view from cognitive neuroscience. *Nature Reviews Neuroscience, 5*, 87–97.

Hess, T. M., & Blanchard-Fields, F. (Eds.). (1999). *Social cognition and aging*. San Diego: Academic Press.

Hofer, S. M., & Sliwinski, M. J. (2006). Design and analysis of longitudinal studies of aging. In J. E. Birren & K. W. Schaie (Eds.), *Handbook of the psychology of aging* (6th ed., pp. 20–38). San Diego: Academic Press.

Hultsch, D. F. (2004). Introduction to special issue on longitudinal studies of cognitive aging. *Aging, Neuropsychology, and Cognition, 11*, 101–103.

Hultsch, D. F., Hertzog, C., Dixon, R. A., & Small, B. J. (1998). *Memory change in the aged.* Cambridge, UK: Cambridge University Press.

Kramer, A. F., Colcombe, S. J., McAuley, E., Scalf, P., & Erickson, K. I. (2005). Fitness, aging and neurocognitive functioning. *Neurobiology of Aging, 26*, 124–127.

Liang, J., Shaw, B. A., Krause, N. M., Bennett, J. M., Blaum, C., Kobayashi, E., et al. (2003). Changes in functional status among older adults in Japan: Successful and usual aging. *Psychology and Aging, 18*, 684–695.

Little, T. D., Bouvaird, J. A., & Card, N. A. (Eds.). (2007). *Modeling contextual effects in longitudinal studies*. Mahwah, NJ: Lawrence Erlbaum Associates, Inc.

MacDonald, S. W. S., Dixon, R. A., Cohen, A. L., & Hazlitt, J. E. (2004). Biological age and 12-year cognitive change in older adults: Findings from the Victoria Longitudinal Study. *Gerontology, 50*, 64–81.

MacDonald, S. W. S., Hultsch, D. F., & Dixon, R. A. (2008). Predicting impending death: Inconsistency in speed is a selective and early marker. *Psychology and Aging, 23*, 595–607.

MacDonald, S. W. S., Nyberg, L., & Bäckman, L. (2006). Intra-individual variability in behavior: Links to brain structure, neurotransmission and neuronal activity. *TRENDS in Neuroscience, 29*, 474–480.

McArdle, J. J., Hamagami, F., Jones, K., Jolesz, F., Kikinis, R., Spiro, A., et al. (2004). Structural modeling of dynamic changes in memory and brain structure using longitudinal data from the Normative Aging Study. *Journal of Gerontology: Psychological Sciences, 59B*, P294–P304.

McDaniel, M. A., Einstein, G. O., & Jacoby, L. L. (2007). New considerations in aging and memory: The glass may be half full. In F. I. M. Craik & T. A. Salthouse (Eds.), *The handbook of aging and cognition* (3rd ed.). Mahwah, NJ: Lawrence Erlbaum Associates, Inc.

Nilsson, L.-G., Adolfsson, R., Bäckman, L., de Frias, C. M., Molander, B., & Nyberg, L. (2004). Betula: A prospective cohort study on memory, health, and aging. *Aging, Neuropsychology, and Cognition, 11*, 134–148.

Nilsson, L.-G., Bäckman, L., Erngrund, K., Nyberg, L., Adolfsson, R., Bucht, G., et al. (1997). The Betula prospective cohort study: Memory, health, and aging. *Aging, Neuropsychology, and Cognition, 4*, 1–32.

Nyberg, L., Maitland, S. B., Rönnlund, M., Bäckman, L., Dixon, R. A., Wahlin, Å., et al. (2003). Selective adult age differences in an age-invariant multifactor model of declarative memory. *Psychology and Aging, 18*, 149–160.

Palmer, K., Wang, H.-X., Bäckman, L., Winblad, B., & Fratiglioni, L. (2002). Differential evolution of cognitive impairment in nondemented older persons: Results from the Kungsholmen Project. *American Journal of Psychiatry, 159*, 436–442.

Park, D. C., Nisbett, R., & Hedden, T. (1999). Aging, culture, and cognition. *Journal of Gerontology: Psychological Sciences, 54*, 75–84.

Perlmutter, M. (Ed.). (1990). *Late-life potential.* Washington, DC: Gerontological Society of America.

Persson, J., & Nyberg, L. (2006). Altered brain activity in healthy seniors: What does it mean? *Progress in Brain Research, 157*, 45–56.

Persson, J., Nyberg, L., Lind, J., Larsson, A., Nilsson, L.-G., Ingvar, M., et al. (2006). Structure-function correlates of cognitive decline in aging. *Cerebral Cortex, 16*, 907–915.

Ram, N., & Nesselroade, J. R. (2007). Modeling intraindividual and intracontextual change: Rendering developmental context operational. In T. D. Little, J. A. Bouvaird, & N. A. Card (Eds.), *Modeling contextual effects in longitudinal studies* (pp. 325–342). Mahwah, NJ: Lawrence Erlbaum Associates, Inc.

Raz, N. (2004). The aging brain: Structural changes and their implications for cognitive aging. In R. A. Dixon, L. Bäckman, & L.-G. Nilsson (Eds.), *New frontiers in cognitive aging.* Oxford, UK: Oxford University Press.

Reuter-Lorenz, P. A., & Lustig, C. (2005). Brain aging: Reorganizing discoveries about the aging mind. *Current Opinion in Neurobiology, 15*, 245–251.

Rowe, J. W., & Kahn, R. L. (1999). *Successful aging.* New York: Dell.

Salthouse, T. A. (1991). *Theoretical perspectives on cognitive aging.* Hillsdale, NJ: Lawrence Erlbaum Associates, Inc.

Scarmeas, N. (2006). Lifestyle patterns and cognitive reserve. In Y. Stern (Ed.), *Cognitive reserve* (pp. 187–206). New York: Psychology Press.

Schaie, K. W. (1996). *Intellectual development in adulthood: The Seattle longitudinal study.* New York: Cambridge University Press.

Schaie, K. W., & Hofer, S. M. (2001). Longitudinal studies in aging research. In J. E. Birren & K. W. Schaie (Eds.), *Handbook of the psychology of aging* (5th ed., pp. 53–77). San Diego: Academic Press.

Siegler, I. C., Bosworth, H. B., & Poon, L. W. (2003). Disease, health, and aging. In R. M. Lerner, M. A. Easterbrooks, & J. Mistry (Eds.), *Handbook of psychology: Vol. 6. Developmental psychology* (pp. 423–442). Hoboken, NJ: Wiley.

Simonton, D. K. (1990). Creativity and wisdom in aging. In J. E. Birren & K. W. Schaie (Eds.), *Handbook of psychology and aging* (3rd ed., pp. 320–329). San Diego: Academic Press.

Small, B. J., Hughes, T. F., Hultsch, D. F., & Dixon, R. A. (2006). Lifestyle activities and late-life changes in cognitive performance. In Y. Stern (Ed.), *Cognitive reserve* (pp. 173–186). New York: Psychology Press.

Staudinger, U. M. (1999). Social cognition and a psychological approach to an art of life. In T. M. Hess & F. Blanchard-Fields (Eds.), *Social cognition and aging* (pp. 343–375). San Diego: Academic Press.

Stern, Y. (Ed.). (2006). *Cognitive reserve.* New York: Psychology Press.

Sternberg, R. J., & Lubart, T. I. (2001). Wisdom and creativity. In J. E. Birren & K. W. Schaie (Eds.), *Handbook of the psychology of aging* (5th ed., pp. 500–522). San Diego: Academic Press.

Tuokko, H., & Hultsch, D. F. (Eds.). (2006). *Mild cognitive impairment: International perspectives*. New York: Psychology Press.

Vaillant, G. E. (2002). *Aging well*. Boston, MA: Little, Brown.

Wahlin, Å. (2004). Health, disease, and cognitive aging. In R. A. Dixon, L. Bäckman, & L.-G. Nilsson (Eds.), *New frontiers in cognitive aging* (pp. 279–302). Oxford, UK: Oxford University Press.

Wahlin, Å., MacDonald, S. W. S., de Frias, C. M., Nilsson, L.-G., & Dixon, R. A. (2006). How do health and biological age influence chronological age and sex differences in cognitive aging: Moderating, mediating or both? *Psychology and Aging*, *21*, 318–322.

Waldstein, S. R. (2000). Health effects on cognitive aging. In P. C. Stern & L. L. Carstensen (Eds.), *The aging mind: Opportunities in cognitive research*. Washington, DC: National Academy Press.

Wang, H.-X., Karp, A., Winblad, B., & Fratiglioni, L. (2002). Late-life engagement in social and leisure activities is associated with a decreased risk of dementia: A longitudinal study from the Kungsholmen Project. *American Journal of Epidemiology*, *155*, 1081–1087.

Winblad, B., Palmer, K., Kivipelto, M., Jelic, V., Fratiglioni, L., Wahlund, L. O., et al. (2004). Mild cognitive impairment – beyond controversies, towards a consensus. *Journal of Internal Medicine*, *256*, 240–246.

10 Decline-induced plastic changes of brain and behaviour in aging

Martin Lövdén

During the last two decades we have witnessed an important body of empirical reports from several longitudinal studies of cognitive aging, such as the Betula study (Nilsson et al., 1997). Thanks to this work, we can now describe the hallmarks of cognitive aging. At the group level, we find accelerating mean negative changes in fluid abilities such as working memory, reasoning, episodic memory, and spatial orientation (e.g., Rönnlund & Nilsson, 2006; Rönnlund, Nyberg, Bäckman, & Nilsson, 2005; Schaie, 1996). These changes are in full view roughly around the age of 65. Different individuals, of course, show substantially different levels of performance, and, more importantly, between-person differences in change appear in old age (DeFrias, Lövdén, Lindenberger, & Nilsson, 2007). Together, these findings draw a chart of the cognitive aging terrain that is depicted in Figure 10.1. During younger adulthood, groups of individuals display normal distribution of individual differences, and individuals travel in parallel. In older age, groups of individuals display mean decline, and individuals starts to display differences among each other in the amount of change in performance. The age at which a functional impairment threshold (e.g., dementia or impairment in everyday functioning; thick black line) is reached is determined by the individual's level of performance when entering adulthood (compare Persons 2 and 3) as well as the individual's amount of change in old age (compare Persons 1 and 2). Prominent potential candidates of brain correlates of these behavioural changes include marked decrements in grey matter volume of, for example, the prefrontal cortex and the hippocampus (Raz et al., 2005), deteriorating white matter integrity that follows an anterior to posterior gradient (Sullivan & Pfefferbaum, 2006), declines in receptor density and concentration of neurotransmitters (e.g., dopamine; Bäckman, Nyberg, Lindenberger, Li, & Farde, 2006; Bäckman & Nyberg, chapter 11, this volume), and negative cerebrovascular alterations (Farkas & Luiten, 2001).

We know today that a healthy lifestyle, rich in terms of mental, physical, and social stimulation, may postpone and slow down cognitive aging (Bäckman, Small, Wahlin, & Larsson, 1999b; Fratiglioni, Paillard-Borg, & Winblad, 2004; Gerstorf, Lövdén, Röcke, Smith, & Lindenberger, 2007; Kramer, Bherer, Colcombe, Dong, & Greenough, 2004; Lövdén, Ghisletta, &

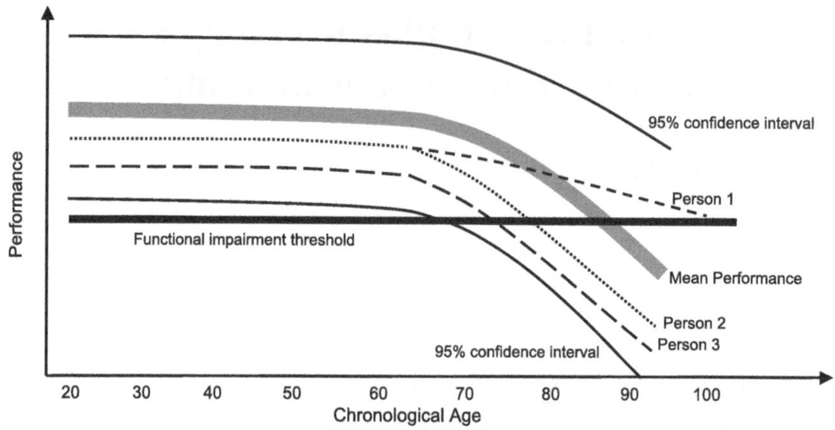

Figure 10.1 Schematic univariate description of the hallmarks of development of fluid abilities in adulthood and aging. Performance at a particular point in time displays normal distribution, with substantial inter-individual differences. During adulthood, until the seventh decade of life, individuals travel to a high degree in parallel. As indicated by comparing the trajectories of Person 1 and Person 2, in older age, inter-individual differences in change appear. The age at which a critical threshold is reached (e.g., dementia; thick black line) is codetermined by level of performance (compare the trajectories of Person 2 and Person 3) and change in performance in old age (compare the trajectories of Person 1 and Person 2).

Lindenberger, 2005a). For example, Lövdén and colleagues (Ghisletta, Bickel, & Lövdén, 2006; Lövdén et al., 2005a) have reported dynamic structural equation modelling of longitudinal data showing that participation in socially relevant activities predicts decline in cognitive capacity in old age (see Figure 10.2). However, we know little about the mechanisms through which these lifestyle factors influence cognitive aging. For example, we do not know whether the positive impact of an engaged lifestyle is best explained by mechanisms involving direct beneficial effects of mental stimulation on cognitive performance or by avoidance of negative effects on cognition (e.g., disuse, depression, and stress). To fill this lacuna, within and across periods of the life span we need to more directly study the interchange of brain, culture, and the behaviours that constitute the building blocks of a healthy lifestyle (Baltes & Singer, 2001; Baltes, Lindenberger, & Staudinger, 2006; S. C. Li, 2003). That is, in order to understand aging of brain and behaviour, we need to study the mechanisms of plasticity.

Plasticity is, however, a highly overused word that permeates most subfields of psychology and neuroscience with multiple connotations. Therefore, in this chapter I first briefly discuss the scientific use of the term "plasticity" in the context of brain and behaviour in aging. Equipped with this background, which distinguishes this review from other recent reviews of the topic (e.g., Greenwood, 2007), I review the empirical literature pertinent to the

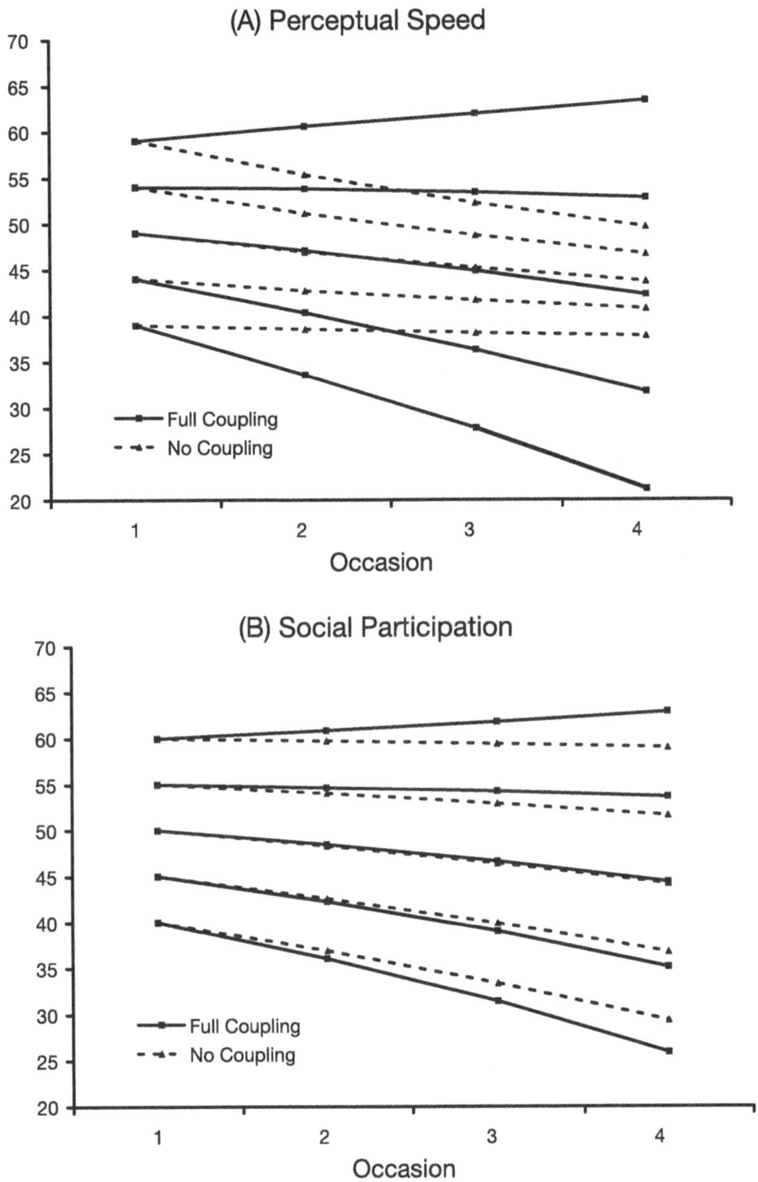

Figure 10.2 Social participation attenuates decline in perceptual speed (Lövdén et al., 2005a). Means for perceptual speed (A) and social participation (B) from a full-coupling model (thick lines) allowing for dynamic lead–lag couplings and from a no-coupling model (dashed lines) not allowing for any coupling between social participation and speed. The means are plotted as a function of time and varied initial (Time 1) means. Allowing for dynamic relations (state influencing change) between the variables has strong impact on the expected development curves for perceptual speed but not for social participation, indicating that social participation drives decline in speed in old age. (Adapted from Lövdén et al., 2005a.)

issue of whether the negative neuronal and behavioural changes that come with aging induce adaptive plastic (or compensatory) changes.

The concept of plasticity

Plasticity denotes the capacity for change, but the scientific use of the term plasticity is typically narrowed down to changes that can be regarded as reactive in some way (e.g., Kelly & Garavan, 2005; Kempermann, 2006; Kolb, 1995; Pascual-Leone, Amedi, Fregni, & Merabet, 2005). For example, in brain injury, the capacity of the brain for change is considered revealed not by the damage *per se*, of course, but by the restoring and compensatory reactions to the damage (e.g., Brion, Demeurisse, & Capon, 1989; Buckner, Corbetta, Schatz, Raichle, & Petersen, 1996). In other words, manifestations of plasticity are typically portrayed as outcomes of some primary change in the neural system that is not a necessary and direct consequence of the primary change.

To further protect the term from overuse, plasticity is typically used for phenomena other than those that can be described as reflecting neuronal and behavioural variability and flexibility. In fact, variability and flexibility must be viewed as the background against which plasticity is studied. Specifically, in contrast to variability, which denotes relatively temporary and reversible fluctuations (adaptive or not) that can be characterized as noise or steady rhythms (Ford, 1987; Nesselroade, 1991), plasticity tends to denote relatively permanent changes from one equilibrium to another (cf. S. C. Li, Huxhold, & Schmiedek, 2004). Flexibility – the neurocognitive system's ability to perform strategic trial-and-error behaviour and to optimize performance through strategic top-down cognitive control and attentional selection – is also associated with less permanent change. Thus, variability, flexibility, and plasticity appear in the bulk of literature as orthogonal concepts (but potential empirically related; e.g., Allaire & Marsiske, 2005; S. C. Li et al., 2004; Lindenberger, Li, & Bäckman, 2006; Siegler, 1994) that describe different types of intra-individual variation. Plasticity thus denotes the capacity of brain and behaviour to undergo relatively permanent changes through reactive processes.

Causes of plastic changes

A feature held in common among reports of plastic change in brain and behaviour is that the workhorse of plasticity is a mismatch between supply in the form of the functioning (nature and performance) of the system and the environmental demands that work on the system through experience (e.g., perceptions, thoughts, and actions; see also Bäckman & Dixon, 1992). Hence, the origin of plastic alterations in brain and behaviour is typically searched for among changes in function or in the experiential demands on function. These changes are sometimes viewed as inducing a movement away from homeostasis, which drives the system to react. To provide some examples, Hihara et al. (2006) trained adult monkeys to use a rake to retrieve food. By injecting anatomical tracers into the intraparietal sulcus and temporo-parietal junction of trained and untrained monkeys, the authors could demonstrate novel and more extensive connections within the intraparietal sulcus as a result of tool-use training. In this example, the environmental conditions demand a skill not initially available, and this mismatch produces functional and structural alterations to meet this demand. Other examples of plastic change in brain and behaviour emanate from direct internal changes in the functioning of the system. The most extreme examples involve brain injuries (e.g., stroke) that may provoke compensatory alterations in response to reduced functioning combined with unaltered environmental demands and behavioural goals (Brion et al., 1989; Buckner et al., 1996; Pascual-Leone et al., 2005). Similar but less perturbing inductions of plastic changes may stem from the negative changes in cognitive performance and brain functioning that occur in aging (Bäckman & Dixon, 1992; Cabeza, 2002; Kolb, 1995). It is on evaluating the viability of the notion of decline-induced plastic changes in aging that I focus in this chapter.

Plastic responses to negative changes in function are, in both lay and academic psychology, typically referred to as compensatory changes. Compensation denotes plastic changes that aim to reinstate some molar level of functioning in response to an objective or perceived serious negative, and irreversible, change (e.g., deficit or loss) in some molecular functional capacity (for review, see Bäckman & Dixon, 1992). Note, however, that compensation is a form of plastic change that is not, in its manifestation, fundamentally different from other forms of plasticity. Rather, it is the origin of the plastic change that determines whether change is labelled compensation (negative change in functional level) or not.

Plasticity, compensation, and reserve

The notion of plastic compensatory changes induced by negative functional changes that come with aging, pathology, and brain injury is related to the popular concept of a reserve against these negative brain changes. The reserve concept stems from empirical observations of inter-individual differences in the behavioural expressions of a particular degree and nature of brain pathology. Two major types of models – passive models and active models – may account for such observations (Stern, 2002). Only the active models evoke the plasticity concept. The passive models (e.g., Satz, 1993) instead define reserve in terms of the degree of brain pathology that can be tolerated before reaching a threshold that produces functional impairments that may motivate clinical diagnosis. Assume that two individuals have two different amounts of reserve before onset of a negative brain change (e.g., pathology in Alzheimer's disease). Reserve may here refer to either macro-level neuroanatomical capacity such as brain volume (i.e., brain reserve; Stern, 2002) or to efficiency of neural and cognitive computations and strategies (i.e., cognitive reserve; Stern, 2002). Pathology of a particular size may result in functional impairment for a person with less reserve. An individual with more reserve could remain unaffected. In other words, the individual with the greatest level of reserve can tolerate a larger pathology burden before the brain's resources that are necessary to maintain a behavioural capacity are depleted. This model is similar to the situation described with Figure 10.1: The level of performance may determine when individuals reach functional impairment thresholds in old age (compare Persons 2 and 3).

In contrast to the passive reserve models, active models postulate that individual differences in the brain's responses to pathology may account for individual differences in the expression of the symptoms. In addition to its definition in the context of the passive reserve models, the term "cognitive reserve" is often assigned such meaning. That is, the notion of cognitive reserve implies individual differences in the latent potentials for improving the nature and efficiency of neural and cognitive computations in response to pathology (i.e., changes in function) and altered environmental (e.g., task) demands (see also Baltes et al., 2006; Kliegl, Smith, & Baltes, 1989). Assume that two individuals have the same current level of neural and cognitive functioning (i.e., reserve as in the passive model). However, because Person 1 can recruit alternative cognitive strategies and brain networks better than can Person 2, Person 1 can tolerate a larger pathology burden before a functional impairment threshold is reached. In other words, Person 1 possesses greater cognitive and brain plasticity than Person 2. Thus, the concept of reserve against negative brain changes that come with aging, pathology, and brain injury is, with its active connotation, identical to the concepts of behavioural (cognitive) and brain plasticity. However, regardless of terminology, the discussion about active reserve models pins down the notion of inter-individual differences in plasticity and its powerful explanatory capacity in brain injury, pathology, and aging. For example, it will become evident below that the concept of inter-individual differences in plasticity generates fruitful predictions in the domain of decline-induced plastic changes with aging.

Decline-induced plastic changes in aging: Empirical review

In this section I review the evidence pertinent to whether aging comes with adaptive compensatory neuronal and behavioural changes. Put in the context of our review of the plasticity concept, the issue concerns whether and how the slowly developing negative changes in brain structure and function (e.g., deteriorating white matter integrity, neurotransmitter depletion, and performance decreases) that slowly unfolds with aging produce plastic, compensatory, changes.

Let's start by pinning down a few empirical patterns of reorganized behavioural and brain functioning that could reflect compensatory changes. First, several authors have reported that sensory functioning (e.g., hearing) and action control (e.g., walking) may involve more higher order controlled cognitive processes with advancing age (Heuninckx, Wenderoth, Debaere, Peeters, & Swinnen, 2005; Huxhold, Li, Schmiedek, & Lindenberger, 2006; Lindenberger, Marsiske, & Baltes, 2000; Lövdén, Schaefer, Pohlmayer, & Lindenberger, 2008; Lövdén, Schellenbach, Grossman-Hutter, Krüger, & Lindenberger, 2005b; Schaefer, Huxhold, & Lindenberger, 2006; Wingfield, Tun, & McCoy, 2005). Second, in the domains of imaging higher order cognition (e.g., working memory and episodic memory), a pattern of increased dorsolateral prefrontal activity with aging has been repeatedly observed, sometimes together with decreased activity in the ventrolateral prefrontal cortex or in posterior regions (Cabeza et al., 2004; Davis, Dennis, Daselaar, Fleck, & Cabeza, 2008; Grady et al., 1994; Grady, McIntosh, & Craik, 2003b; Grossman et al., 2002a) and often in the form of increased activity in the prefrontal cortex contralateral to that primarily activated in younger adults (Bäckman et al., 1999a; Cabeza, 2002; Cabeza et al., 1997; Persson & Nyberg, 2006; Rajah & D'Esposito, 2005; Reuter-Lorenz et al., 2000). Figure 10.3 depicts some examples of these patterns of findings.

These potentially related patterns of findings have been interpreted as manifestations of plasticity. Specifically, in the domain of behavioural data pertinent to sensory functions and action control, it is often argued that top-down and controlled cognitive processes compensate for impairments in low-level, bottom-up, processes that are performed relatively automatically in younger adulthood. For example, the elderly experience problems with hearing and might compensate by recruiting cognitive resources (e.g., logical reasoning and reconstructive recall) that can be used to make sense of degraded stimuli (Alain, McDonald, Ostroff, & Schneider, 2004; Wingfield et al., 2005). Redistribution of activity to dorsal prefrontal regions has been interpreted along the same lines: higher order cognitive processes associated with dorsolateral prefrontal functioning (e.g., organization and inhibition processes) start to operate in response to deficits in posterior brain regions. For example, prefrontal regions might be recruited in an attempt to reconstruct diminished signals from the sensory cortices (Davis et al., 2008). Age-related reductions in asymmetry of prefrontal activity have been argued to arise from compensatory recruitment of homologous or complementary resources (e.g., other strategies) in the contralateral hemisphere in response to some type of neurocognitive decline (Cabeza et al., 1997), much like the pattern often observed in brain injury (Pascual-Leone et al., 2005).

Nevertheless, competing interpretations dismiss plasticity as a mechanism behind these patterns of findings. Specifically, in the domains of sensory functioning and action control, it can be argued that degraded sensory information simply demands cognitive and prefrontal resources that resolve ambiguities in the bottom-up signal. In other words, the increased involvement of higher order controlled processes in the dorsolateral prefrontal

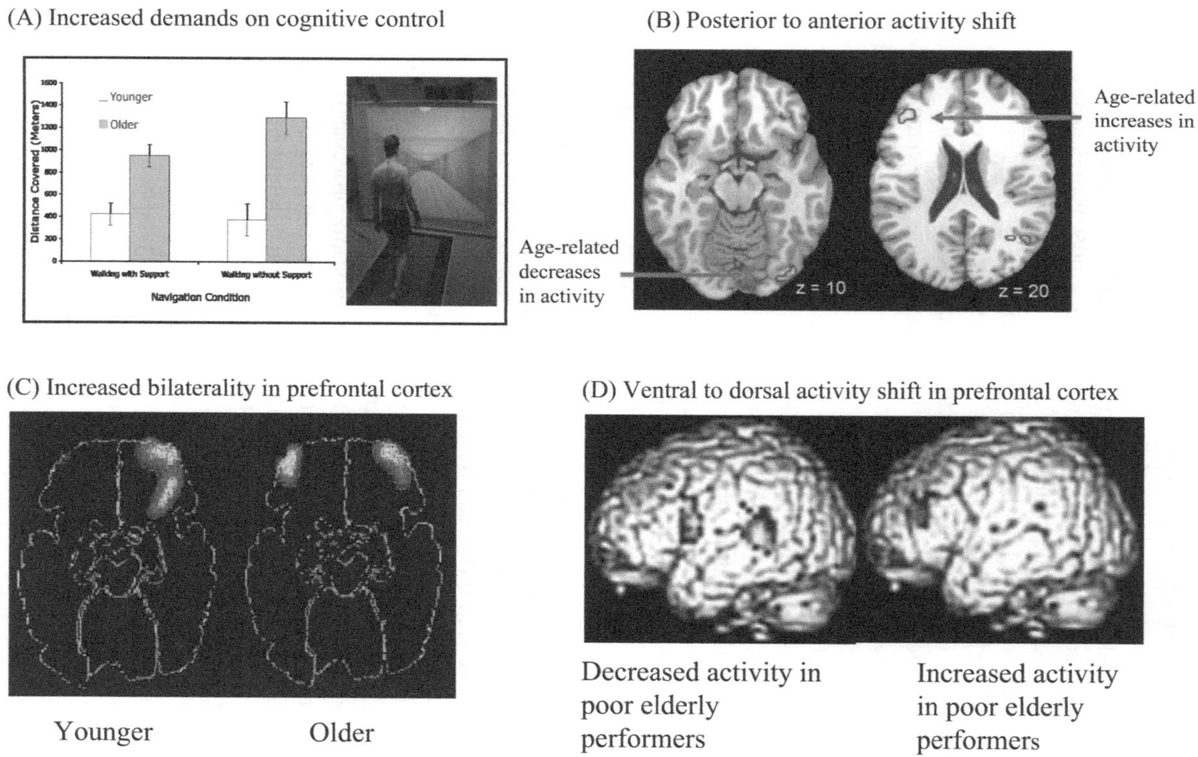

Figure 10.3 (A) Perception and action control is increasingly supported by cognitive control in old age. The figure presents findings from Lövdén et al. (2005b) showing that walking support (holding on to a handrail) significantly reduces age differences in navigation performance while walking in a virtual world. The finding suggests that action control (i.e., walking) in old age requires cognitive resources, which leave fewer resources for other domains of functioning (i.e., navigation). (B) Brain activity during particularly motor and perception tasks are redistributed from posterior areas to the dorsolateral prefrontal cortex. Results from Davis et al. (2008) indicate increased activity in dorsolateral prefrontal cortex and decreased activity in occipital cortex with aging during episodic retrieval and a perceptual task. (C) More bilateral activity appears in aging during episodic encoding and retrieval. Results show a pattern of more bilateral activity in old age during a word-stem cued-recall task. (Adapted with permission from Bäckman et al., 1997.) (D) Redistribution of activity in ventral-to-dorsal prefrontal cortex is common for episodic encoding and working memory tasks. Results show increased activity in dorsolateral prefrontal cortex but decreased activity in ventrolateral prefrontal cortex for healthy elderly poor performers during a comprehension/working memory task. (Adapted with permission from Grossman et al., 2002b.) (This figure is published in colour at http://www.cognitiveneurosciencearena.com/brain-scans/.)

cortices with advancing age may just be a necessary result of impairments in sensory and sensorimotor functions. In a related vein, increased bilaterality of activation patterns may be a direct effect of neurocognitive impairments such as reductions in neurotransmitter levels (S. C. Li, Lindenberger, & Sikström, 2001) and reduced white matter integrity (O'Sullivan et al., 2001). In the neuroimaging literature, this account of increased bilaterality is known as the dedifferentiation account (Cabeza, 2002; S. C. Li et al., 2001). Briefly, the notion is that negative changes with aging produce increases in neuronal noise and reductions in neuronal signalling fidelity. This in turn results in less distinct cortical representations and more diffused activation patterns (S. C. Li et al., 2001; Park et al., 2004).

To synthesize, the critical difference between the two chunks of interpretations can be framed in the core definition of the plasticity concept. Compensation, or decline-induced plastic changes, is a response of the neurocognitive system to a supply–demand mismatch, in this case produced by slowly unfolding sensory, motor, and cognitive impairments. In contrast, the interpretations that do not evoke plasticity as an explanatory concept argue that the patterns of findings reflect a primary change in the neurocognitive system (i.e., dedifferentiation) or are a direct and necessary consequence of such a primary change driven by the flexibility of the neurocognitive system, rather than by more permanent plastic reactions to this change. To exemplify, in the plasticity account, demands arising from the molar goal of comprehending speech in the face of reduced auditory acuity may drive a shift to the involvement of more controlled resources in speech comprehension (Grossman et al., 2002a; Wingfield & Grossman, 2006). The competing interpretations emphasize that the changes are solely produced by reductions on the supply side. For example, dedifferentiation in the auditory system may result in ambiguous auditory signals in the auditory cortex that directly call for the involvement of cognitive control and conflict resolution. Such reduction in auditory acuity are also a common experience for younger adults in situations of low-volume speech or speech embedded in noise, and any adaptive change in how the brain processes the incoming signal in these situations is not a reflection of plasticity – it is a reflection of neurocognitive flexibility. Older adults may simply find themselves more often in such situations of reduced auditory acuity, due to reductions in peripheral and central processing of sounds, and may therefore more often involve top-down processes to resolve ambiguous signals. I refer to these competing interpretations as the plasticity account and the direct account, respectively.

The theoretical differences between the two accounts generate at least two differential predictions. First, if it is possible to induce patterns of redistribution and reorganization in younger adults by simulating the assumed primary plasticity-inducing changes through experimental manipulations such as reducing quality of stimuli, distraction, dual-tasking, and general difficulty, then the notion that the observed changes just reflect the flexibility of the neurocognitive system, rather than a stable and relatively permanent change in the functioning of the system, cannot be excluded. Second, a positive correlation between the extent of the plastic change and performance on the ongoing task may support the plasticity account. Specifically, if a pattern of reorganization is best described by the direct account, then negative or no correlations, but not positive correlations, can be expected. That is, more reorganization can be associated with worse performance (i.e., a negative correlation) if the pattern of redistribution is a direct reflection of the negative changes (e.g., if decreases in neuromodulation cause more widespread brain activation) or if the neural system is not flexible enough to fully restore function in the face of, for example, reduced sensory quality. We may also expect no correlation if the neural system is fully flexible and can restore function in the face of some lower order negative change. However, it is very difficult to explain a positive correlation between the extent of any reorganization and performance on the ongoing task with the direct account: How can something that is a direct reflection, or that stands in direct proportion to something negative, produce better performance?

In contrast, if a pattern of reorganization reflects plasticity, then we cannot predict the correlation between the extent of this reorganization and performance on the ongoing task. That is, a positive correlation is also consistent with a plasticity account. Specifically, we may expect a positive correlation if the plastic response is adaptive and between-person differences in plasticity have a larger impact on performance than the extent of the plasticity-inducing primary change. Negative or no correlations do not, however, exclude a plasticity interpretation. For example, a larger compensatory response will be associated with worse performance (i.e., a negative correlation) if the plasticity-inducing negative change in functioning is larger for individuals that compensate more and if the reactions are not totally successful in compensating for this primary change. This interpretation is isomorphic with the plasticity interpretation of the negative reorganization–performance correlation that will appear, given that it exists, if the sample contains both older and younger adults. However, we may also expect no correlation between the extent of the plastic response and performance if, for example, the plastic reactions are totally balancing out the primary plasticity-inducing change. In sum, findings of a positive correlation between the extents of age-related redistribution support a plasticity account.

Below I review findings pertaining to the mentioned domains of (a) behavioural data on sensory functions and action control and (b) increased dorsal prefrontal activity. I particularly emphasize findings that may inform or have been advanced to enlighten the issue of whether these patterns of data are best described by the plasticity or the direct account, and I critically examine these findings in light of our review of the plasticity concept and the above predictions. More comprehensive overviews of these fields have been published elsewhere (for the sensory and sensorimotor domains, see K. Z. H. Li & Lindenberger, 2002; Schaefer et al., 2006; Schneider & Pichora-Fuller, 2000; Wingfield et al., 2005; Woollacott & Shumway-Cook, 2002; for the neuroimaging literature, see Cabeza, 2002; Davis et al., 2008; Greenwood, 2007; Persson & Nyberg, 2006; Rajah & D'Esposito, 2005).

Behavioural findings: Sensory functions and action control

Several studies indicate that perceptual processing involves a high degree of controlled cognitive processing in old age, in particular when data-driven sensory processing is adversely affected. For example, Gordon-Salant and Fitzgibbons (1997) examined speech understanding among groups of younger and older adults with and without hearing impairments. When final words of spoken sentences were masked with noise, hearing loss was associated with smaller effects on word recognition in highly predictable sentence contexts than in low predictable contexts. This effect was particularly pronounced for the elderly. Thus, in particular elderly listeners used knowledge of the language together with the maintenance of the context emanating from the preceding words to surmount the speech understanding difficulty imposed as a result of hearing loss and noise (see also Pichora-Fuller, Schneider, & Daneman, 1995). This study is important because it shows that the use of contextual support and top-down processes to aid perception may be a particularly common strategy in old age.

The age-related increases in involvement of controlled processes for perception may come at a cost of reducing processing resources otherwise available for other processing, such as encoding of content in memory (Rabbitt, 1968, 1991; Wingfield et al., 2005). This "effortful hypothesis" has been supported in several studies. For example, Rabbitt (1991) reported that older adults with mild hearing loss showed worse immediate recall than those with good hearing, despite perfect word identification accuracy in both groups. In the same vein, Murphy, Craik, Li, and Schneider (2000) tested short-term memory for five word-pairs as a function of serial position for younger and older adults. The words were presented in quiet or in noise. Results showed no significant age-differences on recall performance of the last two word-pairs, but substantial negative effects on recall from the first three positions. Moreover, noise reduced recall of the first three word-pairs for both groups and of the last two words for the group of older adults. These findings have an alternative explanation in that degraded stimuli may be more difficult to encode into long-term memory. However, convergent evidence from several other domains suggests that the effortfulness hypothesis is an explanation that is more generalizable. For example, a similar pattern of negative side effects of the shift to controlled processing is observable in the domain of action control. In a seminal paper in this domain, Lindenberger et al. (2000) trained groups of younger, middle-aged, and older adults in a mnemonic technique for the serial recall of word lists until criterion performance. Individuals were also asked to walk as quickly and accurately as possible on narrow tracks. After training of both tasks under single-task conditions, participants performed the memory task while walking. Age-based increments in dual-task costs (percentage decrease in the dual-task performance relative to single-task performance) were evident among middle-aged adults relative to younger adults, and further increased from middle-aged adults to older age, both with respect to walking and with respect to memory performance.

In sum, impairments in sensory processing and sensorimotor functions that come with aging are associated with increased reliance on the involvement of controlled processing in these domains, which take away resources from other tasks. In the sensory domain, decline in sensory functioning leads to impoverished and inaccurate representation of stimuli, which in turn necessitate top-down processes (e.g., interference resolution and use of context and linguistic knowledge) to recover information lost during sensory processing (Schneider & Pichora-Fuller, 2000). The increased cognitive processing of actions may refer to increased attentional focus, more pronounced processing of sensory information, and more emphasized intersensory integration (Heuninckx et al., 2005).

Several studies have indicated that experimental manipulation may induce similar reorganization in younger non-impaired adults. For example, Rabbitt (1968, Expt. 1) showed worse recall performance for noise-masked strings of spoken digits by normal-hearing younger-to-middle-aged subjects than for strings of digits presented without noise, although the masking still allowed for accurate identification of the digits. In the domain of vision, Dickinson and Rabbitt (1991) examined the effect of induced optical distortion on the ability of normally sighted younger individuals to read and remember text passages. Reading times and comprehension (free and cued recall) were measured. No reading errors were made. Free recall of text was impaired by optical distortion, and this effect increased with text difficulty, but cued recall was unaffected. Reading time was increased by distortion. The results of this study suggest that modest sensory impairment can have significant secondary effects on higher level processes such as memory, because it demands additional information processing capacity that becomes unavailable for inference, rehearsal, and association. Note, however, that the alternative explanation – that degraded stimuli may be more difficult to encode into long-term memory – is difficult to exclude based on these findings. The possibility that such effects of degrading sensory information are restricted to mnemonic processes is further supported by a study reported by Lindenberger, Scherer, and Baltes (2001). They administered cognitive tasks tapping working memory, perceptual speed, reasoning, fluency, and knowledge to middle-aged adults (30–50 years) while simulating old-age reductions in visual and auditory acuity. Visual acuity was manipulated through partial occlusion filters, and auditory acuity through noise protectors. Acuity manipulations reduced visual acuity and auditory acuity to values approximating old-age levels but, with the exception of a small effect of lowered auditory acuity on a working memory task, did not lower cognitive performance. Thus, this study supports the notion that increased reliance on involvement of controlled processing is a phenomenon that is specific for aging and sensory impairments, supporting a plasticity explanation of the shift from automatic to controlled processing of sensory and sensorimotor tasks. That is, the shift may require some time to develop because it is mostly evident in impairment and aging – a conclusion that does not support the interpretation that this shift reflects flexibility of the neurocognitive system.

The evidence from this domain of research suggests that compensatory changes are, at least in some situations, responsible for the shift from more automatic to more controlled processing in sensory and sensorimotor tasks. Notably, these findings are in line with investigations in other behavioural domains and in the expertise literature (Bäckman & Dixon, 1992; Baltes et al., 2006; Salthouse, 1984). The plasticity account is supported in particular by the absence of effects of manipulations of stimuli quality in young adulthood. That is, with the exception of situations when it is likely that degraded stimuli directly cause problems with processing, the effortfulness patterns appear difficult to induce in non-impaired younger adults. Thus, a plasticity account of the cognitive permeation of sensory and sensorimotor function with aging (Lindenberger et al., 2000) appears to be at least weakly supported by the behavioural literature.

Neuroimaging findings: Increased dorsal prefrontal activity

Across functional neuroimaging studies of aging, there is a relatively consistent finding of age-related increases in activity in anterior and dorsal brain regions, notably the dorsolateral prefrontal cortex. This increase in prefrontal activity is often accompanied by age-related reductions, or at least no age differences, in activity in more posterior and ventral regions, including the ventrolateral prefrontal cortex as well as occipital, temporal, and parietal regions (see also Davis et al., 2008; Dennis & Cabeza, 2008). The pattern of redistributed activity to prefrontal cortex is particularly clear for motor tasks (Heuninckx et al., 2005; Ward & Frackowiak, 2003) and visual perception (Grady et al., 1994) tasks. However, with some prominent exceptions (e.g., Madden et al., 2002), there have also been reports of similar redistribution for higher order cognitive tasks, including visuospatial processing (Meulenbroek, Petersson, Voermans, Weber, & Fernandez, 2004), working memory (Grossman et al., 2002a), attention (Cabeza et al., 2004), and episodic encoding (Grady et al., 2003b) and retrieval (Cabeza et al., 1997, 2004).

One form of age-related redistribution of activity has been observed primarily during episodic encoding in the form of age-related reductions or maintenance of activity in the medial temporal lobes and the ventrolateral prefrontal cortex, accompanied by increased activity in the dorsolateral prefrontal cortex (Persson & Nyberg, 2006; Rajah & D'Esposito, 2005). In this vein, Grady et al. (2003b) reported findings for activity during encoding of words and pictures of objects. In young adults, hippocampal activity was correlated with activity in ventral prefrontal and occipitotemporal regions, and increased activity in these regions was associated with better performance. For older adults, there were positive correlations between the dorsolateral prefrontal cortex, hippocampal activity, and performance. It is interesting to note that this ventral-to-dorsal redistribution of activity within the prefrontal cortex can also be observed with working memory tasks (Persson & Nyberg, 2006; Rajah & D'Esposito, 2005), which probably reflects the close overlap in working memory processes and successful episodic memory encoding. Thus, older adults may have shifted processing in these tasks from perceptual and rehearsal processes to using higher order executive processes such as organizational processes in conjunction with posterior regions such as the medial temporal lobe (Grady et al., 2003b).

In contrast to the ventral-to-dorsal shift primarily observed in higher order cognitive tasks, a posterior-to-anterior activity shift is apparent in lower order perceptual and motor tasks. In perhaps the first study of this sort, Grady et al. (1994) showed, with positron emission tomography (PET), that older adults displayed weaker activity in occipitotemporal regions than did younger adults, but more activity in prefrontal cortex when performing a visual perception task. Increased prefrontal activity is also common in motor tasks. For example, Heuninckx et al. (2005) used fMRI to investigate age-related differences in cyclical hand and foot movements as a function of task complexity. The typical motor network was activated in both age groups, but several additional brain areas were involved in the elderly. Specifically, elderly exhibited additional activation in areas involved in sensory processing and integration, such as contralateral anterior insula and secondary somatosensory area. With increasing complexity, age-related differences were additionally observed in areas often involved in cognitive monitoring of motor performance, such as the pre-supplementary motor area and prefrontal cortex. In the most complex movement task, elderly exhibited additional activation in anterior cingulate and dorsolateral prefrontal cortex – areas that are involved in inhibition and cognitive control.

In sum, neuroimaging of perceptual and motor tasks reveals a pattern of activity that is consistent with the interpretations of the behavioural data reviewed above – that is, in old age these tasks come with increased reliance on controlled processing that resides in the dorsolateral prefrontal cortex. The interpretation of increased prefrontal activity during higher order cognitive tasks is typically along similar lines: higher order top-down processes step in to aid impaired lower order, and often data-driven, processes.

To address the interpretation of this shift from posterior to anterior activity in aging, Davis et al. (2008) scanned 12 younger and 12 older adults during visual perception and episodic retrieval tasks. To approximate equal performance across groups, the individuals were matched on performance in the scanner, and the older adults received double the encoding time. Results showed age-related decreases in activity in the occipital, sensorimotor, and parahippocampal cortices and increases in the left dorsolateral prefrontal cortex across both tasks, as well as across subject-performed confidence levels (see Figure 10.3). These findings confirm the pattern of redistribution of activity to the dorsal prefrontal cortex and suggest that this pattern is not associated with task difficulty. Results also revealed a negative correlation between occipital and frontal activity among the old, such that older adults with less occipital activity showed more frontal activity. In addition, the group of older adults displayed a positive correlation between performance and frontal activity. Davis et al. argued that the correlational results indicate that compensatory prefrontal processes can come online in response to degraded functioning in occipital regions. Note that both the direct account and the plasticity account predict that the severity of what is conceived of as the primary change (here, reductions in occipital activity) is correlated with the magnitude of the response (the plasticity account) or with the secondary effect of the primary change (the direct account). For example, the direct account would suggest that diminished signal in the visual cortex would directly call for top-down cognitive control to amplify the signal at later processing stages. However, the positive correlation between activity in the prefrontal cortex and performance on the underlying task speaks against this interpretation. That is, it is difficult to argue that any positive activity-changes (here, in the prefrontal cortex) that stand in direct proportion to negative changes (here, in the occipitotemporal cortex) can produce better performance. In contrast, a positive correlation can be explaining by the plasticity account if the plastic response is adaptive and inter-individual differences in plasticity (i.e., prefrontal activity) have a larger impact on inter-individual differences in performance than the between-person differences in the extent of the plasticity-inducing primary change (i.e., the decrease in occipital activity). In sum, with respect to the anterior to posterior shift in aging, the plasticity account is supported.

Increased bilateral activity is most commonly observed in episodic encoding and retrieval tasks. Specifically, with regard to the prefrontal regions, older adults show less left-sided but more right-sided activation during encoding but more left-sided and less right-sided activation during retrieval (Cabeza, 2002; Persson & Nyberg, 2006; Rajah & D'Esposito, 2005). Several attempts to address the interpretation of this pattern have used the performance logic outlined above. For example, Cabeza, Anderson, Locantore, and McIntosh (2002; see also Rosen et al., 2002) used PET to examine prefrontal cortex activity during a source memory task versus an item memory task. Participants were 12 younger adults, 8 older low-performing adults, and 8 older high-performing adults. Results showed that low-performing older adults activated similar right prefrontal regions to those activated by younger adults, but that high-performing older adults additionally activated the left prefrontal cortex.

Several other papers have also addressed the increased bilateral activation in old age by working with variants of grouping based on performance. In a comprehensive paper, Persson et al. (2006) used longitudinal data to establish two groups of older adults that differed with regard to whether their episodic memory performance remained stable or declined over a decade. Functional

MRI of these participants during semantic categorization revealed left prefrontal cortex activation for both groups and additional activation in the right prefrontal cortex for elderly decliners. In addition, the older group that evinced declining performance also had reduced hippocampal volume and lower fractional anisotropy (a diffusion tensor imaging measure of white matter integrity) in the anterior corpus callosum as compared with the stable performers.

In the same vein, Grady et al. (2003a) reported that individuals in early stages of Alzheimer's disease evinced a more pronounced correlated bilateral network of prefrontal and parietal activations than did controls that displayed a left-sided pattern of activation, during both a semantic memory task and an episodic recognition task. Within the group of demented individuals, performance correlated positively with the level of activation in the bilateral prefrontal–parietal network.

Finally, taking the performance-logic yet another step, Rossi et al. (2004) used repetitive transcranial magnetic stimulation (rTMS) to transiently interfere with processing in the left or right dorsolateral prefrontal cortex during visuospatial recognition memory in 37 younger and 29 older participants. Results showed that rTMS of the right dorsolateral prefrontal cortex interfered with retrieval more than left-sided rTMS in the young. In the older adults, left and right rTMS had similar effects on performance. Results thus suggest that the additional left-sided activation in older adults during retrieval is beneficial for performance.

To sum up, both negative and positive correlations between the extent of bilateral activity in the prefrontal cortex during episodic memory tasks and performance have been reported. Negative correlations have been reported by Persson et al. (2006) and Grady et al. (2003a). Positive correlations have been reported by Rossi et al. (2004), Cabeza et al. (2002), Rosen et al. (2002), and Grady et al. (2003a). The reports of the positive correlations support a plasticity account because we can rule out a direct account based on the unlikelihood that something that is a direct reflection or stands in direct proportion to something negative produces better performance. In contrast, the plasticity account can explain a positive correlation assuming that the plastic response is adaptive and that between-person differences in plasticity have larger impact on performance than do the extent of the plasticity-inducing primary change. Notable, such a pattern of findings is always found in the reviewed studies when the sample can be assumed to be relatively homogenous in terms of the extent of primary change. For example, in the study by Grady et al. (2003a) such a positive correlation is observed within the group of demented individuals, and in Cabeza et al. (2002) such a correlation is observed within a group of healthy elderly. In contrast, negative correlations have been reported when the samples can be assumed heterogeneous in terms of the underlying plasticity-inducing pathology (see also Persson & Nyberg, 2006). For example, Grady et al. (2003a) reported that the group of demented individuals reported by Grady et al. (2003a) and the individuals evincing 10-year decline in performance reported by Persson et al. (2006) displayed more bilateral activation patterns than did healthy controls/non-decliners. These negative correlations can be accounted for by assuming that the plastic reactions are not totally successful in compensating for primary plasticity-inducing changes, which have not taken place at all or to only a small extent in the healthy controls. This interpretation is isomorphic with the plasticity interpretation of the negative redistribution-performance correlation that will appear if the sample contains both older and younger adults. That is, the group differences in the negative changes that come with aging, or some other pathology, overshadows inter-individual differences in the effects of the plastic response on performance.

Concluding remarks

In aging, sensory functioning and action control to a greater extent involve higher order and controlled cognitive processing, and brain activity is redistributed from posterior to anterior brain regions during perceptual and motor tasks, from ventral to dorsal prefrontal cortex during episodic encoding and working memory, and from lateral to contralateral prefrontal cortex during episodic encoding and retrieval. The findings are currently supporting a plasticity account of these changes. In other words, cognitive control functions in the dorsolateral prefrontal cortices may be recruited to compensate for reduction in lower order data-driven processes by finding other ways to achieve acceptable behavioural outcomes. Note that this conclusion and the empirical literature by no means exclude the possibility that some, or even most, phenomena of functional redistribution or reorganization with aging are direct results of pathology. For example, less differentiated activity within the sensory neural systems is more easily explained by the direct account (Park et al., 2004). Several negative changes that come with aging, such as reductions in neuromodulation (S. C. Li, Brehmer, Shing, Werkle-Bergner, & Lindenberger, 2006; S. C. Li et al., 2001) and anterior white matter integrity (O'Sullivan et al., 2001), are likely to produce more distributed activity by themselves. Dedifferentiation, other negative changes, and compensation might also go on at the same time in the same brain region (e.g., prefrontal cortex) or at the same time but in a different brain region (e.g., compensation in prefrontal cortex and dedifferentiation in sensory cortices). In addition, as a negative change for function, dedifferentiation may induce compensation. Thus, and very importantly, the take-home message of this review is only that the current evidence indicates that processes of decline-induced plastic reorganization are operating during aging.

Further teasing apart negative changes that unfold in aging and adaptive reactive changes is a major task for future research. For example, it is not unreasonable to predict decline-induced macro-scale structural plastic changes, in addition to and possibly as a consequence of the reviewed functional changes. In other words, what researchers in many domains of inquiry describe as the aging process may be a result of decline, growth (Baltes et al., 2006), and decline-induced growth. In addition, the concept of maladaptive plasticity (e.g., Pascual-Leone et al., 2005) in aging needs to be considered: Are we witnessing decline-induced decline in aging? Uncovering the mechanisms behind decline-induced plasticity will enlighten the quest for ameliorating and postponing cognitive aging by pinning down factors that not only protect or promote cognitive functions in aging, but also promote adaptive plastic responses in the aging brain. Accepting that behavioural and brain aging come with plastic changes will open up new fields to the study of brain and behaviour in aging individuals.

Acknowledgements

The work on this chapter was supported by the Sofja Kovalevskaja Award, administered by the Alexander von Humboldt foundation and donated by the German Federal Ministry for Education and Research, and by a grant from the Swedish Research Council. Thanks go to Lars Bäckman, Christian Chicherio, Ulman Lindenberger, Lars Nyberg, Sabine Schäfer, Michael Schellenbach, Florian Schmiedek, and Julius Verrel for productive discussions on this topic.

References

Alain, C., McDonald, K. L., Ostroff, J. M., & Schneider, B. (2004). Aging: A switch from automatic to controlled processing of sounds? *Psychology and Aging, 19*, 125–133.

Allaire, J. C., & Marsiske, M. (2005). Intraindividual variability may not always indicate vulnerability in elders' cognitive performance. *Psychology and Aging, 20*, 390–401.

Bäckman, L., Almkvist, O., Anderson, J. R., Nordberg, A., Winblad, B., Rineck, R., et al. (1997). Brain activation in young and old adults during implicit and explicit retrieval. *Journal of Cognitive Neuroscience, 9*, 378–391.

Bäckman, L., Andersson, J. L. R., Nyberg, L., Winblad, B., Nordberg, A., & Almkvist, O. (1999a). Brain regions associated with episodic retrieval in normal aging and Alzheimer's disease. *Neurology, 52*, 1861–1870.

Bäckman, L., & Dixon, R. A. (1992). Psychological compensation: A theoretical framework. *Psychological Bulletin, 112*, 259–283.

Bäckman, L., Nyberg, L., Lindenberger, U., Li, S. C., & Farde, L. (2006). The correlative triad among aging, dopamine, and cognition: Current status and future prospects. *Neuroscience and Biobehavioral Reviews, 30*, 791–807.

Bäckman, L., Small, B. J., Wahlin, Å., & Larsson, M. (1999b). Cognitive functioning in very old age. In F. I. M. Craik & T. A. Salthouse (Eds.), *Handbook of cognitive aging* (Vol. 2, pp. 499–558). Mahwah, NJ: Lawrence Erlbaum Associates, Inc.

Baltes, P. B., Lindenberger, U., & Staudinger, U. (2006). Lifespan theory in developmental psychology. In W. Damon & R. M. Lerner (Eds.), *Handbook of child psychology: Vol. 1. Theoretical models of human development* (6th ed., pp. 569–664). New York: Wiley.

Baltes, P. B., & Singer, T. (2001). Plasticity and the ageing mind: An exemplar of the bio-cultural orchestration of brain and behaviour. *European Review*, *9*, 59–76.

Brion, J.-P., Demeurisse, G., & Capon, A. (1989). Evidence of cortical reorganization in hemiparetic patients. *Stroke*, *20*, 1079–1084.

Buckner, R. L., Corbetta, M., Schatz, J., Raichle, M. E., & Petersen, S. E. (1996). Preserved speech abilities and compensation following prefrontal damage. *Proceedings of the National Academy of Sciences USA*, *93*, 1249–1253.

Cabeza, R. (2002). Hemispheric asymmetry reduction in older adults: The HAROLD model. *Psychology and Aging*, *17*, 85–100.

Cabeza, R., Anderson, N. D., Locantore, J. K., & McIntosh, A. R. (2002). Aging gracefully: Compensatory brain activity in high-performing older adults. *NeuroImage*, *17*, 1394–1402.

Cabeza, R., Daselaar, S. M., Dolcos, F., Prince, S. E., Budde, M., & Nyberg, L. (2004). Task-independent and task-specific age effects on brain activity during working memory, visual attention and episodic retrieval. *Cerebral Cortex*, *14*, 364–375.

Cabeza, R., Grady, C. L., Nyberg, L., McIntosh, A. R., Tulving, E., Kapur, S., et al. (1997). Age-related differences in neural activity during memory encoding and retrieval: A positron emission tomography study. *Journal of Neuroscience*, *17*, 391–400.

Davis, S. W., Dennis, N. A., Daselaar, S. M., Fleck, M. S., & Cabeza, R. (2008). Que pasa? The posterior-anterior shift in aging. *Cerebral Cortex*, *18*(5), 1201–1209.

DeFrias, C. M., Lövdén, M., Lindenberger, U., & Nilsson, L.-G. (2007). Revisiting the dedifferentiation hypothesis with longitudinal multi-cohort data. *Intelligence*, *35*, 381–392.

Dennis, N. A., & Cabeza, R. (2008). Neuroimaging of healthy cognitive aging. In F. I. M. Craik & T. A. Salthouse (Eds.), *The handbook of aging and cognition* (3rd ed., pp. 1–54). Mahwah, NJ: Lawrence Erlbaum Associates, Inc.

Dickinson, C. M., & Rabbitt, P. M. A. (1991). Simulated visual impairment: Effects on text comprehension and reading speed. *Clinical Vision Sciences*, *6*, 301–308.

Farkas, E., & Luiten, P. G. M. (2001). Cerebral microvascular pathology in aging and Alzheimer's disease. *Progress in Neurobiology*, *64*, 575–611.

Ford, D. H. (1987). *Humans as self-constructing living systems: A developmental perspective on behavior and personality*. Hillsdale, NJ: Lawrence Erlbaum Associates.

Fratiglioni, L., Paillard-Borg, S., & Winblad, B. (2004). An active and socially integrated lifestyle in late life might protect against dementia. *Lancet Neurology*, *3*, 343–353.

Gerstorf, D., Lövdén, M., Röcke, C., Smith, J., & Lindenberger, U. (2007). Well-being affects changes in perceptual speed in advanced old age: Longitudinal evidence for a dynamic link. *Developmental Psychology*, *43*, 705–718.

Ghisletta, P., Bickel, J.-F., & Lövdén, M. (2006). Does activity engagement protect against cognitive decline in old age? Methodological and analytical considerations. *Journal of Gerontology: Psychological Sciences*, *61*, 253–261.

Gordon-Salant, S., & Fitzgibbons, P. J. (1997). Selected cognitive factors and speech recognition performance among young and elderly listeners. *Journal of Speech, Language, and Hearing Research*, *40*, 423–431.

Grady, C. L., Maisog, J. M., Horwitz, B., Ungerleider, L. G., Mentis, M. J., Salerno, J. A., et al. (1994). Age-related changes in cortical blood flow activation during visual processing of faces and location. *Journal of Neuroscience*, *14*, 1450–1462.

Grady, C. L., McIntosh, A. R., Beig, S., Keightley, M. L., Burian, H., & Black, S. E.

(2003a). Evidence from functional neuroimaging of a compensatory prefrontal network in Alzheimer's disease. *Journal of Neuroscience, 23*, 986–993.

Grady, C. L., McIntosh, A. R., & Craik, F. I. M. (2003b). Age-related differences in the functional connectivity of the hippocampus during memory encoding. *Hippocampus, 13*, 572–586.

Greenwood, P. M. (2007). Functional plasticity in cognitive aging: Review and hypothesis. *Neuropsychology, 21*, 657–673.

Grossman, M., Cooke, A., DeVita, C., Alsop, D., Detre, J., Chen, W., et al. (2002a). Age-related changes in working memory during sentence comprehension: An fMRI study. *NeuroImage, 15*, 302–317.

Grossman, M., Cooke, A., DeVita, C., Chen, W., Moore, P., Detre, J., et al. (2002b). Sentence processing strategies in healthy seniors with poor comprehension: An fMRI study. *Brain and Language, 80*, 296–313.

Heuninckx, S., Wenderoth, N., Debaere, F., Peeters, R., & Swinnen, S. P. (2005). Neural basis of aging: The penetration of cognition into action control. *Journal of Neuroscience, 25*, 6787–6796.

Hihara, S., Notoya, T., Tanaka, M., Ichinose, S., Ojima, H., Obayashi, S., et al. (2006). Extension of corticocortical afferents into the anterior bank of the intraparietal sulcus by tool-use training in adult monkeys. *Neuropsychologia, 44*, 2636–2646.

Huxhold, O., Li, S.-C., Schmiedek, F., & Lindenberger, U. (2006). Dual-tasking postural control: Aging and the effects of cognitive demand in conjunction with focus of attention. *Brain Research Bulletin, 69*, 294–305.

Kelly, A. M. C., & Garavan, H. (2005). Human functional neuroimaging of brain changes associated with practice. *Cerebral Cortex, 15*, 1089–1102.

Kempermann, G. (2006). *Adult neurogenesis: Stem cells and neuronal development in the adult brain*. Oxford, UK: Oxford University Press.

Kliegl, R., Smith, J., & Baltes, P. B. (1989). Testing-the-limits and the study of adult age differences in cognitive plasticity of a mnemonic skill. *Developmental Psychology, 25*, 247–256.

Kolb, B. (1995). *Brain plasticity and behavior*. Mahwah, NJ: Lawrence Erlbaum Associates, Inc.

Kramer, A. F., Bherer, L., Colcombe, S. J., Dong, W., & Greenough, W. T. (2004). Environmental influences on cognitive and brain plasticity during aging. *Journals of Gerontology. Series A: Biological Sciences and Medical Sciences, 59*, 940–957.

Li, K. Z. H., & Lindenberger, U. (2002). Relations between aging sensory/sensorimotor and cognitive functions. *Neuroscience and Biobehavioral Reviews, 26*, 777–783.

Li, S. C. (2003). Biocultural orchestration of developmental plasticity across levels: The interplay of biology and culture in shaping the mind and behavior across the life span. *Psychological Bulletin, 129*, 171–194.

Li, S. C., Brehmer, Y., Shing, Y. L., Werkle-Bergner, M., & Lindenberger, U. (2006). Neuromodulation of associative and organizational plasticity across the life span: Empirical evidence and neurocomputational modeling. *Neuroscience and Biobehavioral Reviews, 30*, 775–790.

Li, S. C., Huxhold, O., & Schmiedek, F. (2004). Aging and attenuated processing robustness: Evidence from cognitive and sensorimotor functioning. *Gerontology, 50*, 28–34.

Li, S. C., Lindenberger, U., & Sikström, S. (2001). Aging cognition: From neuromodulation to representation. *Trends in Cognitive Sciences, 5*, 479–486.

Lindenberger, U., Li, S.-C., & Bäckman, L. (2006). Delineating brain–behavior mappings across the lifespan: Substantive and methodological advances in developmental neuroscience [Editorial]. *Neuroscience & Biobehavioral Reviews*, *30*, 713–717.

Lindenberger, U., Marsiske, M., & Baltes, P. B. (2000). Memorizing while walking: Increase in dual-task costs from young adulthood to old age. *Psychology and Aging*, *15*, 417–436.

Lindenberger, U., Scherer, H., & Baltes, P. B. (2001). The strong connection between sensory and cognitive performance in old age: Not due to sensory acuity reductions operating during cognitive assessment. *Psychology and Aging*, *16*, 196–205.

Lövdén, M., Ghisletta, P., & Lindenberger, U. (2005a). Social participation attenuates decline in perceptual speed in old and very old age. *Psychology and Aging*, *20*, 423–434.

Lövdén, M., Schaefer, S., Pohlmayer, A., & Lindenberger, U. (2008). Walking variability and working memory load in aging: A dual-process account relating cognitive control to motor control performance. *Journal of Gerontology: Psychological Sciences*, *63*, 121–128.

Lövdén, M., Schellenbach, M., Grossman-Hutter, B., Krüger, A., & Lindenberger, U. (2005b). Environmental topography and postural control demands shape aging-associated decrements in spatial navigation performance. *Psychology and Aging*, *20*, 683–694.

Madden, D. J., Turkington, T. G., Provenzale, J. M., Denny, L. L., Langley, L. K., Hawk, T. C., et al. (2002). Aging and attentional guidance during visual search: Functional neuroanatomy by positron emission tomography. *Psychology and Aging*, *17*, 24–43.

Meulenbroek, O., Petersson, K. M., Voermans, N., Weber, B., & Fernandez, G. (2004). Age differences in neural correlates of route encoding and route recognition. *NeuroImage*, *22*, 1503–1514.

Murphy, D. R., Craik, F. I. M., Li, K. Z. H., & Schneider, B. A. (2000). Comparing the effects of aging and background noise on short-term memory performance. *Psychology and Aging*, *15*, 323–334.

Nesselroade, J. R. (1991). The warp and the woof of the developmental fabric. In R. M. Downs, L. S. Liben, & D. S. Palermo (Eds.), *Vision of aesthetics, the environment and development: The legacy of Joachim F. Wohlwill* (pp. 213–240). Hillsdale, NJ: Lawrence Erlbaum Associates, Inc.

Nilsson, L.-G., Bäckman, L., Erngrund, K., Nyberg, L., Adolfsson, R., Bucht, G., et al. (1997). The Betula prospective cohort study: Memory, health and aging. *Aging, Neuropsychology, and Cognition*, *4*, 1–32.

O'Sullivan, M., Jones, D. K., Summers, P. E., Morris, R. G., Williams, S. C. R., & Markus, H. S. (2001). Evidence of cortical "disconnection" as a mechanism of age-related cognitive decline. *Neurology*, *57*, 632–638.

Park, D. C., Polk, T. A., Park, R., Minear, M., Savage, A., & Smith, M. R. (2004). Aging reduces neural specialization in ventral visual cortex. *Proceedings of the National Academy of Sciences USA*, *101*, 13091–13095.

Pascual-Leone, A., Amedi, A., Fregni, F., & Merabet, L. B. (2005). The plastic human brain cortex. *Annual Review of Neuroscience*, *28*, 377–401.

Persson, J., & Nyberg, L. (2006). Altered brain activity in healthy seniors: What does it mean? *Progress in Brain Research*, *157*, 45–56.

Persson, J., Nyberg, L., Lind, J., Larsson, A., Nilsson, L.-G., Ingvar, M., et al. (2006).

Structure-function correlates of cognitive decline in aging. *Cerebral Cortex*, *16*, 907–915.

Pichora-Fuller, M. K., Schneider, B., & Daneman, M. (1995). How young and old adults listen to and remember speech in noise. *Journal of the Acoustical Society of America*, *97*, 593–607.

Rabbitt, P. M. A. (1968). Channel-capacity intelligibility and immediate memory. *Quarterly Journal of Experimental Psychology*, *20*, 241.

Rabbitt, P. M. A. (1991). Mild hearing-loss can cause apparent memory failures which increase with age and reduce with IQ. *Acta Oto-Laryngologica*, *111*(6), 167–176.

Rajah, M. N., & D'Esposito, M. (2005). Region-specific changes in prefrontal function with age: A review of pet and fMRI studies on working and episodic memory. *Brain*, *128*, 1964–1983.

Raz, N., Lindenberger, U., Rodrigue, K. M., Kennedy, K. M., Head, D., Williamson, A., et al. (2005). Regional brain changes in aging healthy adults: General trends, individual differences and modifiers. *Cerebral Cortex*, *15*, 1679–1689.

Reuter-Lorenz, P. A., Jonides, J., Smith, E. E., Hartley, A., Miller, A., Marshuetz, C., et al. (2000). Age differences in the frontal lateralization of verbal and spatial working memory revealed by pet. *Journal of Cognitive Neuroscience*, *12*, 174–187.

Rönnlund, M., & Nilsson, L.-G. (2006). Adult life-span patterns in WAIS-R block design performance: Cross-sectional versus longitudinal age gradients and relations to demographic factors. *Intelligence*, *34*, 63–78.

Rönnlund, M., Nyberg, L., Bäckman, L., & Nilsson, L.-G. (2005). Stability, growth, and decline in adult life span development of declarative memory: Cross-sectional and longitudinal data from a population-based study. *Psychology and Aging*, *20*, 3–18.

Rosen, A. C., Prull, M. W., O'Hara, R., Race, E. A., Desmond, J. E., Glover, G. H., et al. (2002). Variable effects of aging on frontal lobe contributions to memory. *NeuroReport*, *13*, 2425–2428.

Rossi, S., Miniussi, C., Pasqualetti, P., Babiloni, C., Rossini, P. M., & Cappa, S. F. (2004). Age-related functional changes of prefrontal cortex in long-term memory: A repetitive transcranial magnetic stimulation study. *Journal of Neuroscience*, *24*, 7939–7944.

Salthouse, T. A. (1984). Effects of age and skill in typing. *Journal of Experimental Psychology: General*, *113*, 345–371.

Satz, P. (1993). Brain reserve capacity on symptom onset after brain injury: A formulation and review of evidence for threshold theory. *Neuropsychology*, *7*, 273–295.

Schaefer, S., Huxhold, O., & Lindenberger, U. (2006). Healthy mind in healthy body? A review of sensorimotor-cognitive interdependencies in old age. *European Review of Aging and Physical Activity*, *3*, 45–54.

Schaie, K. W. (1996). *Intellectual development in adulthood: The Seattle longitudinal study*. New York: Cambridge University Press.

Schneider, B. A., & Pichora-Fuller, M. K. (2000). Implications of perceptual deterioration for cognitive aging research. In F. I. M. Craik & T. A. Salthouse (Eds.), *Handbook of aging and cognition* (2nd ed., pp. 155–220). Mahwah, NJ: Lawrence Erlbaum Associates, Inc.

Siegler, R. S. (1994). Cognitive variability: A key to understanding cognitive development. *Current Directions in Psychological Science*, *3*, 1–5.

Stern, Y. (2002). What is cognitive reserve? Theory and research application of the reserve concept. *Journal of the International Neuropsychological Society*, *8*, 448–460.

Sullivan, E. V., & Pfefferbaum, A. (2006). Diffusion tensor imaging and aging. *Neuroscience and Biobehavioral Reviews*, *30*, 749–761.

Ward, N. S., & Frackowiak, R. S. (2003). Age-related changes in the neural correlates of motor performance. *Brain*, *126*, 873–888.

Wingfield, A., & Grossman, M. (2006). Language and the aging brain: Patterns of neural compensation revealed by functional brain imaging. *Journal of Neurophysiology*, *96*, 2830–2839.

Wingfield, A., Tun, P. A., & McCoy, S. L. (2005). Hearing loss in older adulthood: What it is and how it interacts with cognitive performance. *Current Directions in Psychological Science*, *14*, 144–148.

Woollacott, M., & Shumway-Cook, A. (2002). Attention and the control of posture and gait: A review of an emerging area of research. *Gait & Posture*, *16*, 1–14.

11 Dopamine, cognition, and human aging

New evidence and ideas

Lars Bäckman and Lars Nyberg

In this chapter, we discuss research that reveals that the dopamine (DA) system is implicated in cognitive functioning in general (e.g., speed, executive functions, episodic memory) as well as in age-related cognitive deficits. The discussion of DA markers is confined to molecular imaging studies – that is, positron emission tomography (PET) and single positron emission computerized tomography (SPECT). Comparatively large space is devoted to recent studies on DA, cognition, and aging, as well as to prospects for future research.

Aging and dopamine

Much of the work on the relationship between aging and DA neurotransmission has focused on the caudate and the putamen, two major nuclei in the striatal complex with dense dopaminergic innervation from the substantia nigra. Thus, the conditions for reliable analyses of DA biomarkers are particularly favourable in the striatum. There is strong evidence for age-related losses of pre- and postsynaptic biochemical markers of the nigrostriatal DA system. The DA transporter (DAT) is located at nerve terminals and is a commonly used marker for the pre-synaptic neuron. Both PET and SPECT studies (e.g., Erixon-Lindroth et al., 2005; Mozley, Gur, Mozley, & Gur, 2001) indicate marked age-related losses of the DAT in striatum, with the average decline estimated, in cross-sectional studies, to be 5–10% per decade from early to late adulthood.

Several DA receptors have been identified, the most common of which are the D_1 and D_2 receptor subtypes. The D_1 receptor is only expressed in the postsynaptic neuron, whereas the D_2 receptor is to a minor extent also expressed in the presynaptic neuron where it serves as an autoreceptor. Molecular imaging work reveals age-related losses of both striatal D_1 (Suhara et al., 1991; Wang et al., 1998) and D_2 (Antonini et al., 1993; Nordström, Farde, Pauli, Litton, & Halldin, 1992) receptor densities of comparable magnitude as found for the DAT.

A similar downward age trajectory is seen for the mesocortical and mesolimbic dopaminergic pathways. These pathways originate from the ventral tegmentum and project to the limbic system and neocortex, respectively. Thus, marked age-related losses in D_2 receptor binding have been observed throughout the neocortex as well as in hippocampus, amygdala, and thalamus (Inoue et al., 2001; Kaasinen et al., 2000), and there are similar losses for D_1 receptors in frontal cortex (Suhara et al., 1991; Wang et al., 1998).

The general age-related decline of DA systems may have multiple sources, including neuronal loss in substantia nigra, loss of synapses, as well as a decrease of biomarker proteins per neuron with advancing age (for a review, see Bäckman, Nyberg, Lindenberger, Li, & Farde, 2006). The fact that similar age patterns are seen for the DAT and postsynaptic markers suggests that the expression of transporters and receptors may reflect adaptation of major components of the dopaminergic pathways. One possibility is that loss of the DAT initially results in increased DA concentrations; increased DA levels may subsequently lead to down regulation of neurotransmission in postsynaptic neurons (Shinkai, Zhang, Mathias, & Roth, 1997; Zhang, Ravipati, Joseph, & Roth, 1995).

Dopamine and cognition

Data from multiple sources converge in demonstrating a key role of DA in cognitive functioning. First, there is abundant evidence from experimental studies with animals that lesions to the DA system at multiple sites (e.g., prefrontal cortex, nucleus accumbens, subthalamic nucleus) cause impairment in higher order cognitive functions (e.g., attention, memory, inhibition; for a review, see Bäckman & Farde, 2005). Second, studies on patient groups with severe DA alterations – for example, Parkinson's disease (PD) and Huntington's disease (HD) – reveal deficits in several cognitive domains such as executive functioning, episodic memory, and speed (Brandt & Butters, 1986; Brown & Marsden, 1990), and PET studies show strong relations between DA biomarkers and cognitive performance in both PD (Bruck, Aalto, Nurmi, Bergman, & Rinne, 2005) and HD (Bäckman, Robins Wahlin, Lundin, Ginovart, & Farde, 1997).

Third, association studies with genes implicated in dopaminergic neurotransmission provide further support for the DA–cognition link. For example, the catechol-O-methyltransferase (COMT) enzyme degrades DA in prefrontal cortex (Weinshilboum, Otterness, & Szumlanski, 1999). A common valine to methydine (val/met) polymorphism accounts for much of the enzymatic activity (val > met), resulting in less DA availability in D_1 receptors among val carriers (Egan et al., 2001). Consistent with these facts, in executively demanding tasks (e.g., working memory, Wisconsin Card Sorting) a performance advantage of met carriers has been found (for a review, see Goldberg & Weinberger, 2004). Relatedly, variations in the DAT gene (i.e., number of tandem repeats) are associated with DAT availability in the striatum (more repeats > fewer repeats), translating into less synaptic DA for persons with more repeats (Maher, Marazita, Ferrell, & Vanyukov, 2002).

Alleles with 9 or 10 repeats are most common (Mitchell et al., 2000). Behavioural evidence shows lower performance among 10-repeat carriers in tasks assessing speed and attention (Loo et al., 2003) as well as response inhibition (Cornish et al., 2005).

Fourth, pharmacological manipulations of the DA system (i.e., increased activity through agonists or decreased activity through antagonists) have been shown to affect cognition in humans and animals alike. Although the data pattern is somewhat mixed, agonist studies generally indicate performance benefits in cognitive tasks (e.g., working memory, speed, attention), whereas antagonist studies show decrements in the same task domains (e.g., Halliday et al., 1994; Luciana & Collins, 1997; Ramaekers et al., 1999; Sawaguchi & Goldman-Rakic, 1991). However, the effects of these compounds tend to vary with dosage and baseline cognitive capacity (e.g., Kimberg & D'Esposito, 2003; Kimberg, D'Esposito, & Farah, 1997). These findings have been interpreted in terms of an inverted U-shaped function relating DA levels to cognitive performance (Cai & Arnsten, 1997; Knutson & Gibbs, 2007; Li, Lindenberger, & Sikström, 2001; Li & Sikström, 2002).

Evidence in favour of this account was obtained in a study that combined molecular genetics with pharmacology and brain imaging (Mattay et al., 2003). In this study, val carriers of the COMT gene (less frontal DA signalling) had to recruit more frontal tissue than met carriers to achieve the same performance level in a working memory task, a pattern suggesting lower neural efficiency among val carriers. However, under the influence of a DA agonist, the pattern was reversed, with the val carriers showing a more efficient frontal response and the met carriers a less efficient response. This pattern of results provides direct support for the viability of the inverted U-shape account of DA and cognition.

Until recently, in molecular imaging studies, linking DA functions to cognitive performance was assessed outside the scanner, and the biomarker (e.g., DAT binding, receptor densities) was related to the off-line cognitive tasks (for a review, see Cropley, Fujita, Innis, & Nathan, 2006). However, there is emerging evidence for actual release of DA during cognitive activity. A paradigm used to address this issue involves contrasting DA binding under two conditions varying in cognitive load. DA release is inferred if the binding potential is lower under the high-load condition compared with the low-load condition. This is so because binding of the radioligand to the receptor is supposed to compete more fiercely with endogenous DA when conditions are more cognitively challenging. Using this paradigm, Aalto, Brück, Laine, Någren, and Rinne (2005) found evidence for DA release in frontal cortex and hippocampus during working memory performance, whereas Monchi, Ko, and Strafella (2006) reported similar data for striatal DA during a card sorting task.

The correlative triad

We have reviewed evidence indicating that there is a marked negative correlation between adult age and DA functions and that DA is implicated in numerous cognitive domains. With regard to the missing pair in this set of variables, there is strong evidence of a negative relationship between adult age and performance in tasks assessing executive functioning, episodic memory, and speed (for reviews, see Craik & Salthouse, 1999, 2007). The fact that performance in the very same task domains seems to be influenced by DA functions suggests that there might be a correlative triad among age, DA, and cognition. In examining this triad, the key issue is whether alterations in dopaminergic neuromodulation over the life cycle can be empirically linked to age-related cognitive changes. Although relatively few studies have addressed this issue, the data pattern is strikingly consistent.

Wang et al. (1998) reported strong relationships among age, striatal D_1 receptor binding, and performance in a psychomotor test. Similar results were obtained in a study examining the association among age, striatal D_2 receptor binding, and finger-tapping performance (Yang et al., 2003). Although these studies reported bivariate correlations only, the results are important in that they document the correlative triad within the same groups of participants.

In a seminal study, Volkow et al. (1998) assessed striatal D_2 binding in conjunction with testing of executive and motor functioning as well as perceptual speed across the adult life span. In line with earlier studies (e.g., Antonini et al., 1993; Nordström et al., 1992), D_2 receptor binding decreased with advancing age, and there were negative relationships between age and performance in the cognitive tests. Of critical importance, partial correlations revealed moderate-to-strong relationships of D_2 binding to cognitive and motor performance also after controlling for chronological age. These results indicate that age-related decreases in DA function are related to deficits in both cognitive and motor functioning and suggest that DA activity may influence performance, irrespective of age.

These findings were corroborated in a related study (Bäckman et al., 2000), in which we examined striatal D_2 binding and cognitive performance (episodic memory and perceptual speed) in an adult life-span sample. The key finding was that statistical control of D_2 binding effectively eliminated the influence of age on cognitive performance, whereas D_2 binding contributed to performance over and above age (see Table 11.1). These results provide further evidence for the view that DA is implicated in age-related cognitive deficits as well as in cognitive functioning in general.

Other research has extended these findings to presynaptic DA markers such as the DA transporter. Mozley et al. (2001) reported age-related reductions of the DAT in the striatum along with age-related deficits in verbal episodic memory. Importantly, striatal DAT binding was strongly associated with memory performance in both younger and older adults. An age-related

Table 11.1 Amount of variance (R^2) in cognitive performance accounted for by age and dopamine D_2 receptor binding as a function of order of entry

	Perceptual speed		*Episodic memory*	
	Dots	*Trail making*	*Word recognition*	*Face recognition*
Age	.52	.34	.13	.27
D_2	.11	.22	.27	.24
Total	.63	.56	.40	.51
D_2	.61	.55	.38	.48
Age	.02	.01	.02	.03
Total	.63	.56	.40	.51

Adapted from Bäckman et al. (2000).

decrease of DAT density in caudate and putamen was also documented by Erixon-Lindroth et al. (2005). In addition, this study revealed age-related deficits in tests of episodic memory, working memory, and word fluency, but not in a test of general knowledge. As with the Bäckman et al. (2000) study on D_2 receptors, the age-related cognitive deficits were completely mediated by DAT density, although DAT density contributed to the performance variation in memory and fluency independent of age. The latter finding was substantiated by the result that DAT density also was related to performance in the age-insensitive knowledge test (Table 11.2).

Thus, although the database is limited, the available evidence suggests that pre- and postsynaptic markers of the nigrostriatal DA system are strong general correlates of cognitive performance, as well as powerful mediators of the cognitive changes that occur across adulthood and old age.

Novel approaches and data

In a recent review article (Bäckman et al., 2006), we identified several outstanding issues regarding the relationship among aging, DA, and cognition, as well as issues related to the role of DA in cognition irrespective of age. In the remainder of this chapter, we review emerging evidence that speaks to these issues.

Regional selectivity

There is a discrepancy between human and animal research regarding the specificity of the DA–cognition relationship. Studies on aging (e.g., Bäckman et al., 2000; Erixon-Lindroth et al., 2005; Volkow et al., 1998) as well as corresponding research on patients with basal ganglia disorders (e.g., Bäckman et al., 1997; Lawrence et al., 1998) show that markers of D_1, D_2, and DAT binding in both the caudate and the putamen show strong relation-

Table 11.2 Amount of variance (R^2) in cognitive performance accounted for by age and dopamine transporter binding in striatum as a function of order of entry

	Episodic memory		*Executive function*		*Knowledge*	
	Word recall	*Figure recall*	*Face recognition*	*WM*	*Word fluency*	*Information*
Age	.31	.35	.28	.40	.15	.07
DAT	.24	.19	.13	.13	.16	.28
Total	.55	.55	.41	.53	.31	.35
DAT	.46	.49	.40	.49	.30	.31
Age	.09	.06	.01	.04	.01	.04
Total	.55	.55	.41	.53	.31	.35

Adapted from Erixon-Lindroth et al. (2005).

Note: DAT: dopamine transporter; WM: working memory.

ships to each other as well as to cognitive performance. In contrast, dissociative patterns have been found in monkeys with regard to both receptor subtypes as well as regions in the fronto-striatal network. For example, Williams and Goldman-Rakic (1995) showed that a D_1 agonist modulated working memory fields, whereas a D_2 agonist caused changes in the integration of motor and motivational capacities. Wang, Vijayraghavan, and Goldman-Rakic (2004) found that D_2 receptors modulated memory-guided saccades in a working memory task, whereas D_1 receptors modulated persistent memory-related activity. Pasupathy and Miller (2005) demonstrated differential roles for the striatum (rapid, specific, and latency-related neural firing) and the frontal cortex (slow, flexible, accuracy-related neural firing) during conditional association learning.

To be sure, the monkey work is based on acute pharmacological challenges, whereas the human studies deal with inter-individual variability over several decades. The possibility for adaptive regulatory mechanisms (cf. Shinkai et al., 1997; Zhang et al., 1995), reducing the chance of finding selective effects, is obviously greater in the latter case. Also, in contrast to single-cell recordings, one might question whether the measurement devices in human research (e.g., PET) are sensitive enough to detect potential differences between various DA markers regarding their role in cognitive functioning. At the same time, relatively few molecular-imaging studies have addressed the DA–cognition relationship, and the research is characterized by small sample sizes. Thus, the general failure to obtain differential relationships among brain regions as well as different biochemical markers may reflect the limited nature of the database, along with low statistical power in individual studies.

Using a sample of middle-aged adults, Cervenka, Bäckman, Cselényi, Halldin, and Farde (2008) recently examined whether D_2 receptor binding in different regions within the striatal complex are selectively implicated in episodic memory versus knowledge. They subdivided the striatum into ventral (nucleus accumbens, ventral caudate, putamen), associative (mostly caudate, dorsal putamen), and sensorimotor (mostly putamen, dorsolateral caudate) compartments (Alexander, DeLong, & Strick, 1986; Martinez et al., 2003; Parent & Hazrati, 1995; see Figure 11.1). Of chief interest was whether D_2 binding in ventral striatum would be especially critical to episodic memory. Supportive evidence for this hypothesis comes from recent fMRI research showing that coactivation of ventral tegmentum, nucleus accumbens, and hippocampus strongly predicts episodic recall of reward-related items (Adcock, Thangavel, Whitfield-Gabrieli, Knutson, & Gabrieli, 2006; Wittmann et al., 2005); pharmacological fMRI work in rodents suggests a sizable relationship between DA release and blood flow in ventral striatum (Knutson & Gibbs, 2007).

In general, the data from Cervenka et al. (2008) were in agreement with the hypothesis. First, the relationship between D_2 binding in ventral striatum and episodic memory was stronger than for the other striatal compartments. Conversely, D_2 binding in associative and sensorimotor striatum was more strongly related to performance in knowledge-based tasks compared to ventral striatum (Table 11.3). Thus, these findings extend the fMRI observations (Adcock et al., 2006; Wittmann et al., 2005) to the level of neuromodulation and suggest that the striatum, at least in part, may be functionally compartmentalized regarding higher order cognition. This approach could be extended to brain regions outside the striatum. For example, could it be that age-related DA losses in a particular brain area (e.g., putamen) are more

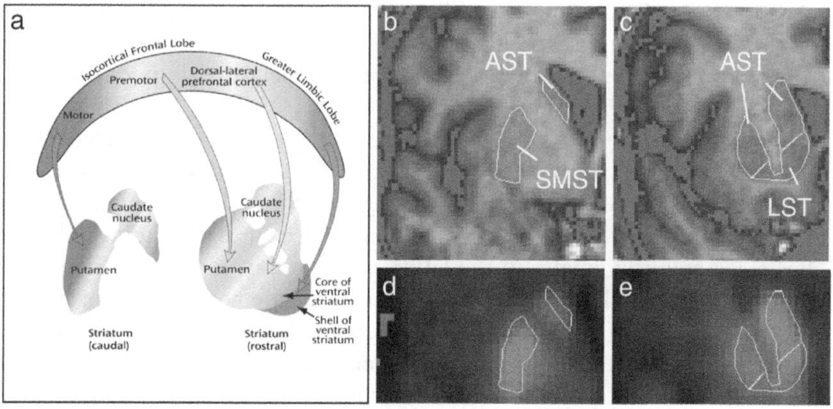

Figure 11.1 (a) Schematic figure of the anatomical connectivity in striatum. (b, c) MRI sections depicting manually drawn regions of interest (ROIs) for striatum in one subject; posterior and anterior to the anterior commissure, respectively. (d, e) Corresponding PET sections showing [^{11}C]raclopride binding in the same subject, with ROIs superimposed. (LST: limbic striatum; AST: associative striatum; SMST: sensorimotor striatum.) (Adapted from Cervenka et al., 2008.) (This figure is published in colour at http://www.cognitiveneurosciencearena.com/brain-scans/.)

Table 11.3 Relationships between D_2 binding potential in striatal subregions and cognitive performance

	Episodic memory						*Knowledge*			
	Paired associate learning		*Word recognition*		*Delayed pattern recognition*		*Information*		*Category fluency*	
	r	*p*	*r*	*p*	*r*	*p*	*r*	*p*	*r*	*p*
Limbic striatum	.67	.01	.56	.02	.47	.04	.33	.11	.42	.06
Associative striatum	.66	.01	.44	.05	.39	.08	.59	.01	.69	.01
Sensorimotor striatum	.50	.03	.29	.15	.24	.20	.48	.04	.72	.01

Adapted from Cervenka et al. (2008).

critical than DA losses in other areas (e.g., frontal cortex, hippocampus) for certain domains of cognitive functioning (e.g., psychomotor speed), whereas the opposite pattern holds for other cognitive domains (e.g., working memory)? Of interest also is whether potential regional selectivity regarding the DA–cognition link remains the same or is attenuated in aging. The latter outcome would suggest dedifferentiation of the DA system in advanced age, a pattern that has often been found for various cognitive and psychometric abilities (e.g., Chen, Myerson, & Hale, 2002; de Frias, Lövdén, Lindenberger, & Nilsson, 2007; Grady, 2002).

COMT genotype and aging

As noted, allelic variations in COMT genotype have been linked to cognitive performance, with met carriers (higher DA availability in prefrontal cortex) outperforming val carriers (lower DA availability in prefrontal cortex; for a review, see Goldberg & Weinberger, 2004). However, in studies with younger adults, effect sizes are small and findings are inconsistent (for overviews, see Barnett, Jones, Robbins, & Müller, 2007; Savitz, Solms, & Ramesar, 2006). Relatively few studies have assessed the effects of COMT genotype on cognition in aging. However, the available evidence suggests a more robust advantage of met carriers in late adulthood (de Frias et al., 2004, 2005; Harris et al., 2005; O'Hara et al., 2006; Starr, Fox, Harris, Deary, & Whalley, 2007). A magnification of COMT gene-related effects on cognitive performance should, in fact, be expected on the basis of the inverted U-shaped function relating DA levels to cognition (e.g., Cai & Arnsten, 1997; Li et al., 2001). Specifically, as aging results in marked DA losses, the inverted U-shaped curve implies that cognitive differences between older met and val carriers of the COMT gene is greater than that between younger met and val carriers (Figure 11.2).

In a recent large-scale study, a direct test of this hypothesis was conducted (Nagel et al., 2008). Using two measures that draw heavily on frontal integrity

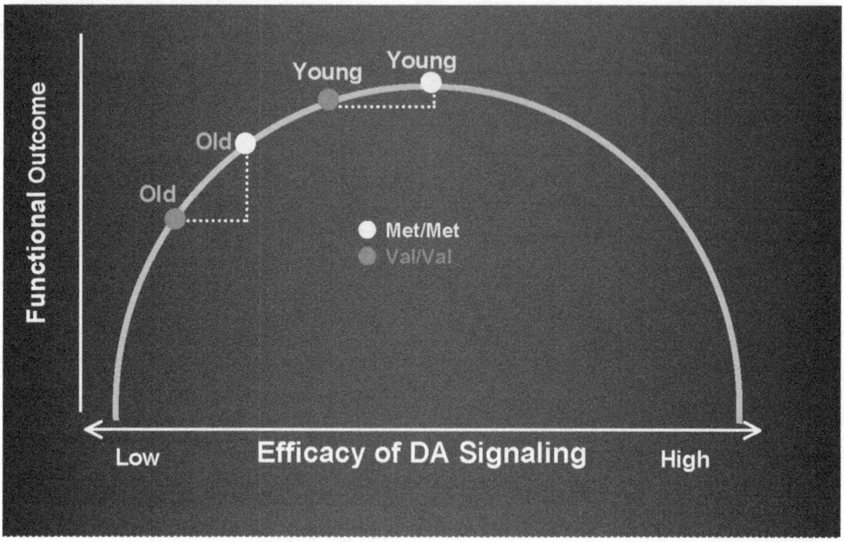

Figure 11.2 Inverted U-shaped function linking a performance outcome to the efficacy of frontal DA signalling in early versus late adulthood. The shape of the curve implies that the difference in performance between older met and val carriers is greater than the difference between younger met and val carriers of the COMT gene. (Adapted from Nagel et al., 2008.) (This figure is published in colour at http://www.cognitiveneurosciencearena.com/brain-scans/.)

– the Wisconsin Card Sorting Test and a test of spatial working memory – we demonstrated clear COMT genotype × Age interactions in the expected direction: Whereas differences between met and val carriers were non-existent in the young sample, a met advantage was observed in the old sample. The point, then, is that although genetic status does not change across adulthood, the functional effects of genotype variation may change because of age-related biological constraints (e.g., DA losses). Future research should extend this approach by examining other genes linked to the DA systems. Of particular interest in this regard is to investigate how potential gene–gene interactions in cognition may be influenced by the human aging process.

Pharmacological intervention

In young adults, DA agonists typically enhance performance (e.g., Luciana & Collins, 1997), whereas DA antagonists impair performance (e.g., Ramaekers et al., 1999) across a variety of cognitive tasks. Furthermore, consistent with the inverted U-shaped function, the effects of DA on cognition and brain activity seem to be modified by COMT genotype, such that val carriers (lower baseline DA levels) show a more efficient frontal response, whereas met carriers (higher baseline DA levels) show a less efficient frontal response following administration of a DA agonist (Mattay et al., 2003). These patterns of data open up a series of interesting research questions regarding the role of DA in cognitive aging. Preliminary answers are emerging for some of these questions.

First, we may ask whether DA antagonists, in addition to lowering performance, would lead to a pattern of brain activation during cognitive performance (e.g., working memory) in young adults that resembles that typically exhibited by older adults under placebo conditions (e.g., more diffuse activation). In an fMRI study, Fischer et al. (2009) addressed this issue by examining whether brain activation patterns in young adults under the influence of a dopaminergic antagonist during a spatial working memory task would resemble those of older adults under normal conditions. Three groups were studied: young-placebo (YP), young-antagonist (YA), and old-placebo (OP). Two initial findings from this study provide support for this assumption: First, the YP group showed greater activity in task-relevant frontal and parietal regions than did the YA and OP groups. Second, the two latter groups showed greater activity in regions outside the load-dependent network (e.g., posterior cingulate). These preliminary findings may reflect the fact that depletion of DA (whether ontogenetically or pharmacologically) decreases the signal-to-noise ratio in relevant networks, resulting in lowered neural efficiency.

We may also ask whether a DA agonist would alter the brain activation patterns of older people in the opposite direction (i.e., more specific and associated with better performance). This research issue may profit from considering COMT gene-related differences in DA signalling. On the basis of the inverted U-shaped relationship between DA levels and cognitive/brain function, older val carriers may be expected to exhibit the largest cognitive improvement and the most pronounced increase in neural efficiency from a DA agonist. Young val carriers and older met carriers may also show some improvement, whereas young met carriers may deteriorate, because their initially high DA levels in conjunction with a DA agonist lead to suboptimally high DA levels. Evidence that speaks to these issues is on its way.

Within-person variability

An interesting observation in neuropsychological research over the past years is that persons who show cognitive deficits also tend to be more variable (e.g., from trial to trial in a reaction time task; from session to session in a memory task). It is vital to note that between-person differences in intra-individual variability (IIV) is not simply an artifact of mean-level differences, for these are routinely partialled out in the analysis of IIV. A wide variety of conditions have been associated with increased IIV, including old age, impending death, ADHD, traumatic brain injury, schizophrenia, Parkinson's disease, and dementia (for a review, see MacDonald, Nyberg, & Bäckman, 2006). At a cognitive level, high IIV is thought to reflect momentary lapses of attention – a failure to exert executive control (West, Murphy, Armilio,

Craik, & Stuss, 2002). Consequently, it has been argued that the frontal lobes may be particularly crucial for maintaining stability, hence minimizing IIV (Stuss, Murphy, Binns, & Alexander, 2003). The fact that patients with fronto-temporal dementia show higher IIV than Alzheimer patients at the same severity level (Murtha, Cismaru, Waechter, & Chertkow, 2002) supports this contention. However, another feature that unites those groups that exhibit high IIV is that they are characterized by alterations in DA functions (MacDonald et al., 2006). Indeed, neurocomputational work on DA, aging, and cognition (Li et al., 2001; Li & Sikström, 2002) suggests that reduced DA activity increases neural noise, resulting in less distinct cortical representations manifest as, among other things, increased IIV (Figure 11.3).

In a first attempt to directly link DA to IIV, MacDonald, Cervenka, Nyberg, Farde, and Bäckman (in press) measured extrastriatal D_2 binding in striatum, anterior cingulate, frontal cortex, and hippocampus in a middle-aged group. IIV was assessed in terms of fluctuations in reaction times during episodic memory retrieval and concept formation. Given that the sample was relatively age-homogeneous, between-person differences in D_2 binding and IIV were relatively small. Nevertheless, there were systematic negative correlations between D_2 binding and IIV across all three extrastriatal brain regions examined (*r*s ranging from –.30 to –.45), although IIV was unrelated to striatal D_2 binding. These data indicate that, even within normal ranges, reduced availability of DA may result in more fluctuating behaviour. Future work along these lines should be extended to other measures of IIV as well as other DA markers and brain regions. In addition, it would be interesting to examine the extent to which the well-established age-related increase in IIV (MacDonald et al., 2006) is mediated by age-related DA losses.

DA release during cognitive activity

The fact that it has been possible to demonstrate DA release in young adults during cognitive activity (e.g., Aalto et al., 2005; Monchi et al., 2006) opens up the possibility of some interesting age-comparative work on this topic. We know that age-related cognitive deficits are especially pronounced in tasks that require active (executive) stimulus processing (Craik & Salthouse, 1999, 2007). We also know that DA markers are strongly related to performance in executively demanding tasks (Bäckman et al., 2000; Erixon-Lindroth et al., 2005; Volkow et al., 1998). Given these observations, we might hypothesize that age differences observed in executively demanding tasks partly reflect the fact that such tasks require excessive DA release to be successfully performed (e.g., Mattay et al., 2003). As a result, relative to less demanding tasks, age-related DA losses should be particularly detrimental.

Karlsson et al. (2009) examined this hypothesis by measuring D_1 receptor binding in young and old adults under two conditions: baseline and cognitive activity. The cognitive task selected was the Multi-Source Interference Task (Bush, Shin, Holmes, Rosen, & Vogt, 2003). This task measures the ability to

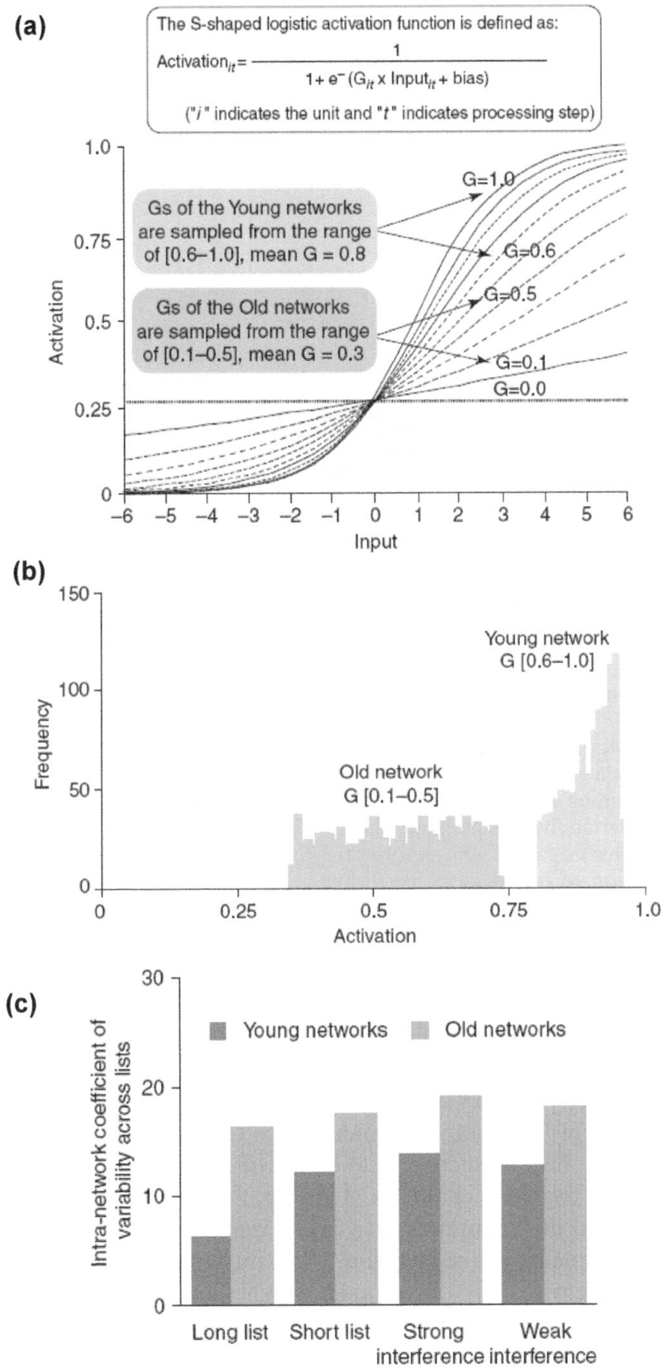

Figure 11.3 (a–c) See over for d–e and figure legend.

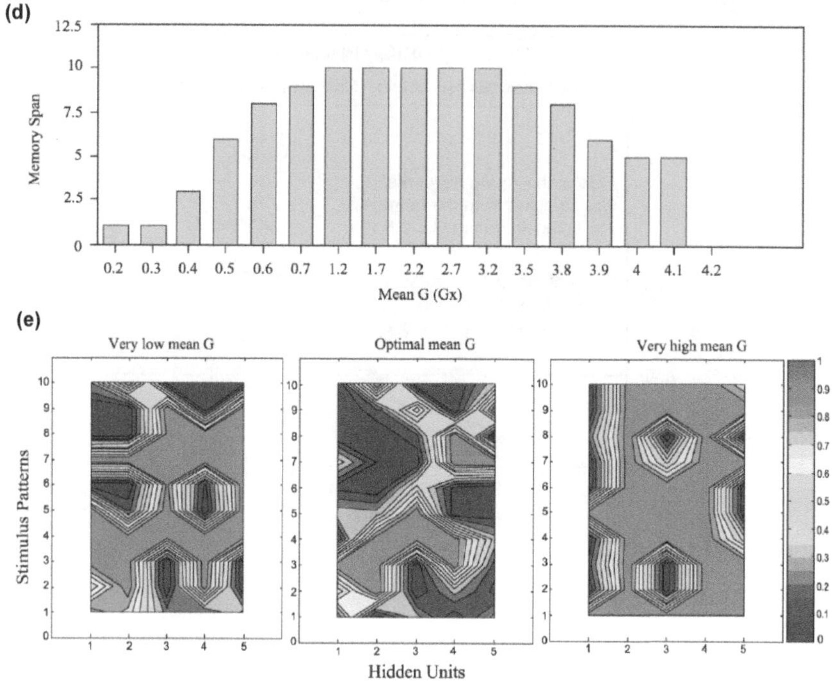

Figure 11.3 Modelling deficient neuromodulation in aging. (a) Simulating aging-related DA modulation by reducing stochastic gain tuning. Reduced gain tuning increases (b) random activation variability and (c) performance variability in simulated old networks (adapted from Li et al., 2001). Stochastic gain tuning captures the inverted-U function relating DA modulation to (d) memory performance, and (e) distinctiveness of activation patterns (adapted from Li & Sikström, 2002). (This figure is published in colour at http://www.cognitiveneurosciencearena.com/brain-scans/.)

inhibit prepotent responses. Although age-group differences were relatively small, the young outperformed the old with regard to both accuracy and latency. In line with corresponding work on D_2 receptors (Aalto et al., 2005; Monchi et al., 2006), the young adults showed less binding of the ligand to striatal D_1 receptors during the interference task compared with baseline. This may reflect displacement due to competition with endogenous DA as a function of the cognitive challenge (Laurelle, 2000). The apparent increased release of DA in the young was seen in the ventral, associative, and sensorimotor compartments of the striatum. Most intriguingly, the pattern of data was very different for the old sample, which showed no differences whatsoever in D_1 receptor binding between the two conditions. This null effect suggests unaltered DA release during executive performance in old adults – a less plastic DA system.

Several outstanding issues remain to be investigated in research on DA and cognitive activity. These include the relationship between DA release and BOLD activation in fMRI studies (Knutson & Gibbs, 2007) and how this relationship might change with advancing age. Furthermore, behavioural studies demonstrate that, although young adults typically benefit more than old adults from cognitive training, there is still a sizable cognitive reserve capacity in aging (e.g., Hill et al., 2000; Nyberg et al., 2003). Towards this end, it would be of interest to examine whether the negative findings for D_1 binding in the old reported by Karlsson et al. (2009) are modifiable through systematic training. Relatedly, investigating training-related changes in transient neurocognitive processes that could be linked to D_2 receptors (Bilder, Volavka, Lachman, & Grace, 2004), such as updating (Dahlin, Stigsdotter-Neely, Larsson, Bäckman, & Nyberg, 2008; O'Reilly & Randall, 2006), constitutes an interesting avenue for future research. How the dynamic relationship between transient (D_2-related) and sustained (D_1-related) DA systems (Grace, Floresco, Goto, & Lodge, 2007) might change with age and is modulated by genetic background (e.g., COMT status; de Frias et al., 2009) will also be a key issue in cognitive DA research in the years to come.

Acknowledgements

Preparation of this chapter was supported by grants from the Swedish Research Council and Swedish Brain Power to Lars Bäckman, and from the Joint Committee for the Nordic Research Councils in the Humanities and the Social Sciences (Center of Excellence in Cognitive Control) to Lars Nyberg.

References

Aalto, S., Brück, A., Laine, M., Någren, K., & Rinne, J. O. (2005). Frontal and temporal dopamine release during working memory and attention tasks in healthy humans: A PET study using the high-affinity dopamine D_2 receptor ligand [^{11}C]-FLB 457. *Journal of Neuroscience*, *25*, 2471–2477.

Adcock, R. A., Thangavel, A., Whitfield-Gabrieli, S., Knutson, B., & Gabrieli, J. D. E. (2006). Reward-motivated learning: Mesolimbic activation precedes memory formation. *Neuron*, *50*, 507–517.

Alexander, G. E., DeLong, M. R., & Strick, P. L. (1986). Parallel organization of functionally segregated circuits linking basal ganglia and cortex. *Annual Review of Neuroscience*, *9*, 357–381.

Antonini, A., Leenders, K. L., Reist, H., Thomann, R., Beer, H. F., & Locher, J. (1993). Effect of age on D_2 dopamine receptors in normal human brain measured by positron emission tomography and [^{11}C]-raclopride. *Archives of Neurology*, *50*, 474–480.

Bäckman, L., & Farde, L. (2005). The role of dopamine functions in cognitive aging. In R. Cabeza, L. Nyberg, & D. C. Park (Eds.), *Cognitive neuroscience of aging: Linking cognitive and cerebral aging* (pp. 58–84). New York: Oxford University Press.

Bäckman, L., Ginovart, N., Dixon, R. A., Robins Wahlin, T. B., Wahlin, Å., Halldin, C., et al. (2000). Age-related cognitive deficits mediated by changes in the striatal dopamine system. *American Journal of Psychiatry*, *157*, 635–637.

Bäckman, L., Nyberg, L., Lindenberger, U., Li, S.-C., & Farde, L. (2006). The correlative triad among aging, dopamine, and cognition: Current status and future prospects. *Neuroscience and Biobehavioral Reviews*, *30*, 791–807.

Bäckman, L., Robins Wahlin, T. B., Lundin, A., Ginovart, N., & Farde, L. (1997). Cognitive deficits in Huntington's disease are predicted by dopaminergic PET markers and brain volumes. *Brain*, *120*, 2207–2217.

Barnett, J. H., Jones, P. B., Robbins, T. W., & Müller, U. (2007). Effects of the catechol-O-methyltransferase Val/158Met polymorphism on executive function: A meta-analysis of the Wisconsin Card Sorting Test in schizophrenia and healthy controls. *Molecular Psychiatry*, *12*, 502–509.

Bilder, R. M., Volavka, J., Lachman, H. M., & Grace, A. A. (2004). The catechol-O-methyltransferase polymorphism: Relations to the tonic-phasic dopamine hypothesis and neuropsychiatric disorders. *Neuropsychopharmacology*, *29*, 1943–1961.

Brandt, J., & Butters, N. (1986). The neuropsychology of Huntington's disease. *Trends in Neurosciences*, *9*, 118–120.

Brown, R. G., & Marsden, C. D. (1990). Cognitive function in Parkinson's disease: From description to theory. *Trends in Neurosciences*, *13*, 21–29.

Bruck, A., Aalto, S., Nurmi, E., Bergman, J., & Rinne, J. O. (2005). Cortical 6-[F-18]fluoro-L-dopa uptake and frontal cognitive functions in early Parkinson's disease. *Neurobiology of Aging*, *26*, 891–898.

Bush, G., Shin, L. M., Holmes, J., Rosen, B. R., & Vogt, B. A. (2003). The Multi-Source Interference Task: Validation study with fMRI in individual subjects. *Molecular Psychiatry*, *8*, 60–70.

Cai, J. X., & Arnsten, A. F. T. (1997). Dose-dependent effects of the dopamine D_1 receptor agonists A77636 or SKF81297 on spatial working memory in aged monkeys. *Journal of Pharmacology and Experimental Therapeutics*, *283*, 183–189.

Cervenka, S., Bäckman, L., Cselényi, Z., Halldin, C., & Farde, L. (2008). Associations between D_2 receptor binding and cognitive performance indicate functional compartmentalization of the human striatum. *NeuroImage*, *40*, 1287–1295.

Chen, J., Myerson, J., & Hale, S. (2002). Age-related dedifferentiation of visuospatial abilities. *Neuropsychologia*, *40*, 2050–2056.

Cornish, K. M., Manly, T., Savage, R., Swanson, J., Morisano, D., Butler, N., et al. (2005). Association of the dopamine transporter (DAT1) 10/10-repeat genotype with ADHD symptoms and response inhibition in a general population sample. *Molecular Psychiatry*, *10*, 686–698.

Craik, F. I. M., & Salthouse, T. A. (Eds.). (1999). *Handbook of aging and cognition* (2nd ed.). Mahwah, NJ: Lawrence Erlbaum Associates, Inc.

Craik, F. I. M., & Salthouse, T. A. (Eds.). (2007). *Handbook of aging and cognition* (3rd ed.). Mahwah, NJ: Lawrence Erlbaum Associates, Inc.

Cropley, V. L., Fujita, M., Innis, R. B., & Nathan, P. J. (2006). Molecular imaging of the dopamine system and its association with human cognitive function. *Biological Psychiatry*, *59*, 898–907.

Dahlin, E., Stigsdotter-Neely, A., Larsson, A., Bäckman, L., & Nyberg, L. (2008). Transfer of learning after updating training mediated by the striatum. *Science*, *320*, 1510–1512.

de Frias, C. M., Annerbrink, K., Westberg, L., Eriksson, E., Adolfsson, R., & Nilsson, L.-G. (2004). COMT gene polymorphism is associated with declarative memory in adulthood and old age. *Behavior Genetics*, *34*, 533–539.

de Frias, C. M., Annerbrink, K., Westberg, L., Eriksson, E., Adolfsson, R., &

Nilsson, L.-G. (2005). Catechol O-methyltransferase Val[158]Met polymorphism is associated with cognitive performance in nondemented adults. *Journal of Cognitive Neuroscience, 17*, 1018–1025.

de Frias, C. M., Lövdén, M., Lindenberger, U., & Nilsson, L.-G. (2007). Revisiting the dedifferentiation hypothesis with longitudinal multi-cohort data. *Intelligence, 35*, 381–392.

de Frias, C. M., Marklund, P., Eriksson, E., Larsson, A., Öman, L., Annerbrink, L., et al. (2009). *Influence of COMT gene polymorphism on fMRI-assessed sustained and transient activity during a working memory task*. Manuscript submitted for publication.

Egan, M. F., Goldberg, T. E., Kolachana, B. S., Callicott, J. H., Mazzanti, C. M., Straub, R. E., et al. (2001). Effect of COMT Val108/158Met genotype on frontal lobe function and risk for schizophrenia. *Proceedings of the National Academy of Sciences USA, 98*, 6917–6922.

Erixon-Lindroth, N., Farde, L., Robins Wahlin, T. B., Sovago, J., Halldin, C., & Bäckman, L. (2005). The role of the striatal dopamine transporter in cognitive aging. *Psychiatry Research: Neuroimaging, 138*, 1–12.

Fischer, H., Nyberg, L., Karlsson, S., Karlsson, P., Rieckmann, A., Brehmer, Y., MacDonald, S. W. S., Farde, L., & Bäckman, L. (2009). *Simulating neurocognitive aging: Effects of a dopaminergic antagonist on brain activation during spatial working memory*. Manuscript submitted for publication.

Goldberg, T. E., & Weinberger, D. R. (2004). Genes and the parsing of cognitive processes. *Trends in Cognitive Sciences, 8*, 325–335.

Grace, A. A., Floresco, S. B., Goto, Y., & Lodge, D. J. (2007). Regulation of firing of dopaminergic neurons and control of goal-directed behaviors. *Trends in Neurosciences, 30*, 220–227.

Grady, C. L. (2002). Age-related differences in face processing: A meta-analysis of three functional neuroimaging experiments. *Canadian Journal of Experimental Psychology, 56*, 208–220.

Halliday, R., Naylor, H., Brandeis, D., Callaway, E., Yano, L., & Herzig, K. (1994). The effect of d-amphetamine, clonidine, and yohimbine on human information processing. *Psychophysiology, 31*, 331–337.

Harris, S. E., Wright, A. F., Hayward, C., Starr, J. M., Whalley, L. J., & Deary, I. J. (2005). The functional COMT polymorphism, Val158Met, is associated with logical memory and the personality trait intellect/imagination in a cohort of healthy 79 year olds. *Neuroscience Letters, 385*, 1–6.

Hill, R. D., Bäckman, L., & Stigsdotter-Neely, A. (Eds.). (2000). *Cognitive rehabilitation in old age*. New York: Oxford University Press.

Inoue, M., Suhara, T., Sudo, Y., Okubo, Y., Yasuno, F., Kishimoto, T., et al. (2001). Age-related reduction of extrastriatal dopamine D_2 receptor measured by PET. *Life Sciences, 69*, 1079–1084.

Kaasinen, V., Vilkman, H., Hietala, J., Någren, K., Helenius, H., Olsson, H., et al. (2000). Age-related D_2/D_3 receptor loss in extrastriatal regions of the human brain. *Neurobiology of Aging, 21*, 683–688.

Karlsson, S., Nyberg, L., Karlsson, P., Fischer, H., Thilers, P., MacDonald, S. W. S., et al. (2009). *Modulation of striatal dopamine* D_1 *binding by cognitive processing*. Manuscript submitted for publication.

Kimberg, D. Y., & D'Esposito, M. (2003). Cognitive effects of the dopamine receptor agonist pergolide. *Neuropsychologia, 41*, 1020–1027.

Kimberg, D. Y., D'Esposito, M., & Farah, M. J. (1997). Effects of bromocriptine on human subjects depend on working memory capacity. *NeuroReport*, *8*, 3581–3585.

Knutson, B., & Gibbs, S. E. B. (2007). Linking nucleus accumbens dopamine and blood oxygenation. *Psychopharmacology*, *191*, 813–822.

Laurelle, M. (2000). Imaging synaptic neurotransmission with in vivo binding competition techniques: A critical review. *Journal of Cerebral Blood Flow and Metabolism*, *20*, 423–451.

Lawrence, A. D., Weeks, R. A., Brooks, D. J., Andrews, T. C., Watkins, L. H. A., Harding, A. E., et al. (1998). The relationship between dopamine receptor binding and cognitive performance in Huntington's disease. *Brain*, *121*, 1343–1355.

Li, S. C., Lindenberger, U., & Sikström, S. (2001). Aging cognition: From neuromodulation to representation to cognition. *Trends in Cognitive Sciences*, *5*, 479–486.

Li, S. C., & Sikström, S. (2002). Integrative neurocomputational perspectives on cognitive aging, neuromodulation, and representation. *Neuroscience and Biobehavioral Reviews*, *26*, 795–808.

Loo, S. K., Specter, E., Smolen, A., Hopper, C., Teale, P. D., & Reite, M. L. (2003). Functional effects of the DAT1 polymorphism on EEG measures in ADHD. *Journal of the American Academy of Child and Adolescent Psychiatry*, *42*, 986–993.

Luciana, M., & Collins, P. F. (1997). Dopamine modulates working memory for spatial but not object cues in normal humans. *Journal of Cognitive Neuroscience*, *9*, 330–347.

MacDonald, S. W. S., Cervenka, S., Nyberg, L., Farde, L., & Bäckman, L. (in press). Extrastriatal dopamine D_2 receptor binding modulates intraindividual variability in episodic recognition and executive functioning. *Neuropsychologia*.

MacDonald, S. W. S., Nyberg, L., & Bäckman, L. (2006). Intra-individual variability in behavior: Links to brain structure, neurotransmission, and neuronal activity. *Trends in Neurosciences*, *29*, 474–480.

Maher, B. S., Marazita, M. L., Ferrell, R. E., & Vanyukov, M. M. (2002). Dopamine system genes and attention deficit hyperactivity disorder: A meta-analysis. *Psychiatric Genetics*, *12*, 207–215.

Martinez, D., Silfstein, M., Broft, A., Mawlawi, O., Hwang, D.-R., Huang, Y., et al. (2003). Imaging human mesolimbic dopamine transmission with positron emission tomography. Part II: Amphetamine-induced dopamine release in the functional subdivisions of the striatum. *Journal of Cerebral Blood Flow and Metabolism*, *23*, 285–300.

Mattay, V. S., Goldberg, T. E., Fara, F., Hariri, A. R., Tessitore, A., Egan, M. F., et al. (2003). Catechol O-methyltransferase val^{158}-met genotype and individual variation in the brain response to amphetamine. *Proceedings of the National Academy of Sciences, USA*, *100*, 6186–6191.

Mitchell, R. J., Howlett, S., Earl, L., McComb, J., Schanfield, M. S., Briceno, I., et al. (2000). Distribution of the 3′ VNTR polymorphism in the human dopamine transporter gene in world populations. *Human Biology*, *72*, 295–304.

Monchi, O., Ko, J. H., & Strafella, A. P. (2006). Striatal dopamine release during performance of executive functions: A [^{11}C]-raclopride PET study. *NeuroImage*, *33*, 907–912.

Mozley, L. H., Gur, R. C., Mozley, P. D., & Gur, R. E. (2001). Striatal dopamine transporters and cognitive functioning in healthy men and women. *American Journal of Psychiatry*, *158*, 1492–1499.

Murtha, S., Cismaru, R., Waechter, R., & Chertkow, H. (2002). Increased variability accompanies frontal lobe damage in dementia. *Journal of the International Neuropsychological Society*, *8*, 360–372.

Nagel, I. E., Chicherio, C., Li, S.-C., von Oertzen, T., Sander, T., Villringer, A., Heekeren, H. R., et al. (2008). Human aging magnifies genetic effects on executive functioning and working memory. *Frontiers in Human Neuroscience*, *2*, 1–8.

Nordström, A. L., Farde, L., Pauli, S., Litton, J. E., & Halldin, C. (1992). PET analysis of [^{11}C]-raclopride binding in healthy young adults and schizophrenic patients: Reliability and age effects. *Human Psychopharmacology*, *7*, 157–165.

Nyberg, L., Sandblom, J., Jones, S., Stigsdotter-Neely, A., Petersson, K. M., Ingvar, M., & Bäckman, L. (2003). Neural correlates of training-related memory improvement in adulthood and aging. *Proceedings of the National Academy of Sciences, USA*, *100*, 13728–13733.

O'Hara, R., Miller, E., Liao, C. P., Way, N., Lin, X. Y., & Hallmayer, J. (2006). COMT genotype, gender, and cognition in community dwelling, older adults. *Neuroscience Letters*, *409*, 205–209.

O'Reilly, R. C., & Randall, C. (2006). Biologically based computational models of high-level cognition. *Science*, *314*, 91–94.

Parent, A., & Hazrati, L. N. (1995). Functional anatomy of the basal ganglia. I. The cortico-basal ganglia-thalamo-cortical loop. *Brain Research Reviews*, *20*, 91–127.

Pasupathy, A., & Miller, E. A. (2005). Different time courses of learning-related activity in the prefrontal cortex and striatum. *Nature*, *433*, 873–876.

Ramaekers, J. G., Louwerens, J. W., Muntjewerff, N. D., Milius, H., de Bie, A., Rosenzweig, P., et al. (1999). Psychomotor, cognitive, extrapyramidal and affective functions of healthy volunteers during treatment with an atypical (amisulpiride) and a classic (haloperidol) antipsychotic. *Journal of Clinical Psychopharmacology*, *19*, 209–221.

Savitz, J., Solms, M., & Ramesar, R. (2006). The molecular genetics of cognition: Dopamine, COMT, and BDNF. *Genes, Brain & Behavior*, *5*, 311–328.

Sawaguchi, T., & Goldman-Rakic, P. S. (1991). D_1 dopamine receptors in prefrontal cortex: Involvement in working memory. *Science*, *251*, 947–950.

Shinkai, T., Zhang, L., Mathias, S. A., & Roth, G. S. (1997). Dopamine induces apoptosis in cultured rat striatal neurons: Possible mechanism of D_2-dopamine receptor neuron loss during aging. *Journal of Neuroscience Research*, *47*, 393–399.

Starr, J. M., Fox, H., Harris, S. E., Deary, I. J., & Whalley, L. J. (2007). COMT genotype and cognitive ability: A longitudinal aging study. *Neuroscience Letters*, *421*, 57–61.

Stuss, D. T., Murphy, K. J., Binns, M. A., & Alexander, M. P. (2003). Staying on the job: The frontal lobes control individual performance variability. *Brain*, *126*, 2363–2380.

Suhara, T., Fukuda, H., Inoue, O., Itoh, T., Suzuki, K., Yamasaki, T., et al. (1991). Age-related changes in human D_1 dopamine receptors measured by positron emission tomography. *Psychopharmacology*, *103*, 41–45.

Volkow, N. D., Gur, R. C., Wang, G. J., Fowler, J. S., Moberg, P. J., Ding, Y. S., et al. (1998). Association between decline in brain dopamine activity with age and cognitive and motor impairment in healthy individuals. *American Journal of Psychiatry*, *155*, 344–349.

Wang, M., Vijayraghavan, S., & Goldman-Rakic, P. S. (2004). Selective D_2 receptor actions on the functional circuitry of working memory. *Science*, *303*, 853–856.

Wang, Y., Chan, G. L. Y., Holden, J. E., Dobko, T., Mak, E., Schulzer, M., et al. (1998). Age-dependent decline of dopamine D_1 receptors in human brain: A PET study. *Synapse*, *30*, 56–61.

Weinshilboum, R. M., Otterness, D. M., & Szumlanski, C. L. (1999). Methylation pharmacogenetics: Catechol-O-methyltransferase, thiopurine methyltransferase, and histamine N-methyltransferase. *Annual Review of Pharmacology and Toxicology*, *39*, 19–52.

West, R., Murphy, K. J., Armilio, M. L., Craik, F. I. M., & Stuss, D. T. (2002). Lapses of intention and performance variability reveal age-related increases in fluctuations of executive control. *Brain and Cognition*, *49*, 402–419.

Williams, G. V., & Goldman-Rakic, P. S. (1995). Modulation of memory fields by dopamine D_1 receptors in prefrontal cortex. *Nature*, *376*, 572–575.

Wittmann, B. C., Schott, B. H., Guderian, S., Frey, J. U., Heinze, H. J., & Duzel, E. (2005). Reward-related fMRI activation of dopaminergic midbrain is associated with enhanced hippocampus-dependent long-term memory formation. *Neuron*, *5*, 459–467.

Yang, Y. K., Chiu, N. T., Chen, C. C., Chen, M., Yeh, T. L., & Lee, I. H. (2003). Correlation between fine motor activity and striatal dopamine D_2 receptor density in patients with schizophrenia and healthy controls. *Psychiatry Research: Neuroimaging*, *123*, 191–197.

Zhang, L., Ravipati, A., Joseph, J., & Roth, G. S. (1995). Aging-related changes in rat striatal D_2 dopamine receptor mRNA-containing neurons: A quantitative nonradioactive in situ hybridization study. *Journal of Neuroscience*, *15*, 1735–1740.

Part III

The brain

12 Post-traumatic fear memories

Analysing a case study of a sexual assault

Arne Öhman

Christianson and Nilsson (1989) described a case of hysterical amnesia in a woman (called CM) who was assaulted and raped when she was out jogging. This highly traumatic event produced an almost complete retrograde amnesia up to the moment in time when she was found by a fellow jogger. When accompanied to the scene of the assault by a police officer four weeks after the assault, the victim "felt very uncomfortable at specific places, but had no recollection of the traumatic evening except that the word 'bricks' crossed her mind" (Christianson & Nilsson, 1989, p. 291). Later they came to a small path covered with crumbled bricks that ran parallel to the running path. When encountering this path, CM "showed an intense emotional stress, and claimed that she associated the unpleasant feelings with the pieces of bricks on the track that she was walking on. She strongly felt that something must have happened at this specific place, although she did not know for certain at this point in time that she had been raped. From the confession by the rapist a few days earlier the policeman knew, however, that this was the place where he had assaulted her and from which she had been forced out onto the small meadow where the actual rape took place" (Christianson & Nilsson, 1989, p. 291). It was only several weeks later, when she was out jogging for the first time after the assault, at a completely different track but one that also was covered by crushed bricks, that images of the assault started to come back to her and she eventually was able to reconstruct the whole episode.

This vignette dramatically demonstrates a dissociation between two types of memories of the same event. There were no accessible traces of the rape and the associated events in CM's conscious memory, yet her emotional responses suggested that her brain and body had recorded the trauma. In this chapter I shall discuss an aspect of this case that was barely touched upon by Christianson and Nilsson (1989), who focused their discussion on its most conspicuous part, the amnesia that was provoked by the trauma. I shall argue that her relatively intact emotional responses in the compete absence of episodic memory is a result of Pavlovian fear conditioning – the operation of a subcortical network for defensive emotional learning that is evolutionarily preserved and independent of conscious cognitive learning. It is this system that results in the emotional responses displayed by CM when she was confronted with stimuli that happened to be present during the trauma.

After having briefly introduced Pavlovian fear conditioning, I shall review data demonstrating that fear can be elicited by stimuli that are experimentally excluded from conscious recognition. These experimental findings provide a centrepiece in explaining CM's emotional responding when she was brought back to the site of the trauma, even though she herself had not even remembered that she had been raped. I then go on to examine a literature that shows that Pavlovian fear conditioning can occur in the absence of awareness, thus explaining that CM could learn to associate aspects of the scene of the rape (crumbled brick) with fear in spite of her being completely unaware of what happened. Finally, I shall review the neuroanatomy of the afferent pathways to the fear network, showing that it is bifurcated into two separate routes – one implicit (unconscious) via the superior colliculi and the pulvinar nucleus of the thalamus, the other an explicit (conscious) route via visual cortical pathways terminating in the inferior temporal cortex.

Pavlovian fear conditioning

Pavlovian fear conditioning is a basic, very general, and evolutionary highly preserved form of learning. It results from the exposure of an organism to a contingency between two stimuli, one that originally is relatively ineffective in evoking responses (the conditioned stimulus, CS; in this case, the location of the assault including the ground covered with crushed bricks), and another stimulus that elicits patterns of defence behaviours and associated physiological changes because it threatens the well-being and survival of the organism (the unconditioned stimulus, US; e.g., a painful stimulus, in this case the assault and the rape). As a result of the forming of an association between the CS and the US there is a transfer of responses between these two stimuli to the effect that the CS comes to elicit fear-related behaviour originally evoked by the US. In this way, the conditioned emotional response can be seen as a lasting scar that will provide reminiscences of the trauma whenever stimuli that are reminders of the CS are encountered, irrespective of the current content of episodic memory.

This response transfer between the CS and the US is commonly taken to mean that an association has been formed between the CS and the US such that the CS prompts retrieval of the US from memory. Because the memory of the US in this way can be retrieved before the actual occurrence of the stimulus, the organism is given the opportunity to expect and prepare for the delivery of the US. The functional advantage of this arrangement should be obvious (see Domjan, 2005). By eliciting defence behaviour (freezing/immobility, flight, fight) in anticipation of a potentially deadly US, the odds of minimizing the damage should be vastly improved. For example, faint cues heralding a predator attack allow the organism to initialize flight before the actual strike, which clearly has survival advantages. Therefore, smells, sounds, and sights produced by the predator are likely to be selected by evolution to serve as particularly effective CSs to warn potential prey of a predatory attack (see, e.g., Öhman, Dimberg, & Öst, 1985; Öhman & Mineka, 2001; Seligman, 1970).

In mammals, there is a multitude of measurable somatic, vegetative, endocrine, and central neural responses that qualify as conditioned responses (CRs) because they originate in conditioned defence behaviour (e.g., Fanselow, 1994; Lang, Bradley, & Cuthbert, 1997). However, particularly among humans, the CS–US contingency is not restricted to storage in implicit memory systems indicated by fear-related responses. In addition, it also gets stored in the explicit, hippocampus-dependent episodic memory system "that allows people to consciously re-experience past experiences" (Tulving, 2002, p. 6). The case of CM provides a dramatic demonstration of the independence between the implicit, emotional memory system and explicit episodic memory. In spite of obvious emotional responses to the location of the assault, her episodic memory did not retrieve the basic fact that she had been raped or anything in the situation except for the crumbled brick on the ground. This dissociation indicates that episodic memory and its neuroanatomical substrate – the hippocampus complex in the medial temporal lobe – is more vulnerable to insults (traumatic or chemical) than the neural circuitry that mediates fear conditioning. For example, intense stress results in a heavy increase of circulating cortisol both peripherally and in the brain, and there are data to suggest that cortisol affects the hippocampus and the retrieval of episodic memories (e.g., de Quervain, Roozendaal, Nitsch, McGaugh, & Hock, 2000; McEwen, 2007).

Bodily responses to feared stimuli

Bodily responses related to fear can be readily measured in the psychophysiological laboratory. Indeed, fear exhibited by individuals diagnosed with phobia when encountering their phobic stimulus can be used a laboratory model of real-life fear responses, such as those displayed by CM when she was brought back to the site of the trauma. These responses include changes in psychophysiological functions mediated by the autonomic nervous system, changes in defensive reflexes such as the startle reflex, and changes in brain activity.

Autonomic responses to phobic stimuli

To examine the activation of autonomically mediated responses to feared stimuli, Globisch, Hamm, Esteves, and Öhman (1999) exposed student volunteers with a phobic-level fear of small animals (snakes or spiders), as well as non-fearful control participants, to pictures of snakes or spiders, household objects, erotica, and cute animals. The fearful participants rated snake/spider pictures as much more unpleasant and arousing than neutral and positive pictures than did the controls. In terms of autonomic responses, the fearful participants showed clearly larger skin conductance responses (SCRs) to animal pictures than did controls, and their responses to animals were larger than their responses to neutral or positive pictures (Figure 12.1, upper panel). Furthermore, fearful participants showed a strong heart-rate acceleration to snake/spider pictures, which was in marked contrast to the deceleration shown by controls to animals, and to the small and indistinguishable response shown by both groups to neutral stimuli (Figure 12.1, middle panel).

Potentiation of the startle reflex to phobic stimuli

The startle reflex is a primary example of an evolutionarily old defence response. It makes us jump to any abrupt, unexpected stimulus, particularly when we are in a state of fear. In humans it is commonly measured by the eyeblink response. "Fear-potentiated startle" denotes enhanced startle reflexes to probes (brief noises with abrupt onset) presented when research participants look at aversive pictures (Lang, Bradley, & Cuthbert, 1997). This effect is mediated by the central nucleus of the amygdala (e.g., see Lang, Davis, & Öhman, 2000).

The startle data for phobic participants examined by Globisch et al. (1999) showed a rapid relative startle potentiation to feared compared to neutral stimuli that was obvious to probes presented as early as 300 ms after picture onset, and it then remained (and even increased) for at least 4 s of picture viewing. Controls, on the other hand, showed a rapid relative startle inhibition to animal stimuli that lasted for more than a second. In concert, these data show that enhanced (phobic) fear to animal stimuli is associated with a distinct psychophysiological response suggesting activation of fight/flight behaviour, which stands in stark contrast to the orienting pattern elicited by these stimuli in non-fearful participants (Figure 12.1, lower panel).

Brain responses to phobic stimuli

Carlsson et al. (2004) recruited participants who were phobic of either snakes or spiders (but not of both) for a brain imaging study. During some positron emission tomography (PET) scans, participants were exposed to repeated brief (but clearly perceivable) presentations of pictures of snakes, spiders, or mushrooms. Confirming the notion of the amygdala as the hub in the fear network of the brain, the results showed strong bilateral amygdala activation to the feared stimulus (e.g., a snake for a snake-phobic participant) compared to the neutral stimulus (mushroom) but not to the fear-relevant but non-feared stimulus (e.g., spiders for a snake-phobic participant) (Figure 12.2, upper panels). Furthermore, the enhanced amygdala response to the feared stimulus was associated with activation of a cortical affective processing network that included the anterior cingulate cortex (ACC), the anterior insula,

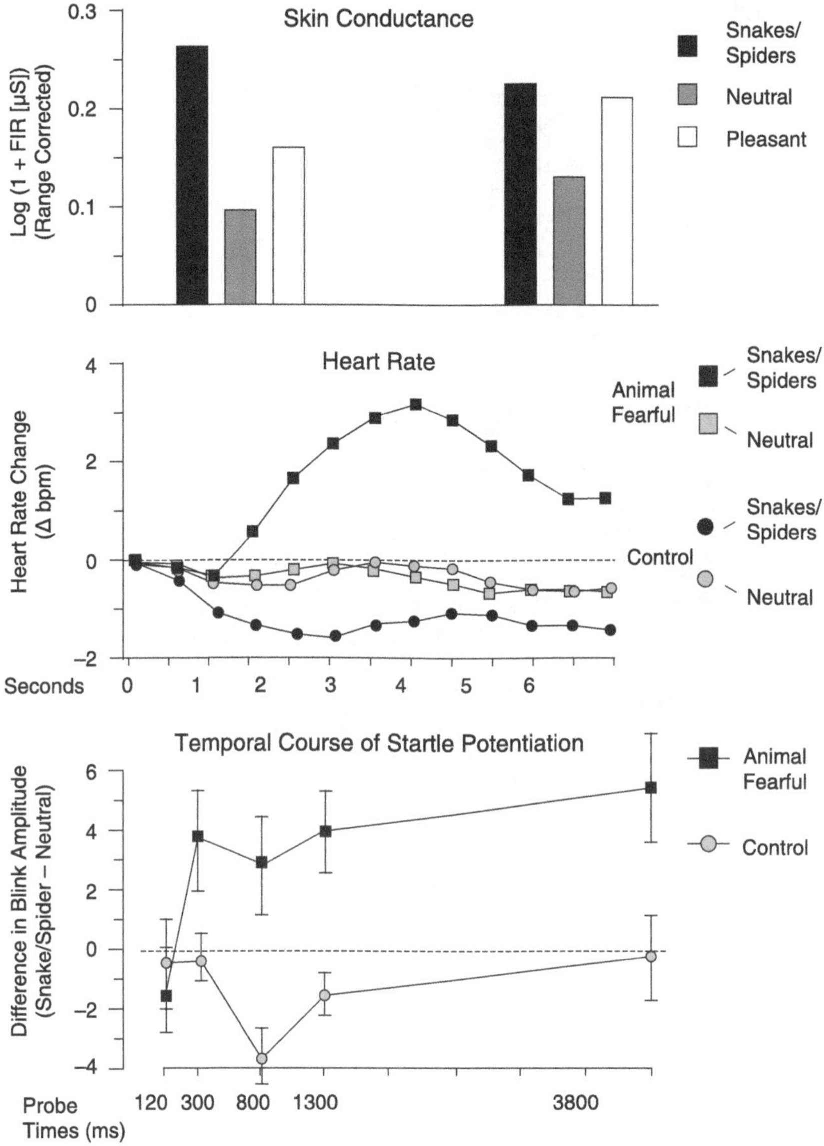

Figure 12.1 Responses of participants highly fearful of snakes or spiders to pictures of phobic and non-phobic content. *Upper panel:* Skin conductance responses to animal, neutral, and positive pictures of fearful (left diagram) and non-fearful (right diagram). *Middle panel:* Heart rate responses to repeated presentations of 6-s pictures of the feared animal and neutral control pictures (as changes from pre-stimulus heart rate level) in animal-fearful and control subjects. *Lower panel:* Difference in startle blink magnitude to brief white noise stimuli presented at different stimulus-onset asynchronies during viewing of animal and neutral stimuli for animal-fearful and control participants. Note the potentiation of startle blinks to feared stimuli and the inhibition of blinks to neutral stimuli. (Data from Globisch, Hamm, Esteves, & Öhman, 1999.)

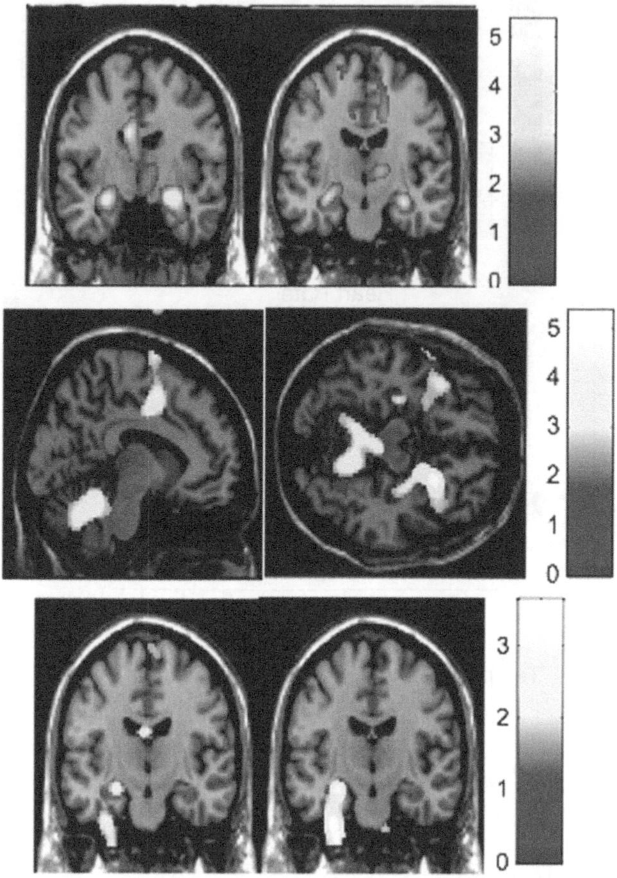

Figure 12.2 *Upper panel:* Coronal views showing bilateral activations in the amygdala/medial temporal lobe in contrasts between a phobic (e.g., a snake) and a neutral stimulus (left brain, $y = -8$), and between the phobic stimulus and a fear-relevant but non-feared animal (e.g., a spider) (right brain, $y = -4$). *Middle panel:* Sagital view ($x = -8$) illustrating activations in the anterior cingulated cortex and the cerebellum in a contrast between feared and non-feared animals (left brain), and a horizontal view ($z = -14$) showing insula/orbitofrontal and periaqueductal grey activations for a contrast between feared and non-feared stimuli (right brain). *Lower panel:* Coronal views ($y = -4$) showing left-sided amygdala/anterior temporal lobe activations for contrast between masked phobic (left brain) and fear-relevant but non-feared animals (right brain), on the one hand, and a neutral control stimulus, on the other. (Data from Carlsson et al., 2004.) (This figure is published in colour at http://www.cognitiveneurosciencearena.com/brain-scans/.)

the orbitofrontal cortex (OFC), as well as the midbrain periaqueductal grey (Figure 12.2, middle panel). Bilateral amygdala activations to snakes in snake-phobics were also reported by Sabatinelli, Bradley, Fitzsimmons, and Lang (2005) and by Dilger et al. (2003). However, Straube, Mentzel, and Miltner (2006) reported left-sided amygdala activation when the participant's task was to identify the phobic stimulus, and bilateral amygdala activations when the task was to report on a superimposed stimulus – that is, when the phobic stimulus was a non-attended, distracting stimulus. The latter study also reported, as did Carlsson et al. (2004) and Dilger et al. (2003), reliable activations of the anterior insula and the prefrontal cortex. However, Sabatinelli et al. (2005), Dilger et al. (2003), and Straube et al. (2006), but not Carlsson et al. (2004), found significant activations of the inferotemporal cortex/fusiform gyrus. Thus, several studies concur in showing amygdala activations to phobic stimulation, as well as activation of both frontal and posterior cortical networks.

Unconscious elicitation of fear responses

CM apparently responded with fear and stress to stimuli that she did not clearly identify. This raises the question of whether fear responses in general can be activated by stimuli that remain inaccessible to conscious perception. To test this notion, it is necessary to develop a methodology that allows stimuli to be presented outside the subject's awareness. Such a method is provided by backward masking, which has been held as the potentially most fruitful avenue to unconscious perception (Holender, 1986; Öhman, 1999). It involves brief presentations of a target stimulus, which is masked from conscious perception by an immediately following masking stimulus (for a methodologically oriented review, see Wiens & Öhman, 2007). Thus if backwardly masked fear stimuli, in the documented absence of conscious recognition, would elicit physiological responses suggesting activation of fear in phobics, we would successfully have modelled CM's responses when returning to the scene of the assault in the psychophysiological laboratory.

Peripheral autonomic responses

Öhman and Soares (1994) selected research participants who feared snakes but not spiders, or vice versa. Participants in the control group feared neither stimulus. In the experiment, participants were exposed to series of pictures of snakes and spiders, with pictures of flowers and mushrooms serving as controls, while SCRs were measured. In the first series, stimulus presentations were effectively masked by pictures that were grossly similar to the target stimuli in colours and texture but lacked any recognizable central object. A pilot experiment using a forced-choice recognition procedure ascertained that both fearful and non-fearful participants consistently failed to identify the target with the masking parameters used. The masks interrupted presentation of the target stimuli after 30 ms of exposure and remained on for 100 ms during the masked presentation series. In the following series of presentations, the stimuli were presented unmasked. After these series, the participants rated the stimuli for arousal, valence, and control/dominance during separately presented masked and nonmasked rating series. Figure 12.3 show SCRs to masked and nonmasked presentations of the stimuli. It is evident that the fearful participants responded specifically to their feared stimulus but did not differ from controls for the other stimulus categories, independently of masking. This enhanced responding to the feared stimulus cannot be attributed to conscious perception. Nevertheless, parallel data were obtained for all three rating dimensions, which suggests that some aspect of the masked stimulation became indirectly available to the conscious system (perhaps through bodily feedback). Thus the fearful participants rated themselves as more disliking, more aroused, and less in control when exposed to masked presentations of their feared stimulus.

Masked activation of the amygdala

Using the same procedure as Öhman and Soares (1994), Carlsson et al. (2004) recruited participants that were fearful of either snakes or spiders (but not of both) for a PET brain imaging study with masked stimuli. The objective of this study was to assess whether the amygdala would respond to

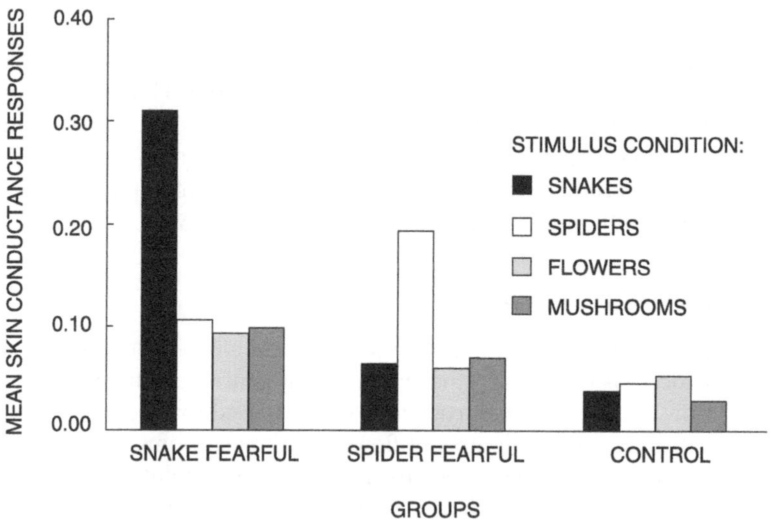

Figure 12.3 Skin conductance responses, in participants selected as fearful to either snakes or spiders, to masked pictures of snakes, spiders, flowers, and mushrooms. Note the elevated responses to the masked feared stimulus in fearful participants. (Data from Öhman & Soares, 1994.)

unconsciously presented stimuli. During different scans, participants were exposed to repeated brief presentation of pictures of snakes, spiders, or mushrooms that were effectively or ineffectively masked, following the procedure of Öhman and Soares (1994). Compared to the effectively masked mushroom control condition, the left amygdala was activated both to the masked feared (e.g., snakes; Figure 12.2, lower left panel) and the masked fear-relevant but non-feared (e.g., spiders; Figure 12.2, lower right panel) condition, with no difference between the two types of fear-relevant stimuli. This implies that the amygdala initially responded to the threat potential of the stimuli rather than to a specifically defined fear stimulus. However, as the processing time was extended to allow conscious perception of the stimuli in a condition with a long target–mask interval, there was strong bilateral amygdala activation to the actually feared stimulus (e.g., snakes; Figure 12.2, upper left panel), but no significant amygdala activation on either side in the fear-relevant but non-feared condition (e.g., spiders for a snake fearful participant; Figure 12.2, upper right panel).

Morris, Öhman, and Dolan (1998) used the masking technique to examine regional cerebral blood flow responses assessed by PET to masked facial stimuli whose emotional impact had been enhanced by Pavlovian fear conditioning. Morris et al. (1998) reported specific activation of the right amygdala to masked conditioned angry faces as compared to masked non-conditioned angry faces. Whalen et al. (1998) also reported larger responses of the amygdala to masked-fearful than to masked-neutral faces.

Binocular rivalry is an alternative method to backward masking for presenting stimuli outside of awareness. If two different stimuli are separately projected onto corresponding retinal locations in the two eyes, rather than being perceived as a mixture they will compete to determine the percept. Given that the two stimuli are roughly matched in salience, the percept will spontaneously shift between them. However, if one stimulus is in some sense more salient than the other, the latter stimulus will be suppressed, which implies that the suppressed stimulus is presented outside of the participant's awareness. Two studies have reported reliable amygdala activation to suppressed pictures of fearful faces in a binocular rivalry paradigm (Pasley, Mayes, & Schultz, 2004; Williams, Morris, McGlone, Abbott, & Mattingley, 2004), thus providing converging evidence with the masking studies to the effect that the amygdala can be activated by consciously non-perceived stimuli.

Fear conditioning to masked stimuli

The findings demonstrating that fear stimuli presented outside of awareness (because of backward masking or binocular rivalry) nonetheless can activate peripheral indices of fear such as SCRs as well as the pivotal central brain nuclei involved in fear activation – the amygdala complex – provide an explanation of CM's dissociation between implicit fear activation and failure of conscious understanding of what was going on. However, a remaining enigma is to explain why she responded in this way. If we assume that her enhanced response to aspects of the context of the rape (e.g., the crumbled brick) was a result of fear conditioning, then the restricted consciousness during, and retroactive amnesia after, the assault would suggest that Pavlovian conditioning does not require awareness.

This possibility was vindicated by Esteves, Parra, Dimberg, and Öhman (1994), who used a neutral face to mask briefly presented (30 ms) angry and happy faces in a differential conditioning procedure with electric shock as the US. For some groups of subjects, one of the masked angry faces served as a CS+ (i.e., was followed by the shock), and the other angry faces served as a CS– (i.e., was not followed by the shock). Other groups had a similar arrangement with happy faces. Control groups received the CSs and the US in unpaired, random order. Half of these groups had a short effective masking interval (30 ms); the other half had a long interval between the CS and the neutral face mask (300 ms), which did not result in perceptual masking. In a subsequent extinction series all subjects had unmasked presentations of the angry and happy faces. Differential responses during extinction were obtained only in subjects conditioned to angry faces, regardless of whether the CS+ had been followed by the short-effective, or the long-ineffective, masking interval between the CS and the masking pictures. Neither subjects conditioned to (masked or non-masked) happy faces nor those who had a random relation between CSs and USs showed any evidence of differential responding during the non-masked extinction trials.

Using a similar procedure, Öhman and Soares (1998) conditioned different groups of subjects to masked pictures of snakes and spiders, or masked pictures of flowers and mushrooms. A differential paradigm was employed in which one of the pictures (the CS+, e.g., a snake) was followed by a shock US, whereas the other picture (the CS–, e.g., a spider) was presented without any USs. Subjects exposed to masked snakes and spiders, but not those exposed to masked flowers and mushrooms, showed reliably larger responses to the CS+ than to the CS– in a subsequent non-masked extinction series (Figure 12.4).

Similar to Esteves et al. (1994), Morris, Büchel, and Dolan (2001a) assessed conditioning to masked faces but used event-related fMRI to assess conditioning. While in the magnet, participants were exposed to a series of trials that included two angry faces either masked by, or masking, two different neutral faces. The noise US consistently followed one of the angry faces when it was masked and none of the other pairs of faces. As in the Esteves et al. (1994) study, the effect of the masked conditioning procedure was assessed by contrasting the non-masked CS+ and CS–. This contrast revealed activations in the ventral and dorsal amygdala that were larger to the CS+ than to the CS–.

Critchley, Mathias, and Dolan (2002) also manipulated awareness by backward masking in a similar procedure to that of Morris et al. (2001a), using two angry and two neutral faces. One of the angry faces (the CS+) was

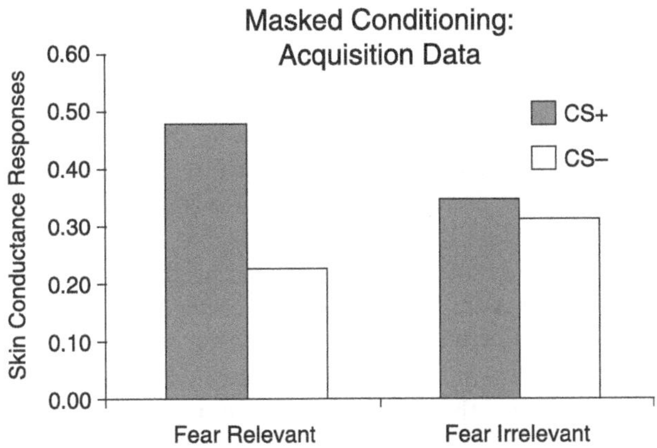

Figure 12.4 Skin conductance responses to one group of participants exposed to masked fear-relevant pictures (snakes and spiders), one of which served as the conditioned stimulus (CS) by being followed by a mild electric shock to the fingers (CS+), whereas the other was not followed by the shock (CS–). A control group had the fear-relevant stimuli exchanged by fear-irrelevant ones (flowers and mushrooms). Note that conditioned differential responding was evident only with fear-relevant CSs. (Data from Öhman & Soares, 1998.)

paired with an aversive noise and was contrasted with the other angry face (the CS–). These stimuli were presented in masking arrangements with neutral faces to assess aware (when the two angry faces masked the neutral faces) and unaware (when the two angry faces were masked by the neutral faces) conditioning. Critchley et al. (2002) reported a main effect of conditioning on the right amygdala that was not modulated by awareness – that is, the conditioning effect was as obvious when the angry CS+ and CS– preceded a neutral face in a masking arrangement (i.e., were unseen) as it was when they followed (i.e., were clearly seen) the neutral face.

This set of studies quite consistently suggests that research participants are able to learn to associate a masked, "non-seen" visual stimulus with an aversive event. Thus, they help us understand the fact that a victim of an assault rape, even though suffering complete amnesia of the event, nevertheless may show evidence of conditioned emotional responding when brought back to the unrecognized context of the trauma.

A direct route to the human amygdala

The apparent unconscious activation and learning of emotion via the amygdala may be attributed to the unique input to this structure. Rodent work by LeDoux (1996, 2000) demonstrated that sensory input can access the amygdala through two distinct anatomical pathways. One is the traditional ventral stream of visual information processing via the lateral geniculate body of the thalamus, to the primary visual cortex in the occipital lobe, and then projecting to the parietal and temporal cortices to end in the inferior temporal cortex, before the amygdala is accessed. The second pathway is a direct monosynaptic route to the amygdala from sensory thalamic nuclei. This conceptualization of the amygdala input was inspired by lesion studies, which demonstrated that fear conditioning in the rat was not affected by lesions in the auditory cortex (with an auditory CSs) but that it required an intact medial geniculate body of the thalamus as well as an intact amygdala (LeDoux, 1987). These findings were then confirmed by neuroanatomical tracing techniques demonstrating a link between the medial geniculate and the amygdala, as well as by molecular studies of fear conditioning demonstrating a critical role for this link in the associative process (LeDoux, 2000).

Data suggesting a direct route to the human amygdala

However, there is a real question of whether findings based on auditory CSs in the rat brain have any bearing on fear conditioning to visual stimuli in the human brain. Thus, at the most basic level, data are required showing that the amygdala can be activated even if cortical processing of visually presented fear stimuli is impossible because of lesions in the relevant sensory cortices. To examine this prediction, Morris, DeGelder, Weiskrantz, and Dolan (2001b) examined a patient with lesions in the primary visual cortex, which resulted in blindsight. Thus, the patient reported no visual sensation for objects presented in the damaged cortical areas. Nevertheless, when exposed to faces in the blind field while fMRI was measured, he showed reliable activation of the right amygdala to fearful as compared to neutral faces. Furthermore, similar results were obtained in a patient whose extensive occipital lesion was associated with total blindness without any signs of residual vision (Pegna, Khateb, Lazeyras, & Seqhier, 2005).

In an ingenious study, DeGelder, Morris, and Dolan (2005) presented emotional faces to the blind right-hemifield of a blindsight patient simultaneously with visual stimuli presented to the intact left visual field, or with emotional voices. The results showed that fearful faces unconsciously presented in the blind field biased conscious perception of emotional faces presented in the intact field, and that these effects were mediated by the amygdala.

In a further analysis of the role of cortex in amygdala activation, Vuilleumier et al. (2002) examined a patient with right inferior parietal lobe damage, which resulted in visual extinction to stimuli presented in the left visual field when another stimulus was simultaneously presented in the right visual field. For example, he failed to notice a picture of a face in the left visual field when a picture of a house was concurrently presented in the right visual field (even though he did perceive the face when it was presented alone in the left visual field). Nevertheless, brain imaging data showed amygdala activation to extinguished faces, particularly when they were fearful. This study showed amygdala activation by fear faces that remained non-perceived because they were presented in spatial locations corresponding to damaged areas in higher order visual areas that failed to be attended because of spatial neglect and extinction (Vuilleumier et al., 2002). Thus, there is consistent data suggesting that the human amygdala can be activated by fear stimuli that are not cortically processed and that are not available to awareness.

The direct route to the amygdala allows rapid priming of visual information processing

Efferent pathways from the amygdala are connected to the primary visual cortex as well as to several later cortical way stations in the sequences of cortical areas in the ventral stream of visual information processing (Emery & Amaral, 2000). This anatomical organization suggests that the rapid amygdala activation occasioned by a fearful encounter may tune subsequent visual processing of the stimulus situation. This notion was tested by Vuilleumier, Richardson, Armony, Driver, and Dolan (2004) in patients with focal amygdala and hippocampal lesions. Vuilleumier et al. (2004) replicated previously demonstrated emotional enhancement of a cortical area involved in vision – the fusiform cortex – to fearful faces (e.g., Vuilleumier, Armony, Driver, & Dolan, 2001) in normal controls and patients with focal hippocampal lesions only. However, such emotional enhancement was not observed in the patients with focused amygdala lesions (with or without hippocampal lesions). Thus, these findings imply that the amygdala is rapidly activated in order to prime the visual cortex for enhanced processing of emotional stimuli, as suggested by LeDoux (1996, 2000).

Phelps, Ling, and Carrasco (2006) reported an experiment in which they briefly cued a perceptual task (judging line orientations as a function of contrast) by fearful or neutral faces. Confirming that emotion facilitates perception of low-level visual features, their data showed improved contrast sensitivity after fearful as opposed to neutral faces. This effect, however, was not obtained with inverted faces, which provides support for the emotional origin of the effect. Furthermore, in a second experiment, Phelps et al. (2006) showed that this enhanced contrast sensitivity was stronger for emotional than for neutral upright (but not inverted) faces both for focused and divided attention conditions, suggesting that it did not depend on attention. However, the emotion effect was larger with focused than with divided attention, which suggested that emotion potentiated the effect of attention.

In concert, these lesion and behavioural data suggest that amygdala activation (consciously or unconsciously) results in improved perceptual performance, thus assisting defence by facilitating detection of potentially important stimuli at basic levels of visual processing.

The structure of the direct route to the amygdala

So far I have reviewed evidence showing that the amygdala appears able to bypass awareness in activating emotional responding and in learning about emotional events. This process, furthermore, appears independent of the relevant sensory cortex, and one of its functions appears to be to rapidly tune perceptual sensitivity for visual stimuli. However, this set of findings raises important questions about the structure of this supposedly direct route to the amygdala. What are the actual pathways and nuclei in the visual system that convey this information?

To examine the route to non-conscious amygdala activation, Morris, Öhman, and Dolan (1999) used the data reported by Morris et al. (1998) to examine the neural connectivity between the amygdala and other brain regions when the amygdala was activated by masked stimuli. Morris et al. (1999) reported that activation of the right amygdala by masked stimuli could be reliably predicted from activation of subcortical way stations in the visual systems such as the superior colliculus and the right pulvinar nucleus of the thalamus, but not from any cortical regions. Both of these subcortical structures are involved in attentional processes – the superior colliculus in eye movement control and shifts of attention, and the pulvinar in attentional salience.

Lidell et al. (2005) examined the effect of masked fearful versus masked neutral faces on anatomically defined regions of interest. Confirming the connectivity data reported by Morris et al. (1999), Lidell et al. found reliable activation to masked fearful faces in the left superior colliculi, the left pulvinar, and the bilateral amygdalae. In addition they found activation in the locus coeruleus and the anterior cingulated cortex.

The resolution that can be achieved by this route is likely to be quite restricted. Vuilleumier, Armony, Driver, and Dolan (2003) suggested that it operates primarily on gross, low-frequency information. Accordingly, they filtered the spatial frequency of pictures of faces to produce facial stimuli that retained only high- or low-frequency spatial information. Their results showed that amygdala responses were larger for low-frequency faces provided that they showed expressions of fear. Moreover, they demonstrated activation of the pulvinar and superior colliculus by low-frequency but not high-frequency fearful faces. Thus, these results suggest that there is a distinct superior colliculus–pulvinar pathway to the amygdala that operates primarily on low-frequency information.

The low-road hypothesis has been controversial (e.g., Pessoa, 2005; Pessoa, Kastner, & Ungerleider, 2002; Rolls, 1999, 2000). In particular it has been claimed that input from the inferior temporal (IT) cortex is necessary for evidence suggesting discriminatory behaviour by the amygdala to facial emotion. It is of considerable interest, therefore, that the study by Pasley et al. (2004), which reported amygdala activation to fearful faces suppressed from awareness by binocular rivalry, demonstrated that areas of the IT that responded to faces under normal viewing did not discriminate faces from objects under conditions of binocular rivalry. Because the primary visual cortex and the IT are the only areas in the ventral visual stream that provide input to the amygdala, these data strongly suggest that there was a subcortical origin of the visual input that allowed the amygdala to discriminate suppressed fearful from suppressed neutral faces.

Concluding comments

My analysis shows that it is possible to provide a quite detailed, neurally based account of CM's emotional responses when she revisited the site of her severe trauma. Deep in our brain there is an evolutionarily old defence system that operates quite independently of more recent evolutionary feats in the primate lineage, which mediate episodic memory and awareness. Not only does this system trigger implicit emotional memory of stimuli of which the victim remains unaware, but there is also good supportive evidence that stimuli in a traumatic situation can become associated with the trauma, later to elicit severe anxiety symptoms, through Pavlovian fear conditioning in the complete absence of awareness of what actually happened. CM may, in fact, have been at least partly unconscious for part of the trauma and, because of the amnesia, she definitely failed to remember anything that happened during the assault. Yet stimuli related to the location of the trauma elicited fear and stress when she was brought back to the scene of the assault.

It is perhaps a reassuring sign of progress that we now are able to provide a convincing scientifically based account of phenomena that a couple of decades ago were not even clearly recognized as problems requiring an explanation. Moreover, this scientifically based account does more than simply explain the fascinating case report by Christianson and Nilsson (1989): It provides an integrated psychobiological framework for understanding many features of several anxiety disorders at a more general level.

References

Carlsson, K., Petersson, K. M., Lundqvist, D., Karlsson, A., Ingvar, M., & Öhman, A. (2004). Fear and the amygdala: Manipulation of awareness generates differential cerebral responses to phobic and fear-relevant (but non-feared) stimuli. *Emotion*, *4*, 340–353.

Christianson, S.-Å., & Nilsson, L.-G. (1989). Hysterical amnesia: A case of aversively motivated isolation of memory. In T. Archer & L.-G. Nilsson (Eds.), *Aversion, avoidance, and anxiety: Perspectives on aversively motivated behavior* (pp. 289–310). Hillsdale, NJ: Lawrence Erlbaum Associates, Inc.

Critchley, H. D., Mathias, C. J., & Dolan, R. J. (2002). Fear conditioning in humans: The influence of awareness and autonomic arousal on functional neuroanatomy. *Neuron*, *33*, 653–663.

de Gelder, B., Morris, J. S., & Dolan, R. J. (2005). Unconscious fear influences emotional awareness of faces and voices. *Proceedings of the National Academy of Science USA*, *102*, 18682–18687.

de Quervain, D. J. F., Roozendaal, B., Nitsch, R. M., McGaugh, J. L., & Hock, C. (2000). Acute cortisone administration impairs retrieval of long-term declarative memory in humans. *Nature Neuroscience, 3*, 313–314.

Dilger, S., Straube, T., Mentzel, H.-J., Fitzek, C., Reichenbach, J. R., Hecht, H., et al. (2003). Brain activation to phobia-related pictures in spider phobic humans: An event-related functional magnetic resonance imaging study. *Neuroscience Letters, 348*, 29–32.

Domjan, M. (2005). Pavlovian conditioning: A functional perspective. *Annual Review of Psychology, 56*, 179–206.

Emery, N. J., & Amaral, D. G. (2000). The role of the amygdala in primate social cognition. In R. D. Lane & L. Nadel (Eds.), *Cognitive neuroscience of emotion* (pp. 156–191). New York: Oxford University Press.

Esteves, F., Parra, C., Dimberg, U., & Öhman, A. (1994). Nonconscious associative learning: Pavlovian conditioning of skin conductance responses to masked fear-relevant facial stimuli. *Psychophysiology, 31*, 375–385.

Fanselow, M. S. (1994). Neural organization of the defensive behavior system responsible for fear. *Psychonomic Bulletin & Review, 1*, 429–438.

Globisch, J., Hamm, A. O., Esteves, F., & Öhman, A. (1999). Fear appears fast: Temporal course of startle reflex potentiation in animal fearful subjects. *Psychophysiology, 36*, 66–75.

Holender, D. (1986). Semantic activation without conscious identification in dichotic listening, parafoveal vision, and visual masking: A survey and appraisal. *Behavioral and Brain Sciences, 9*, 1–66.

Lang, P. J., Bradley, M. M., & Cuthbert, B. N. (1997). Motivated attention: Affect, activation, and action. In P. J. Lang, R. F. Simons, & M. T. Balaban, (Eds.), *Attention and orienting: Sensory and motivational processes* (pp. 97–136). Hillsdale, NJ: Lawrence Erlbaum Associates, Inc.

Lang, P. J., Davis, M., & Öhman, A. (2000). Fear and anxiety: Animal models and human cognitive psychophysiology. *Journal of Affective Disorders, 61*, 137–159.

LeDoux, J. E. (1987). Emotion. In F. Plum (Ed.), *Handbook of physiology: Section 1. The nervous system: Vol. 5. Higher functions of the brain* (pp. 419–460). Bethesda, MD: American Physiological Society.

LeDoux, J. E. (1996). *The emotional brain*. New York: Simon & Schuster.

LeDoux, J. E. (2000). Emotion circuits in the brain. *Annual Review of Neuroscience. 23*, 155–184.

Liddell, B. J., Brown, K. J., Kemp, A. H., Barton, M. J., Das, P., Peduto, A., et al. (2005). A direct brainstem-amygdala-cortical "alarm" system for subliminal signals of fear. *NeuroImage, 24*, 235–243.

McEwen, B. S. (2007). Physiology and neurobiology of stress and adaptation: Central role of the brain. *Physiological Reviews, 87*, 873–904.

Morris, J. S., Büchel, C., & Dolan, R. J. (2001a). Parallel neural responses in amygdala subregions and sensory cortex during implicit fear conditioning. *NeuroImage, 13*, 1044–1052.

Morris, J. S., DeGelder, B., Weiskrantz, L., & Dolan, R. J. (2001b). Differential extra-geniculostriate and amygdala responses to presentation of emotional faces in a cortically blind field. *Brain, 124*, 1241–1252.

Morris, J. S., Öhman, A., & Dolan, R. J. (1998). Conscious and unconscious emotional learning in the human amygdala. *Nature, 393*, 467–470.

Morris, J. S., Öhman, A., & Dolan, R. J. (1999). A subcortical pathway to the right amygdala mediating "unseen" fear. *Proceedings of the National Academy of Sciences USA*, *96*, 1680–1685.

Öhman, A. (1999). Distinguishing unconscious from conscious emotional processes: Methodological considerations and theoretical implications. In T. Dalgleish & M. Power (Eds.), *Handbook of cognition and emotion* (pp. 321–352). Chichester, UK: Wiley.

Öhman, A., Dimberg, U., & Öst, L.-G. (1985). Animal and social phobias: Biological constraints on learned fear responses. In S. Reiss & R. R. Bootzin (Eds.), *Theoretical issues in behavior therapy* (pp. 123–175). New York: Academic Press,.

Öhman, A., & Mineka, S. (2001). Fears, phobias, and preparedness: Toward an evolved module of fear and fear learning. *Psychological Review*, *108*, 483–522.

Öhman, A., & Soares, J. J. F. (1994). "Unconscious anxiety": Phobic responses to masked stimuli. *Journal of Abnormal Psychology*, *103*, 231–240.

Öhman, A., & Soares, J. J. F. (1998). Emotional conditioning to masked stimuli: Expectancies for aversive outcomes following nonrecognized fear-relevant stimuli. *Journal of Experimental Psychology: General*, *127*, 69–82.

Pasley, B. N., Mayes, L. C., & Schultz, R. T. (2004). Subcortical discrimination of unperceived objects during binocular rivalry. *Neuron*, *42*, 163–172.

Pegna, A., Khateb, A., Lazeyras, F., & Seqhier, M. (2005). Discriminating emotional faces without primary visual cortices involves the right amygdala. *Nature Neuroscience*, *8*, 24–25.

Pessoa, L. (2005). To what extent are emotional visual stimuli processed without attention and awareness? *Current Opinion in Neurobiology*, *15*, 188–196.

Pessoa, L., Kastner, S., & Ungerleider, L. G. (2002). Attentional control of the processing of neural and emotional stimuli. *Brain Research: Cognitive Brain Research*, *15*, 31–45.

Phelps, E. A., Ling, S., & Carrasco, M. (2006). Emotion facilitates perception and potentiates the perceptual benefits of attention. *Psychological Science*, *17*, 292–299.

Rolls, E. T. (1999). *Brain and emotion*. Oxford: Oxford University Press.

Rolls, E. T. (2000). Neurophysiology and functions of the primate amygdala, and the neural basis of emotion. In J. P. Aggleton (Eds.), *The amygdala: A functional analysis*. New York: Oxford University Press.

Sabatinelli, D., Bradley, M. M., Fitzsimmons, J. R., & Lang, P. J. (2005). Parallel amygdala and inferotemporal activation reflect emotional intensity and fear relevance. *NeuroImage*, *24*, 1265–1270.

Seligman, M. E. P. (1970). On the generality of the laws of learning. *Psychological Review*, *77*, 406–418.

Straube, T., Mentzel, H.-J., & Miltner, W. H. R. (2006). Neural mechanisms of automatic and direct processing of phobigenic stimuli in specific phobia. *Biological Psychiatry*, *59*, 162–170.

Tulving, E. (2002). Episodic memory: From mind to brain. *Annual Review of Psychology*, *53*, 1–25.

Vuilleumier, P., Armony J. L., Clarke, K., Husain, M., Driver, J., & Dolan, R. J. (2002). Neural response to emotional faces with and without awareness: Event-related fMRI in a parietal patient with visual extinction and spatial neglect. *Neuropsychologia*, *40*, 2156–2166.

Vuilleumier, P., Armony, J. L., Driver, J., & Dolan, R. J. (2001). Effects of attention and emotion on faces processing in the human brain: An event-related fMRI study. *Neuron, 30*, 829–841.

Vuilleumier, P., Armony, J. L., Driver, J., & Dolan, R. J. (2003). Distinct spatial frequency sensitivities for processing faces and emotional expressions. *Nature Neuroscience, 6*, 624–631.

Vuilleumier, P., Richardson, M. P., Armony, J. L., Driver, J., & Dolan, R. J. (2004). Distant influences of amygdala lesion on visual cortical activation during emotional face processing. *Nature Neuroscience, 7*, 1271–1278.

Whalen, P. J., Rauch, S. L., Etcoff, N. L., McInerney, S. C., Lee, M. B., & Jenike, M. A. (1998). Masked presentations of emotional facial expressions modulate amygdala activity without explicit knowledge. *Journal of Neuroscience, 18*, 411–418.

Wiens, S., & Öhman, A. (2007). Probing unconscious emotional processes: On becoming a successful masketeer. In J. A. Coan & J. J. B. Allen (Eds.), *Handbook of emotion elicitation and assessment* (pp. 65–90). New York: Oxford University Press.

Williams, M. A., Morris, A. P., McGlone, F., Abbott, D. F., & Mattingley, J. B. (2004). Amygdala responses to fearful and happy facial expressions under conditions of binocular suppression. *Journal of Neuroscience, 24*, 2898–2904.

13 Environmental influences on autobiographical memory

The mnestic block syndrome

Matthias Brand and Hans J. Markowitsch

Introduction

Human beings live in an environment that changes from moment to moment. For behaving consistently with one's own desires and beliefs, it is fundamentally important to remember the past. In addition, the feeling of having an identity or what is called "personality" is also based on past experiences and associated personal beliefs about one's own self. Remembering events of one's own biography, including a clear relation to time and space, has been referred to as "episodic memory" for a long time. However, the definition of episodic memory has been changed since the term was introduced by Endel Tulving three decades ago (Tulving, 1972, 1987, 1995). In recent reviews (e.g., Tulving, 2002, 2005), he emphasizes that episodic memory is the conjunction of subjective time, autonoetic consciousness, and the experiencing self and that it is not only confined to events with a clear relation to time and space, as other researchers used the term (e.g., for memory measured by laboratory tasks such as learning a word list). In addition to the core facet of autobiographical memory – that is, autobiographical-episodic memory – retrieving facts of one's own history (e.g., the date of birth) also constitutes autobiographical memory. Nevertheless, semantic knowledge related to the biography is not stored in the episodic memory system but is part of the general knowledge system. In this contribution, we focus on autobiographical-episodic memory and its changes linked to environmental influences. After a brief introduction in which we will summarize the brain structures most crucially involved in autobiographical-episodic memory and the processes necessary for building an episodic memory, we will review the main environmental factors influencing autobiographical-episodic memory functioning. Here, we will demonstrate that stress-related and psychogenic factors can severely compromise the ability to remember the past. We will show that even in amnesic conditions without structural brain damage, functional alterations of episodic memory-related brain circuits can be neural correlates of the patients' amnesia.

Brain structures involved in autobiographical-episodic memory

When describing brain correlates of autobiographical-episodic memory, one has to distinguish specific memory processes. First, information has to be encoded and consolidated. Second, memories have to be stored. Last, stored memories can principally be retrieved (cf. Brand & Markowitsch, 2003b; Markowitsch, 1998a, 1998b, 2000a, 2000b). The process of remembering events leads to a "new" encoding of the memory, a process frequently referred to as re-encoding. Re-encoding can strengthen the storage and the ability to remember the information, but it can also result in falsification of details and therefore produce false memories (Ciaramelli & Ghetti, 2007; Geng et al., 2007; Ladowsky-Brooks & Alcock, 2007; Loftus, 2003).

The processes of encoding and consolidation of episodic memories depend on the integrity of brain circuits that involve structures and fibre connections from nearly all parts of the brain, primarily parts of the prefrontal cortex, the medial temporal lobe, and the medial diencephalon (e.g., Brand & Markowitsch, 2003b). Medial temporal lobe, diencephalic, and further limbic structures principally engaged in encoding and consolidation of episodic memories (and at least partially also in semantic memory) are the hippocampal formation, the mammillary bodies, the anterior thalamic nuclei, and the cingulate gyrus. These structures – together with connecting tracts such as the fornix, the mammillothalamic tract, thalamic pedunculi, and the cingulum – build the so-called Papez circuit (Papez, 1937). In addition to the Papez circuit, the amygdala and surrounding structures are critically involved in encoding and consolidation whenever information to be learned is emotionally coloured. The amygdala is exceptionally linked to evaluating emotional sensory stimuli (e.g., Phelps, 2006; Phelps & LeDoux, 2005) and to binding the emotional relevance of information during memory building in general (Cahill, 2000; Cahill et al., 2001; Fujiwara & Markowitsch, 2006; Markowitsch, 2000a). As autobiographical-episodic memories have an emotional connotation by definition (see above), both the Papez circuit and the amygdala together with other structures of the so-called basolateral-limbic loop (mediodorsal nucleus of the thalamus, subcallosal area) are necessarily engaged in the formation of an autobiographical-episodic memory (Markowitsch, 2000a; Markowitsch et al., 1994; Zald, 2003).

Evidence for the critical role of both medial temporal and diencephalic structures in encoding and consolidation comes from recent studies with functional imaging techniques as well as from descriptions of patients who suffer from memory deficits following damage to specific brain areas (cf. Brand & Markowitsch, 2003a). The disastrous consequences of hippocampal lesions for memory acquisition are well known since Scoville and Milner (1957) described the severe anterograde memory impairments of patient HM following bilateral medial temporal lobe resection (though such consequences had been described in German language literature since 1900; cf. Markowitsch, 1992). Moreover, there are several other single- or multiple-case reports that confirm the critical function of the hippocampal formation for anterograde memory (cf. Aggleton & Brown, 1999; Broman, Rose, Hotson, & Casey, 1997; Cipolotti & Bird, 2006; Gilboa et al., 2006; Kapur et al., 1997; Markowitsch, 2000b, 2003a; Mayes, 1995; Park, Seo, & Yoon, 2007; Tulving & Markowitsch, 1998; Vargha-Khadem et al., 1997, 2003). Examples for patients with anterograde amnesia in the course of diencephalic damage are patients with alcoholic Korsakoff's syndrome (Brand, Kalbe, Fujiwara, Huber, & Markowitsch, 2003; Fujiwara, Brand, Borsutzky, Steingass, & Markowitsch, 2008a; Kopelman, 1995; Kopelman, Stanhope, & Kingsley, 1999; Krabbendam et al., 2000; Labudda, Todorovski, Markowitsch, & Brand, 2008), even though in these patients other brain pathologies, such as frontal abnormalities, may also contribute to the amnesic condition (Brand et al., 2005; Brokate et al., 2003; Reed et al., 2003) and potentially a hippocampal involvement (Sullivan & Marsh, 2003). Patients with selective bilateral damage to the amygdalae suffer from deficits in emotional memory, as demonstrated in patients with Urbach-Wiethe disease (Markowitsch et al., 1994; Siebert, Markowitsch, & Bartel, 2003; Tranel & Hyman, 1990), although these patients may also show additional dysfunctions – for example, impairments in decision-making (Bechara, Damasio, Damasio, & Lee, 1999; Brand, Grabenhorst, Starcke, Vandekerckhove, & Markowitsch, 2007).

The findings in brain-damaged patients that indicate that the structures mentioned above are important for memory acquisition are principally supported by recent neuroimaging investigations with healthy subjects and different patient populations (e.g., Binder, Bellgowan, Hammeke, Possing, & Frost, 2005; Cabeza, Dolcos, Graham, & Nyberg, 2002; Cabeza & Nyberg, 2000; Cabeza & St Jacques, 2007; Cabeza et al., 1997; Greicius et al., 2003; Kircher et al., 2007; Kumaran & Maguire, 2006; Nyberg et al., 1996; Rand-Giovannetti et al., 2006; Uncapher & Rugg, 2005a, 2005b).

Even though the limbic structures mentioned are often regarded as the key structures in memory encoding and consolidation, the prefrontal cortex is definitively not less significant for a successful memory acquisition (and retrieval). The dorsolateral portion of the prefrontal cortex (mainly comprising Brodmann's areas 9 and 46 as well as the posterior part of 10) supports encoding of new material. This is primarily based on its important function in organizing and categorizing the items to be learned, at least when the learning situation is complex and requires strategic memory processes (Miotto et al., 2006) and effort (e.g., Buckner, Koutstaal, Schacter, Wagner, & Rosen, 1998; Gerton et al., 2004; Jansma, Ramsey, de Zwart, van Gelderen, & Duyn, 2007). In addition, the dorsolateral part supports a specific encoding strategy – namely, the learning of associations between items (Addis & McAndrews, 2006; Blumenfeld & Ranganath, 2006; Staresina & Davachi, 2006; Summerfield et al., 2006). This predominant function of the dorsolateral prefrontal area also reflects its key role in a network providing the neural basis for higher order executive functions (e.g., Elliott, 2003; Fuster, 2006; Kane & Engle, 2002; Roberts, Robbins, & Weiskrantz, 1998). It is also important for working memory (Cabeza et al., 2002; Cabeza & Nyberg, 2000; Fletcher & Henson, 2001). However, also discussed is how specific the dorsolateral part is engaged in direct encoding processes (Ranganath & Blumenfeld, 2008). Beyond the general involvement of executive functions supported by the dorsolateral section, it is also linked to reflective processes that necessarily contribute to encoding (and also to retrieval) of memories (Ranganath, Johnson, & D'Esposito, 2003). On the basis of its connections with other prefrontal regions (e.g., the orbitofrontal cortex) and limbic structures (e.g., amygdala), the dorsolateral part is also associated with the integration of stimuli processed by various sensory and motor systems and with linking the information to emotional and motivational aspects of behaviour.

Other parts of the prefrontal cortex are also involved in encoding of episodic memories – for example, the orbitofrontal cortex (Brodmann's areas 11 and 47) – when information to be learned has an emotional connotation, such as faces (Herholz et al., 2001) or other visual (Frey & Petrides, 2000) or auditory material (Frey, Kostopoulos, & Petrides, 2004).

Nevertheless, the prefrontal regions are generally more strongly associated with retrieval of information. Within the recall of autobiographical episodes, the dorsolateral section was found inconsistently activated (Piolino et al., 2004; Vandekerckhove, Markowitsch, Mertens, & Woermann, 2005) with potential sex differences (more intensely activated in females compared with male volunteers; Piefke, Weiss, Markowitsch, & Fink, 2005) and depending on the methods applied to retrieve autobiographical events (Cabeza & St Jacques, 2007). It is more likely activated when the retrieval condition is difficult and requires effort (Buckner, 2003; Lepage, Ghaffar, Nyberg, & Tulving, 2000; Rugg, Otten, & Henson, 2002; Velanova et al., 2003). In contrast, the orbitofrontal cortex seems to be more likely retrieval-specific and was consistently found activated when the episodes that are recalled have an emotional tone (e.g., Cabeza et al., 2004; Conway et al., 1999; Levine et al., 2004; Maguire, Henson, Mummery, & Frith, 2001; Markowitsch, Vandekerckhove, Lanfermann, & Russ, 2003; Piefke, Weiss, Zilles, Markowitsch, & Fink, 2003; Ryan et al., 2001; Svoboda, McKinnon, & Levine, 2006).

As outlined in the introduction to this chapter, episodic memories have a relation to one's own self (Tulving, 2002, 2005). Processing self-relevant information is also regarded as a crucial element of autobiographical memory's social and directive function (Conway, 2003; Conway & Pleydell-Pearce, 2000). Accordingly, the neural correlates of "the self" – that is, the dorsomedial prefrontal cortex together with other midline structures, such as the anterior cingulate gyrus (cf. Johnson et al., 2002; Northoff et al., 2006; Zysset, Huber, Samson, Ferstl, & von Cramon, 2003) – are associated with remembering autobiographical events (Fossati et al., 2004; Svoboda et al., 2006).

Beyond the critical role of prefrontal areas for remembering one's own past, it is under debate (e.g., Conway et al., 1999) to what degree the limbic structures described earlier in this chapter are necessary for retrieval in addition to their main function during memory acquisition. A hippocampal contribution to successful retrieval was demonstrated for recent, in contrast to remote, memories in an fMRI study with healthy volunteers by Piefke et al. (2003). In addition, an involvement of the hippocampal formation and other limbic structures in remembering the autobiography was also shown by other previous studies (e.g., Fink et al., 1996; Haist, Bowden Gore, & Mao, 2001; Levine et al., 2004; Moscovitch et al., 2005; Piefke et al., 2005; Steinvorth, Levine, & Corkin, 2005; Svoboda et al., 2006; Vandekerckhove et al., 2005). Although there is some evidence suggesting that the contribution of the hippocampal formation in autobiographical remembering is moderated by age and gender (Piefke & Fink, 2005; Piefke et al., 2005), there are also studies that found a general involvement of the hippocampal formation in retrieving personal events independent of the age of the memories and other variables (Viard et al., 2007). Previous reports also indicate an engagement of the hippocampal region (in addition to the amygdala) in emotional intensity ratings of autobiographical memories (Daselaar et al., 2008) and that the (left) hippocampus is linked to constructing both past and future events (Addis, Wong, & Schacter, 2007). Neuroimaging results on the impact of the hippocampal formation and surrounding structures in recalling one's own biography are confirmed by studies with brain-damaged subjects in whom lesions involved primarily the medial temporal lobe (Addis, Moscovitch, & McAndrews, 2007; Bell & Giovagnoli, 2007; Buchanan, Tranel, & Adolphs, 2006; Geffen, Isles, Preece, & Geffen, 2008; Noulhiane et al., 2007). It should, however, be noted that neurological patients have much more widespread brain damage than usually assumed, and that methodological limitations frequently underestimate lesion extents and lesion loci (cf. Markowitsch, Weber-Luxenburger, Ewald, Kessler, & Heiss, 1997c). For HM this was exemplified by Corkin, Amaral, Gonzalez, Johnson, and Hyman (1997).

In summary, evidence suggests that the prefrontal cortex and limbic structures are the key neural correlates of remembering personal events having an emotional connotation and a relation to the self (see Figure 13.1, in which the cerebral structures related to the retrieval of episodic events and semantic facts are depicted and compared indicating that right hemispheric limbic and prefrontal regions are more strongly related to retrieval of autobiographical-episodic memories than are left hemispheric structures; cf. LaBar & Cabeza, 2006; Markowitsch, 2003b). In the following paragraphs we will show that limbic and prefrontal regions are specifically vulnerable to stress-induced changes of neural plasticity and neural functioning and are therefore candidates for key structures relevant for autobiographical memory disorders linked to environmental influences, such as long-term stress and trauma.

Stress and memory

Several factors can substantially influence brain functions and, accordingly, autobiographical memory. Beyond various idiopathic conditions that reduce

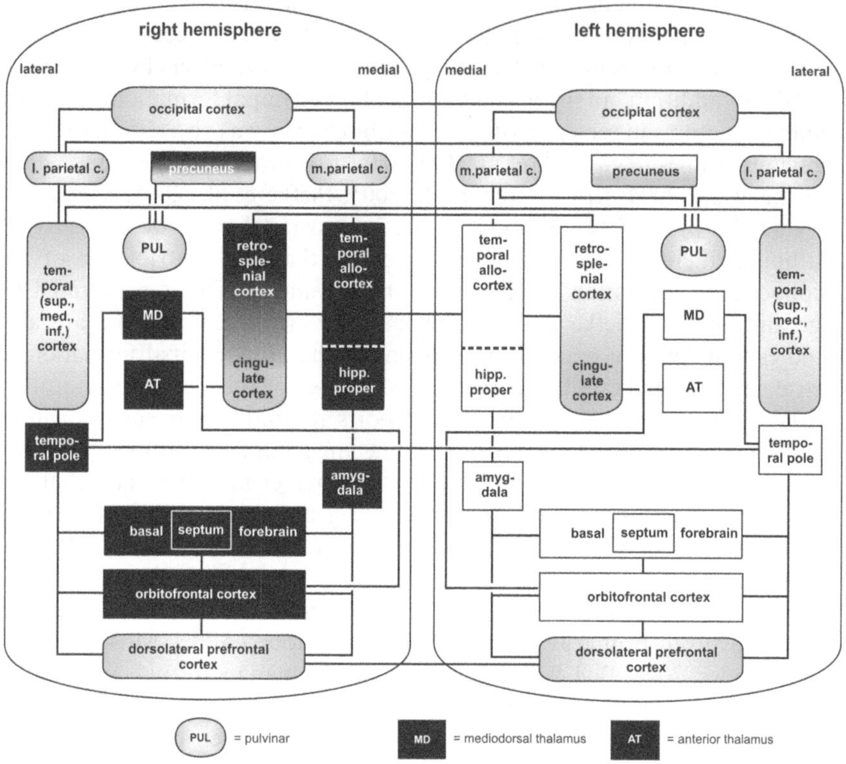

Figure 13.1 Structures of the right and the left hemisphere linked to retrieval of stored information. Limbic structures of the right hemisphere are most likely more strongly engaged in remembering autobiographical-episodic information than are homologous structures of the left hemisphere. (Modified from Markowitsch, 2003b, Fig. 3.)

autobiographical memory functioning (e.g., neurodegenerative diseases, vascular processes, tumours, and encephalitis), environmental factors can also compromise encoding and retrieval of autobiographical-episodic memories. One of the most common environmental influences on autobiographical memory is long-lasting and/or excessive stress. Here, primarily subjectively perceived negative stress with high intensity may alter the integrity of neurons, resulting in brain abnormalities. While short-term and positive stress may enhance neural plasticity and therefore brain functioning, a long-term dysregulation of stress hormones (i.e. glucocorticoids such as cortisol) can also diminish the neurobiological basis of learning and memory (primarily the synaptic plasticity). The short-term positive (and at least partially also negative) effects of stress on learning memory was demonstrated imposingly by a series of studies with animals (McGaugh, 2004; Roozendaal, Okuda, de Quervain, & McGaugh, 2006; Roozendaal, Okuda, Van der Zee, & McGaugh, 2006).

For human beings, both the positive and the negative effects of short-term stress could be replicated and concretized (cf. LaBar & Cabeza, 2006). While encoding of information may be positively influenced by stress (Buchanan & Lovallo, 2001; Putman, Van Honk, Kessels, Mulder, & Koppeschaar, 2004), recall of memories seems to be compromised by a higher level of stress induced with either a psychological stress intervention or application of glucocorticoids (cortisol) (Kuhlmann, Kirschbaum, & Wolf, 2005; Kuhlmann, Piel, & Wolf, 2005). Primarily, the information central for the content seems to be affected by stress, while peripheral information is almost unaffected (Payne et al., 2006). Administration of high-dose glucocorticoids may also lead to impaired memory functions in patients with neurological disorders (e.g., with multiple sclerosis), while other cognitive functions, such as attention and executive functioning, seem to be unaffected (Brunner et al., 2006). In a recent study by Buss, Wolf, Witt, and Hellhammer (2004), it was also shown that healthy subjects generate less specific autobiographical memories in an autobiographical memory interview after administration of hydrocortisone (10 mg). This finding further emphasizes the relationship between stress and a tendency of overgeneralized memory in patients with massive or long-lasting stress experiences (e.g., post-traumatic stress disorder, PTSD) (see next section).

Further evidence for the negative impact of stress and associated altered levels of stress hormones comes from a recent study by Wolf, Fujiwara, Luwinski, Kirschbaum, and Markowitsch (2005), in which reduced cortisol levels in patients with retrograde amnesia of organic origin were found. Potentially, in individuals who suffer from massive or chronic stress experiences, the baseline cortisol level is decreased over time as a response to very high rates of cortisol release. This might also explain the disparate findings of glucocorticoid levels in young and old patients with PTSD (see de Quervain, 2006; Grossman et al., 2006). For instance, it was reported recently that administration of cortisol may enhance episodic and working memory functioning in aged patients with PTSD (Yehuda, Harvey, Buchsbaum, Tischler, & Schmeidler, 2007).

As pointed out earlier in this chapter, stress can change neural functioning, at least at the level of synaptic transmission and plasticity (Alfarez, Wiegert, & Krugers, 2006). Although discussed controversially, stress may also increase neural aging and, accordingly, cell death (Epel et al., 2004; Raz & Rodrigue, 2006; Susman, 2006; Szeszko et al., 2006). Higher cortisol levels seem to play an important role in stress-related neural decline, as proposed by Porter and Landfield (1998). They argue that a higher cortisol release primarily interacts with pyramidal cells of the hippocampal formation (Figure 13.2), resulting in an increase of excitatory synaptic transmissions. These are linked to an increase of intracellular calcium, which may be linked to synthesis of free radicals. These free radicals can affect the neuron's functioning and can be neurotoxic. This model explains why long-term and excessive stress can lead to decrease of neural density and – most importantly – why some

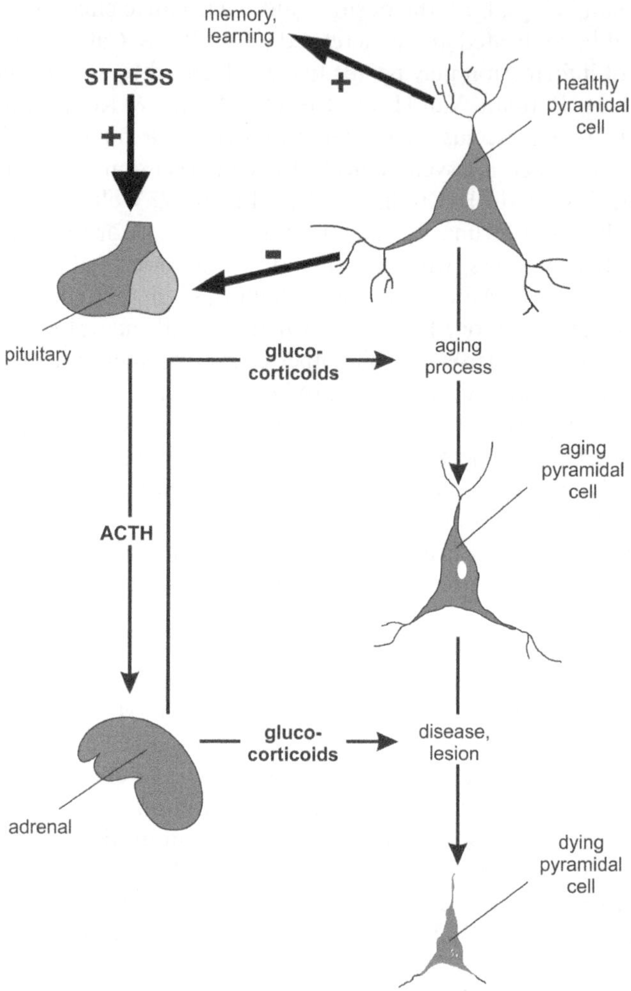

Figure 13.2 Summary of the steps of stress-related damage to hippocampal neurons as proposed by Porter and Landfield (1998). It is assumed that stress activates the pituitary gland, which delivers adenocorticotrope hormone (ACTH). In the adrenal cortex, ACTH triggers the release of glucocorticoids (e.g., cortisol), which can influence hippocampal neurons as they have a high density of glucocorticoid receptors. An excessive activation of these receptors may initiate intracellular mechanisms, resulting in acceleration of the cell's age and finally in the neuron's death.

brain regions are more vulnerable to stress-related cell death than are others (but see the critical review by Jelicic & Merckelbach, 2004).

On the other hand, there are also studies demonstrating that stress-induced hippocampal changes are less stable than previously assumed (Hibberd, Yau, & Seckl, 2000; McEwen, Magariños, & Reagan, 2002) and that beyond the level of glucocorticoids, plasticity of the *N*-methyl-D-aspartate receptors is also involved in hippocampal neural cell loss (McEwen, 1997, 1999).

Post-traumatic stress disorder

A psychological syndrome that is associated with stress is post-traumatic stress disorder. In such patients, hippocampal volume loss has been reported commonly (Bremner, 2001; Bremner, Elzinga, Schmahl, & Vermetten, 2007; Bremner et al., 2003; Elzinga & Bremner, 2002; Li et al., 2006). There is also evidence for structural or functional changes of other limbic structures (e.g., amygdala and insula) in patients with PTSD, as recently demonstrated by several studies (e.g., Bremner, 2007b; Bremner et al., 2007; Chen et al., 2006). In particular, there is convincing evidence for a greater amygdala activity in patients with PTSD that is comparable to that observed in patients with anxiety disorders (e.g., social or specific phobia) (Etkin & Wager, 2007; Gilboa et al., 2004; Phan, Britton, Taylor, Fig, & Liberzon, 2006; Stein, Simmons, Feinstein, & Paulus, 2007).

For instance, Shin et al. (2004) investigated hippocampal functioning in a group of 16 firefighters, 8 of whom had PTSD. Shin et al. used positron emission tomography (^{15}O-PET) measuring regional cerebral blood flow and a standard experimental design (a word stem completion task). The PTSD group showed stronger activations in the hippocampal formation bilaterally and in the left amygdala compared with the group of firefighters without PTSD. Within the PTSD group, the hippocampal formation was the stronger activated the more the participants had higher symptom severity. Shin et al. concluded that this abnormal pattern of hippocampal activation during recollection of non-emotional material may reflect that the hippocampal formation is less effective in patients with PTSD, resulting in an overactivation even in less complex or less personal and emotional tasks. It may contribute to a less effective inhibition of the amygdala, which was found abnormally activated in patients with PTSD or anxiety disorders (Paquette et al., 2003; Shin, Rauch, & Pitman, 2006; Straube, Glauer, Dilger, Mentzel, & Miltner, 2006).

A limbic dysregulation in patients with PTSD was also recently reported by Driessen et al. (2004). They used fMRI to investigate retrieval of traumatic, and of negative but non-traumatic, autobiographical episodes in two samples: one with borderline personality disorder (BPD) and a second group of individuals with both BPD and PTSD. In the fMRI paradigm applied, individual keywords were displayed to induce remembering of specific autobiographical events (obtained from a semi-structured interview prior to the scans). Two out of four episodes described by the participants had a negative valence but were rated as non-traumatic. These events did not meet the *DSM-IV* criteria for traumatic events, although they were personally relevant and negatively coloured. The other two episodes were rated as traumatic by the participants and fulfilled *DSM-IV* criteria for traumatic events (APA, 1994; see the criteria for diagnosis of PTSD). Interestingly, in the sample of patients with both BPD and PTSD, activations were found in sensorimotor and temporal regions as well as of the amygdala (bilateral) when comparing traumatic with non-traumatic events. In patients with BPD but without PTSD symptoms, activation of the bilateral orbitofrontal cortex preponderated.

In addition to hippocampal and amygdalar volume reductions (e.g., Vermetten, Schmahl, Lindner, Loewenstein, & Bremner, 2006) and an exaggerated amygdala activity in patients with PTSD, the medial prefrontal cortex and its control function on amygdala activity seems to be diminished (Shin et al., 2005). In summary, dysregulations within a network consisting of hippocampal formation, amygdala, cingulate gyrus, and medial prefrontal cortex most likely contribute to the stress-related symptoms in patients with PTSD (Bremner, 2007b, 2007c; Bremner et al., 2007). It is also very likely that these structural and functional brain alterations are responsible for the memory deficits seen in patients with PTSD (Bremner, 2007a; Wessa, Jatzko, & Flor, 2006). These deficits mainly comprise autobiographical memory changes characterized by a tendency to overgeneralization as well as intrusive or involuntary memories and rumination (Brewin, 2007; Bryant, Sutherland, & Guthrie, 2007; Evans, Ehlers, Mezey, & Clark, 2007; Moore & Zoellner, 2007; Schönfeld & Ehlers, 2006; Schönfeld, Ehlers, Böllinghaus, & Rief, 2007; Speckens, Ehlers, Hackmann, Ruths, & Clark, 2007). However, this phenomenon was also seen in individuals who experienced a trauma but who did not develop PTSD symptoms (Raes, Hermans, Williams, & Eelen, 2005). This type of autobiographical memory disorder in PTSD may affect other cognitive functions, such as social problem solving (Sutherland & Bryant, 2008) and may therefore contribute to the course of PTSD symptoms (Sutherland & Bryant, 2007).

In summary, there is growing evidence for functional brain changes in patients with PTSD beyond the described structural alterations of limbic structures. Both volume reductions in medial temporal structures and functional changes of amygdala activity most likely contribute to the patients' autobiographical memory alterations. The phenomena described provide insightful examples for the significant impact of environmental influences on autobiographical memory functioning, as they demonstrate that stress and trauma experiences may go along with specific brain responses and associated functional dysregulations. Nonetheless, the influence of environmental factors (trauma experiences) on autobiographical memory integrity can be even more pronounced than is seen in patients with PTSD. Trauma experiences can be followed by a complete loss of the ability to remember the personal past. This is the issue discussed in the next section.

The mnestic block syndrome

Beyond amnesia caused by focal or more general (degenerative) brain damage, retrograde memory impairments can also occur in the absence of observable structural brain changes. As outlined above, stress and stress-related syndromes (e.g., PTSD) can affect autobiographical memory functioning. One of these syndromes is referred to as dissociative amnesia, a condition that is characterized by reduced retrograde memory, primarily for personal events, in the absence of a neurological causation (Brandt & van Gorp, 2006; Kopelman, 2000). Other terms used to describe this condition are "functional" or "psychogenic" amnesia, although all these terminologies are discussed controversially. Markowitsch introduced the term "mnestic block syndrome" in order to describe the phenomenon of autobiographical amnesia without referring to a clear causation, but highlighting the role of massive or long-lasting stress or traumas in the development of amnesic symptoms in these patients (e.g., Markowitsch, 2002; Markowitsch et al., 1999b, 2000). In this chapter, however, we use the terms "mnestic block syndrome" and "dissociative" or "psychogenic" amnesia interchangeably. We will show that even in patients with this type of amnesia, functional brain alterations can be demonstrated using modern functional imaging techniques.

Clinical features of the mnestic block syndrome: Examples

Even though severe reductions in remembering autobiographical-episodic content are the most common symptoms in patients with mnestic block syndrome (Markowitsch, 2003b), the amnesia can additionally affect personal semantic facts as well as general semantic knowledge (Fujiwara et al., 2008b). Nevertheless, even in cases with both autobiographical-episodic and semantic memory impairments, the episodic domain is affected much more severely (Brandt & van Gorp, 2006; Markowitsch, 2003b). Amnesia comprises either the whole lifespan or specific time periods. In addition, on a content-based level, deficits can affect all autobiographical memories or distinct contents such as business-related episodes or other purposes in life.

The predominant role of stress or stressful life events in the causation of a mnestic block syndrome can be seen in several cases reported. One example is the case DO described by Markowitsch, Thiel, Kessler, von Stockhausen, and Heiss (1997b). DO was a 59-years-old female patient who suffered from selective memory loss covering the age between 10 and 16 years. Over this period of time, she was presumably abused repeatedly. During psychotherapeutic interventions, DO painted different scenes related to the abuse but without having conscious access to these scenes. Markowitsch et al. (1997b) conducted a functional imaging investigation (^{15}O-PET) in which these pictures were presented. In addition, as a control condition, more neutral pictures to which DO had conscious access were shown. Both conditions led to an increased activation of the right anterior temporal cortex, but the increase was stronger in the "unconscious" or "semi-conscious" condition than in the "neutral" or "conscious" condition. Results indicate that the scenes related to the abuse were processed in an emotional way, even though she did not have full awareness for the emotions and details related to the events presented in the paintings. The findings emphasize that even traumas that happened many years ago can be linked to specific functional brain changes and can alter the neural correlates of emotional memory retrieval.

Another interesting case of mnestic block syndrome described by Markowitsch, Fink, Thöne, Kessler, and Heiss (1997a) is that of a 37-year-old male patient who left his house in the morning to buy rolls for breakfast. Instead of coming home, he continued cycling for five days along the Rhine River. During this time, as revealed retrospectively, he had no idea about who he was and did not recognize himself in display windows. This condition is referred to as "dissociative fugue" (e.g., Loewenstein, 1996; Serra, Fadda, Buccione, Caltagirone, & Carlesimo, 2007), formerly known as *Wanderlust* (wandering) (Markowitsch, 1992), characterized by sudden loss of autobiographical memory accompanied by travelling away from home. After the patient described by Markowitsch et al. (1997a) was found and accommodated in a psychiatric clinic, he was examined neuropsychologically and with neurological and neuroradiological techniques. No signs of brain abnormalities were detected, although he persistently suffered from amnesia for personal events prior to the onset of the fugue. In a ^{15}O-PET investigation with an autobiographical-episodic memory task (on the basis of the design by Fink et al., 1996), in which the patient was asked to imagine scenes of his own life (collected from his wife and other relatives and triggered by sentences) or scenes taken from the life of others, respectively, the patient activated predominantly left hemispheric regions during both conditions. In the study by Fink et al. (1996), healthy volunteers had primarily right hemispheric activations during processing autobiographical events and left hemispheric activations during processing scenes taken from other persons. The finding in the patient reported by Markowitsch et al. (1997a) may therefore reflect that he processed his own biography in a more neutral and verbal way, as healthy individuals do when they imagine scenes that are unrelated to their biographies.

More recently, Glisky et al. (2004) described another case of a male patient with dissociative fugue, who travelled from Germany to the United States and "forgot" his biography and his native German-language capacities. While the patient could not retrieve explicitly knowledge about his personal past, he apparently used implicit information about autobiographical facts and some semantic or associative language aspects, as revealed by several neuropsychological, psychophysiological, and functional imaging examinations. In summary, the cases reported by Markowitsch et al. (1997a) as well as by Glisky et al. (2004) demonstrate that memory loss associated with the relatively rare syndrome of dissociative fugue may have neuropsychological and neuroimaging correlates. In addition, amnesia is not restricted to personal autobiographical memories but can also affect basic abilities, such as the first language. In both patients, exposure to stress prior to the onset of amnesia could be revealed retrospectively, emphasizing the critical role of stressful or traumatic events in the causation of dissociative amnesic syndromes.

A further patient who suffered from retrograde amnesia following a traumatic event is case AMN (Markowitsch, Kessler, Van der Ven, Weber-Luxenburger, & Heiss, 1998). AMN, a 23-year-old male patient, became retrogradely amnesic following a fire in his house. He suddenly lost his autobiographical memories of the last six years (age between 17 and 23 years). Any organic causation (e.g., hypoxia) was excluded by excessive neurological and neuroradiological examinations (MRI, EEG, blood investigation). In addition to the retrograde memory impairments, AMN also suffered from anterograde amnesia and executive deficits, while his general intellectual abilities were preserved. Markowitsch et al. (1998) conducted a PET investigation – [^{18}F]-fluorodeoxyglucose-PET (FDG-PET) – revealing metabolic reductions in temporofrontal regions. The metabolic decrease was comparable to patients with organic retrograde amnesia (e.g., in the course of hypoxia). The question remained as to why the fire in AMN's house initiated the autobiographical memory loss. During extensive psychotherapeutic interventions, AMN reported that he was traumatized during childhood (at the age of 4 years), as he had to follow a man dying in a burning car. Therefore, the fire in his house at the age of 23 years was interpreted as a re-traumatization linked to a massive release of stress hormones that blocked the retrieval of autobiographical memories (O'Brien, 1997). The time gradient (memory loss covering the last six years) may result from the life events happening during this time period (e.g., severe conflicts with his parents, leaving both home and school). After one year of extensive psychotherapy and psychopharmacological interventions, AMN recovered from both retrograde and anterograde amnesia. In the course of recovering from memory impairments, his brain metabolism also normalized, as shown by a second FDG-PET scan twelve months after onset of amnesia (Markowitsch et al., 2000). This case demonstrates two important issues: First, functional brain correlates of autobiographical retrograde amnesia can be revealed even in the absence of observable structural brain damage. Functional changes can be comparable to those of patients with an organic causation of amnesic syndrome. Second, brain dysfunctions linked to memory loss in patients with mnestic block syndrome can normalize in the course of recovery from memory impairments. Recovering from mnestic block syndrome associated with normalization of metabolic brain dysfunctions was also reported by Yasuno et al. (2000).

Neuropsychological profile in patients with mnestic block syndrome: Are there commonalities?

The most prominent symptom of mnestic block syndrome is without doubt a disproportionate deficit of retrograde memory compared to other neuropsychological alterations. As the amnesia can comprise several days, months, or years or the whole lifespan, a temporal gradient of preserved and deteriorated retrograde memory can substantially differ across patients. Beyond the autobiographical-episodic memory domain, most of the patients may additionally suffer from semantic memory reductions, either restricted to the autobiographical-semantic memory or to both personal and general semantic memory (Barbarotto, Laiacona, & Cocchini, 1996; Fujiwara et al., 2004; Fujiwara et al., 2008b; Kritchevsky, Chang, & Squire, 2004; Markowitsch, 2003b). Nevertheless, in patients with mnestic block syndrome, an implicit use of "forgotten" information can be demonstrated when tasks implicitly assess remote memory (Kopelman, Christensen, Puffett, & Stanhope, 1994) (a detailed discussion of this point can be found in the article by Fujiwara et al., 2008b).

Whether or not retrograde amnesia of dissociative origin is accompanied by anterograde memory deficits, as seen in patient AMN, is still a matter of debate, and previous findings are disparate. In some cases, clear evidence for additional anterograde amnesic symptoms were reported (Kritchevsky et al., 2004; Markowitsch et al., 1998). However, there are also other patients without anterograde memory reductions (De Renzi, Lucchelli, Muggia, & Spinnler, 1997; Fujiwara, 2008b; Glisky et al., 2004). Unfortunately, multiple-case and group studies with patients suffering from dissociative amnesia appear very seldomly, given that the syndrome is relatively rare. In a first group study by Kritchevsky et al. (2004), including 9 patients with dissociative amnesia (note that 1 out of the 10 initially examined patients reported that he had simulated the amnesic symptoms), 5 patients showed signs of verbal anterograde memory reductions, while 4 patients performed normally. In a recent study by Brand et al. (in press), 14 patients with dissociative amnesia were investigated neuropsychologically and with FDG-PET. All patients had severe autobiographical-episodic memory deficits covering either the whole lifespan or several days or weeks to years. Semantic memory (both personal semantic and general semantic information) was affected in 8 patients. Regarding potential accompanying neuropsychological deficits, results were mixed. Moderate to severe anterograde memory impairments were present in 6 patients, and 7 patients had symptoms of executive dysfunctions. The majority of patients with severe executive problems also had more pronounced retrograde memory deficits than those with normal executive functioning. However, this was not the case in a convergent manner for those with additional anterograde amnesia. The finding of a relationship between executive functions and retrograde amnesia is in accordance with previous studies indicating that cognitive flexibility, categorization, and problem solving are important basic functions for a successful recall of autobiographical-episodic memories (see above). It also emphasizes the assumptions by Kopelman (2000) that executive deteriorations contribute to retrieval deficits in patients with dissociative amnesia (see also the case reported by Glisky et al., 2004).

In a multiple-case study, Fujiwara et al. (2008b) examined neuropsychological functions in 5 patients (3 men, 2 women) with mnestic block syndrome. They used an extensive test battery assessing retrograde memory (autobiographical-episodic, autobiographical-semantic, and general semantic memory) and the main neuropsychological functions (intelligence, verbal and figural anterograde memory, executive functions, attention and concentration, speed of information processing). Beyond these standard neuropsychological domains, they also used several tasks assessing emotional processing and theory-of-mind/perspective-taking functions and assessed personality and psychological–psychiatric symptoms with standardized instruments. As a result, the patients differed regarding several aspects. The age range was between 17 and 35 years. The critical life events that were followed by the onset of amnesia also differed across subjects: unconsciousness for unknown reasons during an apprenticeship, car accident, falling down under the shower, following anaesthesia, and in the course of travelling away from home for unknown reasons (see *Wanderlust*, mentioned above). Also, the time for which the patients had amnesia differed between 12 years prior to the incident and the whole lifespan. Given this heterogeneity, one might also expect differences in the patients' neuropsychological profile. This was, in fact, observed for the anterograde memory domain: 2 patients had mild impairments while the other 3 subjects performed normally. In the other domains assessed, no systematic impairments across the subjects were found, with two exceptions: All 5 patients had deficits in at least one task assessing executive functions. In addition, 3 of 4 patients in whom theory-of-mind functions were examined by the "Reading the mind in the eyes" test (Baron-Cohen, Wheelwright, Hill, Raste, & Plumb, 2001) showed reductions in processing the facial emotional expression of other people.

The importance of emotional and self-related processing in retrieving autobiographical memories was pointed out by Tulving in his definition of episodic memory (Tulving, 2005). Evidence for the link between disturbances in both remembering personal episodes and processing emotional stimuli comes from two female adolescent patients with probable psychogenic amnesia reported recently by Reinhold and Markowitsch (2007). The patients suffered from severe amnesia covering the whole lifespan following stressful events. While they performed normally on all standard neuropsychological tasks (including anterograde memory, intelligence, executive functions), they showed reductions in basic emotional processing (facial affect discrimination) and in theory-of-mind functions, measured by the "Reading the mind in the eyes" test (Baron-Cohen et al., 2001) and theory-of-mind stories. In addition to the test results, both patients were described by themselves and their relatives as being emotionally detached as they were unable to perceive changes in emotionality in others and to react adequately (*la belle indifference*). The authors concluded that emotional dysregulations, in combination with changes in autonoetic awareness, can disrupt successful retrieval of autobiographical memories that – as stated above – have a strong link to emotions and the self.

The results by Reinhold and Markowitsch (2007) are in accordance with other recent investigations indicating that theory-of-mind deficits may be a core phenomenon in patients with dissociative or psychogenic amnesia (e.g., the study, summarized above, by Fujiwara et al., 2008b). The association of perspective-taking capacities and autobiographical memory has already been described by Corcoran and Frith (2003) in patients with schizophrenia. The results indicate that patients with schizophrenia are reduced in the application of contextual information to retrieve specific information embedded in a socially relevant situation. This "general" deficit may result in autobiographical memory impairments (when information about personal events and situations has to be retrieved). It may also explain the more basic autobiographical memory reductions in schizophrenia – that is, the difference between autonoetic remembering and noetic knowing (e.g., Sonntag et al., 2003). Also, emotional judgments, as required in theory-of-mind tasks, may also be affected by a disability to recall emotionally coloured personal events previously experienced, as remembering feelings can trigger the perception and attribution of emotional states in others.

In summary, recent reports of patients with mnestic block syndrome show a high range of inter-individual differences with respect to neuropsychological reductions that may accompany the retrograde amnesia. Given the complexity of the syndrome, consisting of different clinical facets and neuropsychological profiles, a multidimensional approach in diagnosing dissociative amnesia is most appropriate (Serra et al., 2007). Nevertheless, there are also some commonalities across patients. The findings summarized emphasize a relationship between executive functioning, emotional processing, autonoetic consciousness, and autobiographical memory, as proposed by Tulving (2002, 2005), and demonstrate that disruptions in any of these components may affect the others (see also Kopelman, 2000).

Neuroimaging findings in patients with mnestic block syndrome

General considerations

In the previous paragraphs of this chapter, we already summarized some results of neuroimaging investigations in patients with probable mnestic block syndrome. It is apparent that findings are disparate in detail and that it is hardly possible to argue convincingly for one single brain structure being responsible for the patients' memory disorders. When summarizing potential neural correlates of the mnestic block syndrome, one has to keep in mind that the core of this condition is that the patients have no structural brain damage, at least to a degree detectable by current structural imaging techniques (e.g., low-Tesla MRI). As described in the case reports summarized above, brain changes were found on a functional level (e.g., in glucose metabolism, or cerebral blood flow), as demonstrated by functional imaging techniques. When trying to figure out commonalities of mnestic block syndrome's neural correlates, it is important to consider differential sensitivities of the specific methods used (PET and fMRI), as parameters measured by these methods differ with respect to several aspects. For instance, glucose utilization and cerebral blood flow (PET measures) or blood oxygen level dependent signals (fMRI) have distinct time resolutions and are not directly comparable.

In addition, the parameters measured by the techniques mentioned are indirect indicators for neural activity only, and they have differential validity and reliability for measuring neural responses. This might, at least partially, explain the heterogeneity of findings described in previous studies. Furthermore, some studies measured neural activity (indirectly) during resting-state, while other investigations used an activation design, meaning that they studied neural correlates of the patients' retrieval attempt. Here, the activation designs used also differ across studies (e.g., pictures or sentences as triggers for autobiographical-episodic retrieval). Therefore, one has to be very cautious in comparing single findings of previous studies. This is also important to bear in mind as the mnestic block syndrome is a very rare condition, and, until now, no group studies have been available that analysed both neuropsychological and neuroimaging data in patients with this condition.

Considering the limitations mentioned above, we nonetheless summarize some neuroimaging studies with patients suffering from mnestic block syndrome, pointing out that prefrontal regions (together with medial temporal areas) might be candidates for being critically involved in the symptoms of retrograde autobiographical-episodic memory deficits. Before we try to make inferences on neural correlates of this amnesic condition, we will start with a further description of a patient with dissociative amnesia in order to comment on different methodological aspects that need attention.

An example of a neuroimaging investigation in a patient with mnestic block syndrome and methodological constraints

In a recently published review on neuroimaging in memory disturbances (Reinhold, Kühnel, Brand, & Markowitsch, 2006), we described a female patient who was amnesic for the whole lifespan, including her name and other personal facts. The patient, KL, a 43-year-old woman, fell down a staircase at work two years prior to the investigation (at the age of 41 years). She became unconscious for a few minutes and thereafter did not recognize any person around her (e.g., her colleagues who found her). She was disoriented with respect to time, place, and situation. KL was admitted to a local hospital, where she recognized neither her husband nor her son who visited her. In addition, she was unable to remember her name and was completely amnesic regarding her whole life. Medical investigations including structural MRI did not find any brain abnormality. The amnesic condition was still unchanged two years after the onset of amnesia. In addition, she developed severe symptoms of depression. A few months prior to our neuropsychological investigation, she attempted suicide.

In the neuropsychological test battery conducted two years after onset of amnesia, KL showed normal to above-average performance in standard anterograde memory tests, as well as normal intelligence, executive functioning, and information processing. Her retrograde amnesia was still present with a focus on autobiographical-episodic and autobiographic-semantic memories. Her general semantic memory was also lower than average. However, she was able to re-learn her biography within the last two years, but she did not have emotional access to the events, which were described in an almost neutral way. In addition, she was very insecure about whether or not the events re-learned were really true, as all information about her life was dependent on descriptions given by her relatives. For instance, she was insecure whether her son was really her son.

In order to investigate potential neural correlates of her autobiographical-episodic amnesia, we conducted a ^{15}O-PET examination using (A) photographs of herself that were made during the time for which she was amnesic (amnesia condition), (B) pictures of herself made within the last two years (after amnesia onset) for which she was not amnesic (non-amnesia condition), and (C) photographs of unknown women comparable with respect to the visual input (i.e., women in situations comparable to the situations of Conditions A and B – e.g., a woman drinking a cup of coffee). Examples of the material used are shown in Figure 13.3. The photographs of KL were not seen by herself prior to the PET scan (we obtained the pictures from her husband, who received them from other relatives and friends). During the PET investigation, KL should try to remember the situation in which each photograph was made. After the scan, we did a debriefing, asking KL whether or not she could recognize herself on the pictures during the scan and whether or not she was able to recall the specific situation shown in the pictures. In summary, she recognized herself on each photo of both conditions (A and B) but could remember the situations presented on photographs of Condition B only (the non-amnesic condition consisting of photos after the onset of amnesia).

The activation pattern in KL when subtracting Condition B from Condition A comprised the right dorsolateral prefrontal section and the left cerebellum. In the reverse contrast (non-amnesic minus amnesic condition), the right medial frontal region and the right cingulate gyrus were activated. Results suggest that retrieval attempt of episodes for which she was amnesic was associated with regions classically linked to retrieval effort (Buckner, 2003; Lepage et al., 2000; Rugg et al., 2002; Velanova et al., 2003). In contrast, activations found when she (successfully) remembered episodes from the non-amnesic time period were comparable to those frequently shown in healthy subjects (Markowitsch et al., 2003; Piefke et al., 2003, 2005) (medial frontal and limbic regions – see description above of the relevance of limbic and medial frontal circuits for autobiographical memory retrieval). In conclusion, the differential activation pattern demonstrated in KL may be interpreted as distinct neural correlates of her autobiographical retrograde amnesia in the absence of structural brain damage.

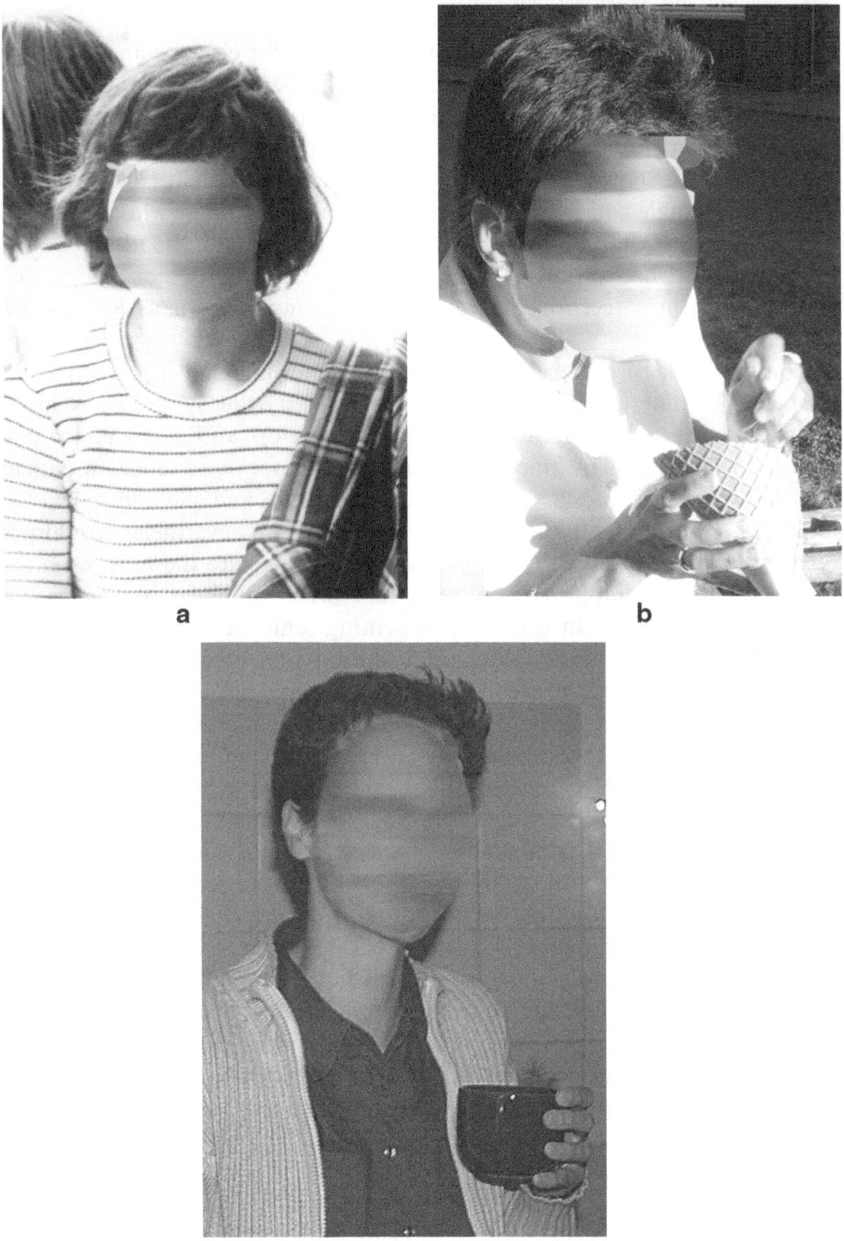

Figure 13.3 Stimuli used in the PET investigation of KL's autobiographical memory disturbance. The pictures of Condition A show KL in situations before the onset of amnesia (events that were not retrievable = amnesic time period). Pictures of Condition B were taken after onset of amnesia (episodes that are retrievable = non-amnesic time period), and Condition C consists of pictures of unknown women in situations comparable to those of Conditions A and B. (For more details, see the text and the description in Reinhold et al., 2006.)

One has to keep in mind that there are also other circumstances that go along with difficulties in remembering specific personal situations on the basis of personal photographs. For instance, it is documented that patients with Alzheimer's disease may have a temporal gradient in recognizing themselves in photos. For instance, Hehman, German, and Klein (2005) recently described a female patient with late-stage Alzheimer's disease who was able to recognize herself on pictures from the very past (e.g., childhood and young adulthood) but had problems remembering recent episodes or recognizing herself in pictures recently made – a phenomenon known as Ribot's law (Ribot, 1892).

Coming back to more general aspects of neuroimaging in patients with dissociative amnesia, one has to consider that as the syndrome is interindividually very heterogeneous, one must develop and apply individual activation paradigms in functional imaging studies. For instance, in patient KL, the onset of amnesia was two years previously, and she had re-learned most of her autobiography. As mentioned above, she nevertheless could not re-experience the events, though she was able to narrate the most essential events of her biography (all episodes had been explained to her by her relatives and friends). In this case, presenting sentences that describe such "milestones" of her life could have triggered remembering the situation in which she re-learned the events (e.g., "My husband has told me that I had a moped accident at the age of 17 years"). Therefore, a design was developed consisting of stimuli (the photos) that were more concrete, not verbal but visual, and had not been seen or discussed before. (A comprehensive review of various techniques to study autobiographical memory and to collect information about a person's biography and building adequate items for a functional imaging investigation can be found in the article by Cabeza & St Jacques, 2007.) Although we think that applying such an experimental design was fruitful in patient KL, it is not applicable to all patients. Given that we need to obtain photographs from both the amnesic and the non-amnesic time period, it would be very difficult to collect pictures from distinct episodes when the onset of amnesia has occurred more recently. It is also not principally possible to conduct the same paradigm with PET or fMRI, as typically more stimuli are needed for an fMRI investigation than for a PET design. While fMRI, in principle, has a higher resolution with respect to time (at least event-related designs) and space, which is a clear advantage compared to PET, some patients cannot be scanned by MRI as they, for example, have metal in their bodies, suffer from claustrophobia, have vision disorders that have to be compensated for by glasses, and so on.

These few examples of constraints in the context of neuroimaging investigations with patients suffering from mnestic block syndrome emphasize the remarkableness of considering the individually most adequate technique in combination with developing a design that fits best with the subject's symptoms and course of the amnesia.

Synthesis of previous functional imaging studies in patients with mnestic block syndrome

Considering the limitations mentioned at the beginning of this section, and given that previous functional brain abnormalities described in these patients differ across studies (see the review by Reinhold et al., 2006) and that there is no consensus as yet about the most critical neural correlate of the patients' memory dysfunction in the literature, some regions seem more likely to be linked to dissociative amnesia than are others. Some studies that measured brain responses to stimuli triggering autobiographical memory retrieval found abnormal activation patterns mainly within limbic and prefrontal regions (Fujiwara et al., 2004; Markowitsch et al., 1997b; Yasuno et al., 2000). To the best of our knowledge, the recent study by Fujiwara et al. (2004) is the first one that investigated neural correlates of the autobiographical retrieval blockade in a sample of at least three patients with mnestic block syndrome using the same activation design for all subjects. They interviewed the patients' relatives about the patients' lives and asked them to report specific events that had happened in the patients' lives prior to the critical incident (before onset of amnesia = amnesic time period). The relatives also described episodes from the time after onset of amnesia (= non-amnesic time period). Based on this information, Fujiwara et al. constructed sentences describing the different episodes obtained from the interviews. In the fMRI experiments, the sentences describing events from the amnesic and those referring to episodes from the non-amnesic time period were presented to the patients (in a block design in accordance with the paradigm used by Piefke et al., 2003). In addition, fictitious episodes were also presented, as control items. The patients were asked to remember the distinct episodes described by the sentences, if possible. In the three patients studied by Fujiwara et al., differential activation patterns were found for successful retrieval of events from the non-amnesic time period (after onset of amnesia) and retrieval attempts (events from the amnesic time period). The retrieval success was measured by post-scanning debriefing, which indicated that the subjects indeed remembered the events from the non-amnesic, but not from the amnesic, time. Comparing the patterns across patients showed several individual activities. Nevertheless, there was evidence for a contribution of the (left) prefrontal cortex when differentiating between true and fictitious events, even within the amnesic time period. Most likely, the activation of the prefrontal cortex during retrieval attempt may reflect retrieval effort and retrieval mode (Buckner, 2003; Lepage et al., 2000; Rugg et al., 2002; Velanova et al., 2003), which was stronger for the events that were not retrievable. Results are also in accordance with other previous single-case studies emphasizing that frontal (and temporal) regions show functional alterations in patients with dissociative amnesia when they are confronted with an autobiographical memory task (e.g., Markowitsch et al., 1997a, 1997b).

Given that there is little consistency in the functional imaging designs used in studying neural correlates of the mnestic block syndrome (see comments above), and given that patients with this syndrome may also have more general functional brain abnormalities in the absence of structural damage, it seems to be worth examining general brain functioning independently from performing a memory task. For instance, patients may show reductions in glucose utilization even in a "resting-state" paradigm. Glucose metabolism was assessed in several patients with mnestic block syndrome using FDG-PET. Results are somewhat disparate. In some patients glucose utilization was normal compared to the healthy population (Dalla Barba, Mantovan, Ferruzza, & Denes, 1997; De Renzi & Lucchelli, 1993; De Renzi, Lucchelli, Muggia, & Spinnler, 1995; Kessler et al., 1997; Markowitsch, Kessler, Kalbe, & Herholz, 1999a; Markowitsch et al., 1999b; Reinvang & Gjerstad, 1998) (see also case EF in Fujiwara et al., 2008b). By contrast, in other patients, reductions of brain glucose metabolism (or hypoperfusion, measured by single photon emission computed tomography) were found, mainly within temporal, prefrontal, or (other) limbic regions (Costello, Fletcher, Dolan, Frith, & Shallice, 1998; Lucchelli, Muggia, & Spinnler, 1995; Markowitsch, 1996; Markowitsch et al., 1997a, 1998; Sellal, Manning, Seegmuller, Scheiber, & Schoenfelder, 2002). An example of reduced glucose utilization within the medial temporal lobe (bilaterally) in a male patient with mnestic block syndrome is shown in Figure 13.4.

As outlined above, medial temporal and prefrontal regions are necessarily engaged in retrieving autobiographic-episodic memories. Patients with mnestic block syndrome frequently have emotional alterations – seen, for instance, in theory-of-mind tasks, as summarized above. For processing emotions and self-relevant information in the context of episodic retrieval, prefrontal and limbic structures are crucial (Keenan, Wheeler, & Ewers, 2003; Tulving, 2002; Wheeler & Stuss, 2003). Given these considerations, patients with mnestic block syndrome may show functional abnormalities in these areas. This hypothesis was confirmed by Piolino et al. (2005). Their case of a patient with dissociative retrograde amnesia showed reduced glucose utilization in a FDG-PET investigation within the ventrolateral (or inferolateral) prefrontal cortex. Further evidence for dysfunctions of the ventral prefrontal area in patients with mnestic block syndrome comes from a recent study in which we analysed the brain glucose metabolism in a sample of 14 patients suffering from this amnesia type (Brand et al., in press). While there was a clear variability across the patients with respect to regions found hypometabolic in comparison with normative data, the group analysis (patients vs. a sample of 19 healthy control participants) revealed a significant metabolic reduction in the right ventrolateral prefrontal cortex. The glucose metabolism in this region was also significantly reduced in 10 of the 14 patients in individual comparisons with the control group. Although the results are preliminary and need replication, we argue that the finding of a hypometabolism in this right prefrontal area most likely reflects the patients' deficits to integrate

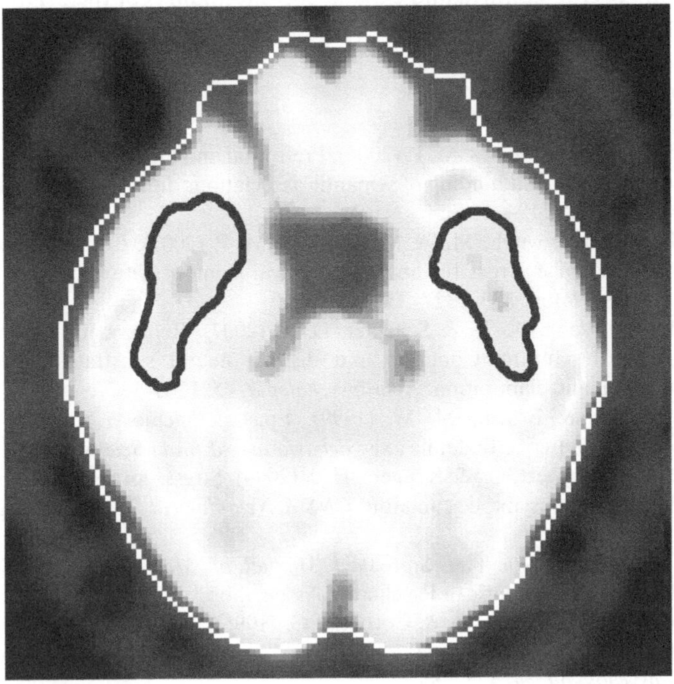

Figure 13.4 FDG-PET examination (measuring glucose utilization) in a male patient with mnestic block syndrome (horizontal view). The medial temporal lobe (bilaterally) was hypometabolic (indicated by the darker grey, framed). The other brain regions showed normal glucose utilization. (This figure is published in colour at http://www.cognitiveneurosciencearena.com/brain-scans/.)

autobiographical memories related to the self and the subjective emotional connotation (see the definition of autobiographical memory as proposed by Tulving in his recent articles, 2002, 2005).

Conclusion

Stress-related memory disorders can have different forms and accentuations (e.g., overgeneral memory and intrusions in PTSD, retrograde amnesia in mnestic block syndrome). Even though the clinical features of the mnestic block syndrome can vary across patients, there are some commonalities that concern executive reductions and abnormalities in emotional processing. In patients with mnestic block syndrome, functional brain changes can be demonstrated in the absence of structural damage. Temporal and prefrontal regions are most likely candidates for neural correlates of the patients' autobiographical memory retrieval disturbances. Further research – especially group studies with patients suffering from mnestic block syndrome – are needed in order to confirm and expand current findings of the brain–amnesia interaction in this condition.

References

Addis, D. R., & McAndrews, M. P. (2006). Prefrontal and hippocampal contributions to the generation and binding of semantic associations during successful encoding. *NeuroImage*, *33*, 1194–1206.

Addis, D. R., Moscovitch, M., & McAndrews, M. P. (2007). Consequences of hippocampal damage across the autobiographical memory network in left temporal lobe epilepsy. *Brain*, *130*, 2327–2342.

Addis, D. R., Wong, A. T., & Schacter, D. L. (2007). Remembering the past and imagining the future: Common and distinct neural substrates during event construction and elaboration. *Neuropsychologia*, *45*, 1363–1377.

Aggleton, J. P., & Brown, M. W. (1999). Episodic memory, amnesia, and the hippocampal-anterior thalamic axis. *Behavioral and Brain Sciences*, *22*, 425–444.

Alfarez, D. N., Wiegert, O., & Krugers, H. J. (2006). Stress, corticosteroid hormones and hippocampal synaptic function. *CNS & Neurological Disorders Drug Targets*, *5*, 521–529.

APA. (1994). *Diagnostic and Statistical Manual of Mental Disorders* (4th ed.). Washington, DC: American Psychiatric Association.

Barbarotto, R., Laiacona, M., & Cocchini, G. (1996). A case of simulated, psychogenic or focal pure retrograde amnesia: Did an entire life become unconscious? *Neuropsychologia*, *34*, 575–585.

Baron-Cohen, S., Wheelwright, S., Hill, J., Raste, Y., & Plumb, I. (2001). The "Reading the Mind in the Eyes" Test revised version: A study with normal adults, and adults with Asperger syndrome or high-functioning autism. *Journal of Child Psychology and Psychiatry*, *42*, 241–251.

Bechara, A., Damasio, H., Damasio, A. R., & Lee, G. P. (1999). Different contributions of the human amygdala and ventromedial prefrontal cortex to decision-making. *Journal of Neuroscience*, *19*, 5473–5481.

Bell, B. D., & Giovagnoli, A. R. (2007). Recent innovative studies of memory in temporal lobe epilepsy. *Neuropsychology Review*, *17*, 455–476.

Binder, J. R., Bellgowan, P. S., Hammeke, T. A., Possing, E. T., & Frost, J. A. (2005). A comparison of two FMRI protocols for eliciting hippocampal activation. *Epilepsia*, *46*, 1061–1070.

Blumenfeld, R. S., & Ranganath, C. (2006). Dorsolateral prefrontal cortex promotes long-term memory formation through its role in working memory organization. *Journal of Neuroscience*, *26*, 916–925.

Brand, M., Eggers, C., Reinhold, N., Fujiwara, E., Kessler, J., Heiss, W.-D., & Markowitsch, H. J. (in press). Functional brain imaging in fourteen patients with psychogenic amnesia reveals right inferolateral prefrontal hypometabolism. *Psychiatry Research: Neuroimaging*.

Brand, M., Fujiwara, E., Borsutzky, S., Kalbe, E., Kessler, J., & Markowitsch, H. J. (2005). Decision-making deficits of Korsakoff patients in a new gambling task with explicit rules: Associations with executive functions. *Neuropsychology*, *19*, 267–277.

Brand, M., Grabenhorst, F., Starcke, K., Vandekerckhove, M. M. P., & Markowitsch, H. J. (2007). Role of the amygdala in decisions under ambiguity and decisions under risk: Evidence from patients with Urbach-Wiethe disease. *Neuropsychologia, 45*, 1305–1317.

Brand, M., Kalbe, E., Fujiwara, E., Huber, M., & Markowitsch, H. J. (2003). Cognitive estimation in patients with probable Alzheimer's disease and alcoholic Korsakoff patients. *Neuropsychologia, 41*, 575–584.

Brand, M., & Markowitsch, H. J. (2003a). Amnesia: Neuroanatomic and clinical issues. In T. Feinberg & T. Farah (Eds.), *Behavioral neurology and neuropsychology* (pp. 431–443). New York: McGraw-Hill.

Brand, M., & Markowitsch, H. J. (2003b). The principle of bottleneck structures. In R. H. Kluwe, G. Lüer, & F. Rösler (Eds.), *Principles of learning and memory* (pp. 171–184). Basel: Birkhäuser.

Brandt, J., & van Gorp, W. G. (2006). Functional ("psychogenic") amnesia. *Seminars in Neurology, 26*, 331–340.

Bremner, J. D. (2001). Hypotheses and controversies related to effects of stress on the hippocampus: An argument for stress-induced damage to the hippocampus in patients with posttraumatic stress disorder. *Hippocampus, 11*, 75–81.

Bremner, J. D. (2007a). Functional neuroimaging in post-traumatic stress disorder. *Expert Review of Neurotherapeutics, 7*, 393–405.

Bremner, J. D. (2007b). Neuroimaging in posttraumatic stress disorder and other stress-related disorders. *Neuroimaging Clinics of North America, 17*, 523–538.

Bremner, J. D. (2007c). Traumatic stress: Effects on the brain. *Dialogues in Clinical Neuroscience, 8*, 445–461.

Bremner, J. D., Elzinga, B., Schmahl, C., & Vermetten, E. (2007). Structural and functional plasticity of the human brain in posttraumatic stress disorder. *Progress in Brain Research, 167*, 171–186.

Bremner, J. D., Vythilingam, M., Vermetten, E., Southwick, S. M., McGlashan, T., Nazeer, A., et al. (2003). MRI and PET study of deficits in hippocampal structure and function in women with childhood sexual abuse and posttraumatic stress disorder. *American Journal of Psychiatry, 160*, 924–932.

Brewin, C. R. (2007). Autobiographical memory for trauma: Update on four controversies. *Memory, 15*, 227–248.

Brokate, B., Hildebrandt, H., Eling, P., Fichtner, H., Runge, K., & Timm, C. (2003). Frontal lobe dysfunctions in Korsakoff's syndrome and chronic alcoholism: Continuity or discontinuity? *Neuropsychology, 17*, 420–428.

Broman, M., Rose, A. L., Hotson, G., & Casey, C. M. (1997). Severe anterograde amnesia with onset in childhood as a result of anoxic encephalopathy. *Brain, 120*, 417–433.

Brunner, R., Schaefer, D., Hess, K., Parzer, P., Resch, F., & Schwab, S. (2006). Effect of high-dose cortisol on memory functions. *Annals of the New York Academy of Sciences, 1071*, 434–437.

Bryant, R. A., Sutherland, K., & Guthrie, R. M. (2007). Impaired specific autobiographical memory as a risk factor for posttraumatic stress after trauma. *Journal of Abnormal Psychology, 116*, 837–841.

Buchanan, T. W., & Lovallo, W. R. (2001). Enhanced memory for emotional material following stress-level cortisol treatment in humans. *Psychoneuroendocrinology, 26*, 307–317.

Buchanan, T. W., Tranel, D., & Adolphs, R. (2006). Memories for emotional autobiographical events following unilateral damage to medial temporal lobe. *Brain, 129*, 115–127.

Buckner, R. L. (2003). Functional-anatomic correlates of control processes in memory. *Journal of Neuroscience, 23*, 3999–4004.

Buckner, R. L., Koutstaal, W., Schacter, D. L., Wagner, A. D., & Rosen, B. R. (1998). Functional-anatomic study of episodic retrieval using fMRI. I. Retrieval effort versus retrieval success. *NeuroImage, 7*, 151–162.

Buss, C., Wolf, O. T., Witt, J., & Hellhammer, D. H. (2004). Autobiographic memory impairment following acute cortisol administration. *Psychoneuroendocrinology, 29*, 1093–1096.

Cabeza, R., Dolcos, F., Graham, R., & Nyberg, L. (2002). Similarities and differences in the neural correlates of episodic memory retrieval and working memory. *NeuroImage, 16*, 317–330.

Cabeza, R., Grady, C. L., Nyberg, L., McIntosh, A. R., Tulving, E., Kapur, S., et al. (1997). Age-related differences in neural activity during memory encoding and retrieval: A positron emission tomography study. *Journal of Neuroscience, 17*, 391–400.

Cabeza, R., & Nyberg, L. (2000). Imaging cognition II: An empirical review of 275 PET and fMRI studies. *Journal of Cognitive Neuroscience, 12*, 1–47.

Cabeza, R., Prince, S. E., Daselaar, S. M., Greenberg, D. L., Budde, M., Dolcos, F., et al. (2004). Brain activity during episodic retrieval of autobiographical and laboratory events: An fMRI study using a novel photo paradigm. *Journal of Cognitive Neuroscience, 16*, 1583–1594.

Cabeza, R., & St Jacques, P. (2007). Functional neuroimaging of autobiographical memory. *Trends in Cognitive Sciences, 11*, 219–227.

Cahill, L. (2000). Emotional modulation of long-term memory storage in humans: Adrenergic activation and the amygdala. In J. P. Aggleton (Ed.), *The amygdala: A functional analysis*. Oxford, UK: Oxford University Press.

Cahill, L., Haier, R. J., White, N. S., Fallon, J., Kilpatrick, L., Lawrence, C., et al. (2001). Sex-related differences in amygdala activity during emotionally influenced memory storage. *Neurobiology of Learning and Memory, 75*, 1–9.

Chen, S., Xia, W., Li, L., Liu, J., He, Z., Zhang, Z., et al. (2006). Gray matter density reduction in the insula in fire survivors with posttraumatic stress disorder: A voxel-based morphometric study. *Psychiatry Research, 146*, 65–72.

Ciaramelli, E., & Ghetti, S. (2007). What are confabulators' memories made of? A study of subjective and objective measures of recollection in confabulation. *Neuropsychologia, 45*, 1489–1500.

Cipolotti, L., & Bird, C. M. (2006). Amnesia and the hippocampus. *Current Opinion in Neurology, 19*, 593–598.

Conway, M. A. (2003). Commentary: Cognitive-affective mechanisms and processes in autobiographical memory. *Memory, 11*, 217–224.

Conway, M. A., & Pleydell-Pearce, C. W. (2000). The construction of autobiographical memories in the self-memory system. *Psychological Review, 107*, 261–288.

Conway, M. A., Turk, D. J., Miller, S. L., Logan, J., Nebes, R. D., Cidis Meltzer, C., et al. (1999). A positron emission tomography (PET) study of autobiographical memory retrieval. *Memory, 7*, 679–702.

Corcoran, R., & Frith, C. D. (2003). Autobiographical memory and theory of mind: Evidence of a relationship in schizophrenia. *Psychological Medicine, 33*, 897–905.

Corkin, S., Amaral, D. G., Gonzalez, R. G., Johnson, K. A., & Hyman, B. T. (1997). H.M.'s medial temporal lobe lesion: Findings from magnetic resonance imaging. *Journal of Neuroscience, 17*, 3964–3979.

Costello, A., Fletcher, P. C., Dolan, R. J., Frith, C. D., & Shallice, T. (1998). The origins of forgetting in a case of isolated retrograde amnesia following a haemorrhage: Evidence from functional imaging. *Neurocase*, *4*, 437–446.

Dalla Barba, G., Mantovan, M. C., Ferruzza, E., & Denes, G. (1997). Remembering and knowing the past: A case study of isolated retrograde amnesia. *Cortex*, *33*, 143–154.

Daselaar, S. M., Rice, H. J., Greenberg, D. L., Cabeza, R., LaBar, K. S., & Rubin, D. C. (2008). The spatiotemporal dynamics of autobiographical memory: Neural correlates of recall, emotional intensity, and reliving. *Cerebral Cortex*, *18*, 217–229.

de Quervain, D. J. (2006). Glucocorticoid-induced inhibition of memory retrieval: Implications for posttraumatic stress disorder. *Annals of the New York Academy of Sciences*, *1071*, 216–220.

De Renzi, E., & Lucchelli, F. (1993). Dense retrograde amnesia, intact learning capability and abnormal forgetting rate: A consolidation deficit? *Cortex*, *29*, 449–466.

De Renzi, E., Lucchelli, F., Muggia, S., & Spinnler, H. (1995). Persistent retrograde amnesia following a minor trauma. *Cortex*, *31*, 531–542.

De Renzi, E., Lucchelli, F., Muggia, S., & Spinnler, H. (1997). Is memory without anatomical damage tantamount to a psychogenic deficit? The case of pure retrograde amnesia. *Neuropsychologia*, *35*, 781–794.

Driessen, M., Beblo, T., Mertens, M., Piefke, M., Rullkoetter, N., Silva-Saavedra, A., et al. (2004). Posttraumatic stress disorder and fMRI activation patterns of traumatic memory in patients with borderline personality disorder. *Biological Psychiatry*, *55*, 603–611.

Elliott, R. (2003). Executive functions and their disorders. *British Medical Bulletin*, *65*, 49–59.

Elzinga, B. M., & Bremner, J. D. (2002). Are the neural substrates of memory the final common pathway in posttraumatic stress disorder (PTSD)? *Journal of Affective Disorders*, *70*, 1–17.

Epel, E. S., Blackburn, E. H., Lin, J., Dhabhar, F. S., Adler, N. E., Morrow, J. D., & Cawthon, R. M. (2004). Accelerated telomere shortening in response to life stress. *Proceedings of the National Academy of Sciences USA*, *101*, 17312–17315.

Etkin, A., & Wager, T. D. (2007). Functional neuroimaging of anxiety: A meta-analysis of emotional processing in PTSD, social anxiety disorder, and specific phobia. *American Journal of Psychiatry*, *164*, 1476–1488.

Evans, C., Ehlers, A., Mezey, G., & Clark, D. M. (2007). Intrusive memories and ruminations related to violent crime among young offenders: Phenomenological characteristics. *Journal of Traumatic Stress*, *20*, 183–196.

Fink, G. R., Markowitsch, H. J., Reinkemeier, M., Bruckbauer, T., Kessler, J., & Heiss, W.-D. (1996). Cerebral representation of one's own past: Neural networks involved in autobiographical memory. *Journal of Neuroscience*, *16*, 4275–4282.

Fletcher, P. C., & Henson, R. N. A. (2001). Frontal lobes and human memory: Insights from functional neuroimaging. *Brain*, *124*, 849–881.

Fossati, P., Hevenor, S. J., Lepage, M., Graham, S. J., Grady, C., Keightley, M. L., et al. (2004). Distributed self in episodic memory: Neural correlates of successful retrieval of self-encoded positive and negative personality traits. *NeuroImage*, *22*, 1596–1604.

Frey, S., Kostopoulos, P., & Petrides, M. (2004). Orbitofrontal contribution to auditory encoding. *NeuroImage*, *22*, 1384–1389.

Frey, S., & Petrides, M. (2000). Orbitofrontal cortex: A key prefrontal region for encoding information. *Proceedings of the National Academy of Sciences USA, 97*, 8723–8727.

Fujiwara, E., Brand, M., Borsutzky, S., Steingass, H.-P., & Markowitsch, H. J. (2008a). Cognitive performance of detoxified alcoholic Korsakoff syndrome patients remains stable over two years. *Journal of Clinical and Experimental Neuropsychology, 30*, 576–587.

Fujiwara, E., Brand, M., Kracht, L., Kessler, J., Diebel, A., Netz, J., & Markowitsch, H. J. (2008b). Functional retrograde amnesia: A multiple case study. *Cortex, 44*, 29–45.

Fujiwara, E., & Markowitsch, H. J. (2006). Brain correlates of binding processes of emotion and memory. In H. Zimmer, A. M. Mecklinger, & U. Lindenberger (Eds.), *Binding in human memory: A neurocognitive perspective* (pp. 379–410). Oxford, UK: Oxford University Press.

Fujiwara, E., Piefke, M., Lux, S., Fink, G. R., Kessler, J., Kracht, L., et al. (2004). Brain correlates of functional retrograde amnesia in three patients. *Brain and Cognition, 54*, 135–136.

Fuster, J. M. (2006). The cognit: A network model of cortical representation. *International Journal of Psychophysiology, 60*, 125–132.

Geffen, G., Isles, R., Preece, M., & Geffen, L. (2008). Memory systems involved in professional skills: A case of dense amnesia due to herpes simplex viral encephalitis. *Neuropsychological Rehabilitation, 18*, 89–108.

Geng, H., Qi, Y., Li, Y., Fan, S., Wu, Y., & Zhu, Y. (2007). Neurophysiological correlates of memory illusion in both encoding and retrieval phases. *Brain Research, 1136*, 154–168.

Gerton, B. K., Brown, T. T., Meyer-Lindenberg, A., Kohn, P., Holt, J. L., Olsen, R. K., & Berman, K. F. (2004). Shared and distinct neurophysiological components of the digits forward and backward tasks as revealed by functional neuroimaging. *Neuropsychologia, 42*, 1781–1787.

Gilboa, A., Shalev, A. Y., Laor, L., Lester, H., Louzoun, Y., Chisin, R., & Bonne, O. (2004). Functional connectivity of the prefrontal cortex and the amygdala in posttraumatic stress disorder. *Biological Psychiatry, 55*, 263–272.

Gilboa, A., Winocur, G., Rosenbaum, R. S., Poreh, A., Gao, F., Black, S. E., et al. (2006). Hippocampal contributions to recollection in retrograde and anterograde amnesia. *Hippocampus, 16*, 966–980.

Glisky, E. L., Ryan, L., Reminger, S., Hardt, O., Hayes, S. M., & Hupbach, A. (2004). A case of psychogenic fugue: I understand, aber ich verstehe nichts. *Neuropsychologia, 42*, 1132–1147.

Greicius, M. D., Krasnow, B., Boyett-Anderson, J. M., Eliez, S., Schatzberg, A. F., Reiss, A. L., & Menon, V. (2003). Regional analysis of hippocampal activation during memory encoding and retrieval: fMRI study. *Hippocampus, 13*, 164–174.

Grossman, R., Yehuda, R., Golier, J., McEwen, B., Harvey, P., & Maria, N. S. (2006). Cognitive effects of intravenous hydrocortisone in subjects with PTSD and healthy control subjects. *Annals of the New York Academy of Sciences, 1071*, 410–421.

Haist, F., Bowden Gore, J., & Mao, H. (2001). Consolidation of human memory over decades revealed by functional magnetic resonance imaging. *Nature, 4*, 1139–1145.

Hehman, J. A., German, T. P., & Klein, S. B. (2005). Impaired self-recognition from recent photographs in a case of late-stage Alzheimer's disease. *Social Cognition, 23*, 118–123.

Herholz, K., Ehlen, P., Kessler, J., Strotmann, T., Kalbe, E., & Markowitsch, H. J. (2001). Learning face-name associations and the effect of age and performance: A PET activation study. *Neuropsychologia, 39*, 643–650.

Hibberd, C., Yau, J. L., & Seckl, J. R. (2000). Glucocorticoids and the ageing hippocampus. *Journal of Anatomy, 4*, 553–562.

Jansma, J. M., Ramsey, N. F., de Zwart, J. A., van Gelderen, P., & Duyn, J. H. (2007). fMRI study of effort and information processing in a working memory task. *Human Brain Mapping, 28*, 431–440.

Jelicic, M., & Merckelbach, H. (2004). Traumatic stress, brain changes, and memory deficits: A critical note. *Journal of Nervous and Mental Disease, 192*, 548–553.

Johnson, S. C., Baxter, L. C., Wilder, L. S., Pipe, J. G., Heiserman, J. E., & Prigatano, G. P. (2002). Neural correlates of self-reflection. *Brain, 125*, 1808–1814.

Kane, M. J., & Engle, R. W. (2002). The role of prefrontal cortex in working-memory capacity, executive attention, and general fluid intelligence: An individual-differences perspective. *Psychonomic Bulletin & Review, 9*, 637–671.

Kapur, N., Millar, J., Colbourn, C., Abbott, P., Kennedy, P., & Docherty, T. (1997). Very long-term amnesia in association with temporal lobe epilepsy: Evidence for multiple-stage consolidation process. *Brain and Cognition, 35*, 58–70.

Keenan, J., Wheeler, M. A., & Ewers, M. (2003). The neural correlates of self-awareness and self-recognition. In T. Kircher & A. David (Eds.), *The self in neuroscience and psychiatry* (pp. 166–179). Cambridge, UK: Cambridge University Press.

Kessler, J., Markowitsch, H. J., Huber, M., Kalbe, E., Weber-Luxenburger, G., & Kock, P. (1997). Massive and persistent anterograde amnesia in the absence of detectable brain damage: Anterograde psychogenic amnesia or gross reduction in sustained effort? *Journal of Clinical and Experimental Neuropsychology, 19*, 604–614.

Kircher, T. T., Weis, S., Freymann, K., Erb, M., Jessen, F., Grodd, W., et al. (2007). Hippocampal activation in patients with mild cognitive impairment is necessary for successful memory encoding. *Journal of Neurology, Neurosurgery, and Psychiatry, 78*, 812–818.

Kopelman, M. D. (1995). The Korsakoff syndrome. *British Journal of Psychiatry, 166*, 154–173.

Kopelman, M. D. (2000). Focal retrograde amnesia and the attribution of causality: An exceptionally critical review. *Cognitive Neuropsychology, 17*, 585–621.

Kopelman, M. D., Christensen, H., Puffett, A., & Stanhope, N. (1994). The great escape: A neuropsychological study of psychogenic amnesia. *Neuropsychologia, 32*, 675–691.

Kopelman, M. D., Stanhope, N., & Kingsley, D. (1999). Retrograde amnesia in patients with diencephalic, temporal lobe or frontal lesions. *Neuropsychologia, 37*, 939–958.

Krabbendam, L., Visser, P. J., Derix, M. M. A., Verhey, F., Hofman, P., Verhoeven, W., et al. (2000). Normal cognitive performance in patients with chronic alcoholism in contrast to patients with Korsakoff's syndrome. *Journal of Neuropsychiatry and Clinical Neurosciences, 12*, 44–50.

Kritchevsky, M., Chang, J., & Squire, L. R. (2004). Functional amnesia: Clinical description and neuropsychological profile of 10 cases. *Learning and Memory, 11*, 213–226.

Kuhlmann, S., Kirschbaum, C., & Wolf, O. T. (2005). Effects of oral cortisol treatment in healthy young women on memory retrieval of negative and neutral words. *Neurobiology of Learning and Memory, 83*, 158–162.

Kuhlmann, S., Piel, M., & Wolf, O. T. (2005). Impaired memory retrieval after psychosocial stress in healthy young men. *Journal of Neuroscience*, *25*, 2977–2982.

Kumaran, D., & Maguire, E. A. (2006). The dynamics of hippocampal activation during encoding of overlapping sequences. *Neuron*, *49*, 617–629.

LaBar, K. S., & Cabeza, R. (2006). Cognitive neuroscience of emotional memory. *Nature Reviews Neuroscience*, *7*, 54–64.

Labudda, K., Todorovski, S., Markowitsch, H. J., & Brand, M. (2008). Judgment and memory performance for emotional stimuli in patients with alcoholic Korsakoff syndrome. *Journal of Clinical and Experimental Neuropsychology*, *30*, 224–235.

Ladowsky-Brooks, R., & Alcock, J. E. (2007). Semantic-episodic interactions in the neuropsychology of disbelief. *Cognitive Neuropsychiatry*, *12*, 97–111.

Lepage, M., Ghaffar, O., Nyberg, L., & Tulving, E. (2000). Prefrontal cortex and episodic memory retrieval mode. *Proceedings of the National Academy of Sciences USA*, *97*, 506–511.

Levine, B., Turner, G. R., Tisserand, D., Hevenor, S. J., Graham, S. J., & McIntosh, A. R. (2004). The functional neuroanatomy of episodic and semantic autobiographical remembering: A prospective functional MRI study. *Journal of Cognitive Neuroscience*, *16*, 1633–1646.

Li, L., Chen, S., Liu, J., Zhang, J., He, Z., & Lin, X. (2006). Magnetic resonance imaging and magnetic resonance spectroscopy study of deficits in hippocampal structure in fire victims with recent-onset posttraumatic stress disorder. *Canadian Journal of Psychiatry*, *51*, 431–437.

Loewenstein, R. J. (1996). Dissociative amnesia and dissociative fugue. In L. K. Michelson & W. J. Ray (Eds.), *Handbook of dissociation: Theoretical, empirical, and clinical perspectives* (pp. 307–336). New York: Plenum Press.

Loftus, E. (2003). Our changeable memories: Legal and practical implications. *Nature Reviews Neuroscience*, *4*, 231–234.

Lucchelli, F., Muggia, S., & Spinnler, H. (1995). The "Petites Madeleines" phenomenon in two amnesic patients: Sudden recovery of forgotten memories. *Brain*, *118*, 167–183.

Maguire, E. A., Henson, R. N., Mummery, C. J., & Frith, C. D. (2001). Activity in prefrontal cortex, not hippocampus, varies parametrically with the increasing remoteness of memories. *NeuroReport*, *12*, 441–444.

Markowitsch, H. J. (1992). *Intellectual functions and the brain: An historical perspective*. Toronto: Hogrefe & Huber.

Markowitsch, H. J. (1996). Organic and psychogenic retrograde amnesia: Two sides of the same coin? *Neurocase*, *2*, 357–371.

Markowitsch, H. J. (1998a). The biological basis of memory. In A. I. Tröster (Ed.), *Memory in neurodegenerative disease: Biological, cognitive and clinical perspective* (pp. 140–153). New York: Cambridge University Press.

Markowitsch, H. J. (1998b). Cognitive neuroscience of memory. *Neurocase*, *4*, 429–435.

Markowitsch, H. J. (2000a). The anatomical bases of memory. In M. S. Gazzaniga (Ed.), *The new cognitive neurosciences* (2nd ed., pp. 781–795). Cambridge, MA: MIT Press.

Markowitsch, H. J. (2000b). Memory and amnesia. In M.-M. Mesulam (Ed.), *Principles of behavioral and cognitive neurology* (pp. 257–293). New York: Oxford University Press.

Markowitsch, H. J. (2002). Functional retrograde amnesia – mnestic block syndrome. *Cortex*, *38*, 651–654.

Markowitsch, H. J. (2003a). Memory: Disturbances and therapy. In T. Brandt, L. Caplan, J. Dichgans, H. C. Diener, & C. Kennard (Eds.), *Neurological disorders: Course and treatment* (2nd ed., pp. 287–302). San Diego: Academic Press.

Markowitsch, H. J. (2003b). Psychogenic amnesia. *NeuroImage*, *20*, S132–S138.

Markowitsch, H. J., Calabrese, P., Würker, M., Durwen, H. F., Kessler, J., Babinsky, R., et al. (1994). The amygdala's contribution to memory: A study on two patients with Urbach-Wiethe disease. *NeuroReport*, *5*, 1349–1352.

Markowitsch, H. J., Fink, G. R., Thöne, A., Kessler, J., & Heiss, W.-D. (1997a). A PET study of persistent psychogenic amnesia covering the whole life span. *Cognitive Neuropsychiatry*, *2*, 135–158.

Markowitsch, H. J., Kessler, J., Kalbe, E., & Herholz, K. (1999a). Functional amnesia and memory consolidation: A case of persistent anterograde amnesia with rapid forgetting following whiplash injury. *Neurocase*, *5*, 189–200.

Markowitsch, H. J., Kessler, J., Russ, M. O., Frölich, L., Schneider, B., & Maurer, K. (1999b). Mnestic block syndrome. *Cortex*, *35*, 219–230.

Markowitsch, H. J., Kessler, J., Van der Ven, C., Weber-Luxenburger, G., & Heiss, W.-D. (1998). Psychic trauma causing grossly reduced brain metabolism and cognitive deterioration. *Neuropsychologia*, *36*, 77–82.

Markowitsch, H. J., Kessler, J., Weber-Luxenburger, G., Van der Ven, C., Albers, M., & Heiss, W. D. (2000). Neuroimaging and behavioral correlates of recovery from mnestic block syndrome and other cognitive deteriorations. *Neuropsychiatry, Neuropsychology, and Behavioral Neurology*, *13*, 60–66.

Markowitsch, H. J., Thiel, A., Kessler, J., von Stockhausen, H.-M., & Heiss, W.-D. (1997b). Ecphorizing semi-conscious episodic information via the right temporopolar cortex: A PET study. *Neurocase*, *3*, 445–449.

Markowitsch, H. J., Vandekerckhove, M. M., Lanfermann, H., & Russ, M. O. (2003). Engagement of lateral and medial prefrontal areas in the ecphory of sad and happy autobiographical memories. *Cortex*, *39*, 643–665.

Markowitsch, H. J., Weber-Luxenburger, G., Ewald, K., Kessler, J., & Heiss, W.-D. (1997c). Patients with heart attacks are not valid models for medial temporal lobe amnesia: A neuropsychological and FDG-PET study with consequences for memory research. *European Journal of Neurology*, *4*, 178–184.

Mayes, A. R. (1995). Memory and amnesia. *Behavioural Brain Research*, *66*, 29–36.

McEwen, B. S. (1997). Possible mechanisms for atrophy of the human hippocampus. *Molecular Psychiatry*, *2*, 255–262.

McEwen, B. S. (1999). Stress and hippocampal plasticity. *Annual Review of Neuroscience*, *22*, 105–122.

McEwen, B. S., Magariños, A. M., & Reagan, L. P. (2002). Studies of hormone action in the hippocampal formation: Possible relevance to depression and diabetes. *Journal of Psychosomatic Research*, *53*, 883–890.

McGaugh, J. L. (2004). The amygdala modulates the consolidation of memories of emotionally arousing experiences. *Annual Review of Neuroscience*, *27*, 1–28.

Miotto, E. C., Savage, C. R., Evans, J. J., Wilson, B. A., Martins, M. G., Iaki, S., et al. (2006). Bilateral activation of the prefrontal cortex after strategic semantic cognitive training. *Human Brain Mapping*, *27*, 288–295.

Moore, S. A., & Zoellner, L. A. (2007). Overgeneral autobiographical memory and traumatic events: An evaluative review. *Psychological Bulletin*, *133*, 419–437.

Moscovitch, M., Rosenbaum, R. S., Gilboa, A., Addis, D. R., Westmacott, R., Grady, C., et al. (2005). Functional neuroanatomy of remote episodic, semantic and spatial memory: A unified account based on multiple trace theory. *Journal of Anatomy*, *207*, 35–66.

Northoff, G., Heinzel, A., de Greck, M., Bermpohl, F., Dobrowolny, H., & Panksepp, J. (2006). Self-referential processing in our brain: A meta-analysis of imaging studies on the self. *NeuroImage*, *31*, 440–457.

Noulhiane, M., Piolino, P., Hasboun, D., Clemenceau, S., Baulac, M., & Samson, S. (2007). Autobiographical memory after temporal lobe resection: Neuropsychological and MRI volumetric findings. *Brain*, *130*, 3184–3199.

Nyberg, L., McIntosh, A. R., Cabeza, R., Habib, R., Houle, S., & Tulving, E. (1996). General and specific brain regions involved in encoding and retrieval of events: What, where, and when. *Proceedings of the National Academy of Sciences USA*, *93*, 11280–11285.

O'Brien, J. T. (1997). The "glucocorticoid cascade" hypothesis in man. *British Journal of Psychiatry*, *170*, 199–201.

Papez, J. W. (1937). A proposed mechanism of emotion. *Archives of Neurology and Psychiatry*, *38*, 725–743.

Paquette, V., Levesque, J., Mensour, B., Leroux, J. M., Beaudoin, G., Bourgouin, P., & Beauregard, M. (2003). "Change the mind and you change the brain": Effects of cognitive-behavioral therapy on the neural correlates of spider phobia. *NeuroImage*, *18*, 401–409.

Park, K. W., Seo, J. H., & Yoon, G. U. (2007). Selective anterograde amnesia with thalamus and hippocampal lesions in neuro-Behcet's disease. *Clinical Neurology and Neurosurgery*, *109*, 470–473.

Payne, J. D., Jackson, E. D., Ryan, L., Hoscheidt, S., Jacobs, J. W., & Nadel, L. (2006). The impact of stress on neutral and emotional aspects of episodic memory. *Memory*, *14*, 1–16.

Phan, K. L., Britton, J. C., Taylor, S. F., Fig, L. M., & Liberzon, I. (2006). Corticolimbic blood flow during nontraumatic emotional processing in posttraumatic stress disorder. *Archives of General Psychiatry*, *63*, 184–192.

Phelps, M. E. (2006). Emotion and cognition: Insights from studies of the human amygdala. *Annual Review of Psychology*, *57*, 27–53.

Phelps, M. E., & LeDoux, J. E. (2005). Contributions of the amygdala to emotion processing: From animal models to human behavior. *Neuron*, *48*, 175–187.

Piefke, M., & Fink, G. R. (2005). Recollections of one's own past: The effects of aging and gender on the neural mechanisms of episodic autobiographical memory. *Anatomy and Embryology*, *210*, 497–512.

Piefke, M., Weiss, P. H., Markowitsch, H. J., & Fink, G. R. (2005). Gender differences in the functional neuroanatomy of emotional episodic autobiographical memory. *Human Brain Mapping*, *24*, 313–324.

Piefke, M., Weiss, P. H., Zilles, K., Markowitsch, H. J., & Fink, G. R. (2003). Differential remoteness and emotional tone modulate the neural correlates of autobiographical memory. *Brain*, *126*, 650–668.

Piolino, P., Giffard-Quillon, G., Desgranges, B., Chételat, G., Baron, J. C., & Eustache, F. (2004). Re-experiencing old memories via hippocampus: A PET study of autobiographical memory. *NeuroImage*, *22*, 1371–1383.

Piolino, P., Hannequin, D., Desgranges, B., Girard, C., Beaunieux, H., Giffard, B., et al. (2005). Right ventral frontal hypometabolism and abnormal sense of self in a case of disproportionate retrograde amnesia. *Cognitive Neuropsychology*, *22*, 1005–1034.

Porter, N., & Landfield, P. W. (1998). Stress hormones and brain ageing: Adding injury to insult. *Nature Neuroscience*, *1*, 3–4.

Putman, P., Van Honk, J., Kessels, R. P., Mulder, M., & Koppeschaar, H. P. (2004). Salivary cortisol and short and long-term memory for emotional faces in healthy young women. *Psychoneuroendocrinology*, *29*, 953–960.

Raes, F., Hermans, D., Williams, J. M., & Eelen, P. (2005). Autobiographical memory specificity and emotional abuse. *British Journal of Clinical Psychology*, *44*, 133–138.

Rand-Giovannetti, E., Chua, E. F., Driscoll, A. E., Schacter, D. L., Albert, M. S., & Sperling, R. A. (2006). Hippocampal and neocortical activation during repetitive encoding in older persons. *Neurobiology of Aging*, *27*, 173–182.

Ranganath, C., & Blumenfeld, R. S. (2008). Prefrontal cortex and human memory: An integrated account of results from neuropsychological and neuroimaging studies of working- and long-term memory. In H. Eichenbaum (Ed.), *Learning and memory: A comprehensive reference* (pp. 189–201). Oxford, UK: Elsevier.

Ranganath, C., Johnson, M. K., & D'Esposito, M. (2003). Prefrontal activity associated with working memory and episodic long-term memory. *Neuropsychologia*, *41*, 378–389.

Raz, N., & Rodrigue, K. M. (2006). Differential aging of the brain: Patterns, cognitive correlates and modifiers. *Neuroscience and Biobehavioral Reviews*, *30*, 730–748.

Reed, L. J., Lasserson, D., Marsden, P., Stanhope, N., Stevens, T., Bello, F., et al. (2003). FDG-PET findings in the Wernicke-Korsakoff syndrome. *Cortex*, *39*, 1027–1045.

Reinhold, N., Kühnel, S., Brand, M., & Markowitsch, H. J. (2006). Functional brain imaging in memory and memory disorders. *Current Medical Imaging Reviews*, *2*, 35–57.

Reinhold, N., & Markowitsch, H. J. (2007). Emotion and consciousness in adolescent psychogenic amnesia. *Journal of Neuropsychology*, *1*, 53–64.

Reinvang, I., & Gjerstad, L. (1998). Focal retrograde amnesia associated with vascular headache. *Neuropsychologia*, *36*, 1335–1341.

Ribot, T. (1892). *Diseases of memory*. New York: D. Appleton and Co.

Roberts, A. C., Robbins, T. W., & Weiskrantz, L. (Eds.). (1998). *The prefrontal cortex: Executive and cognitive functions*. Oxford, UK: Oxford University Press.

Roozendaal, B., Okuda, S., de Quervain, D. J., & McGaugh, J. L. (2006). Glucocorticoids interact with emotion-induced noradrenergic activation in influencing different memory functions. *Neuroscience*, *138*, 901–910.

Roozendaal, B., Okuda, S., Van der Zee, E. A., & McGaugh, J. L. (2006). Glucocorticoid enhancement of memory requires arousal-induced noradrenergic activation in the basolateral amygdala. *Proceedings of the National Academy of Sciences USA*, *103*, 6741–6746.

Rugg, M. D., Otten, L. J., & Henson, R. N. A. (2002). The neural basis of episodic memory: Evidence from functional neuroimaging. *Philosophical Transactions of the Royal Society of London, Series B, Biological Sciences*, *357*, 1097–1110.

Ryan, L., Nadel, L., Keil, K., Putnam, K., Schnyer, D., Trouard, T., & Moscovitch, M. (2001). Hippocampal complex and retrieval of recent and very remote autobiographical memories: Evidence from functional magnetic resonance imaging in neurologically intact people. *Hippocampus*, *11*, 707–714.

Schönfeld, S., & Ehlers, A. (2006). Overgeneral memory extends to pictorial retrieval cues and correlates with cognitive features in posttraumatic stress disorder. *Emotion, 6*, 611–621.

Schönfeld, S., Ehlers, A., Böllinghaus, I., & Rief, W. (2007). Overgeneral memory and suppression of trauma memories in post-traumatic stress disorder. *Memory, 15*, 339–352.

Scoville, W. B., & Milner, B. (1957). Loss of recent memory after bilateral hippocampal lesions. *Journal of Neurology, Neurosurgery and Psychiatry, 20*, 11–21.

Sellal, F., Manning, L., Seegmuller, C., Scheiber, C., & Schoenfelder, F. (2002). Pure retrograde amnesia following mild head trauma: A neuropsychological and metabolic study. *Cortex, 38*, 499–509.

Serra, L., Fadda, L., Buccione, I., Caltagirone, C., & Carlesimo, G. A. (2007). Psychogenic and organic amnesia: A multidimensional assessment of clinical, neuroradiological, neuropsychological and psychopathological features. *Behavioural Neurology, 18*, 53–64.

Shin, L. M., Rauch, S. L., & Pitman, R. K. (2006). Amygdala, medial prefrontal cortex, and hippocampal function in PTSD. *Annals of the New York Academy of Sciences, 1071*, 67–79.

Shin, L. M., Shin, P. S., Heckers, S., Krangel, T. S., Macklin, M. L., Orr, S. P., et al. (2004). Hippocampal function in posttraumatic stress disorder. *Hippocampus, 14*, 292–300.

Shin, L. M., Wright, C. I., Cannistraro, P. A., Wedig, M. M., McMullin, K., Martis, B., et al. (2005). A functional magnetic resonance imaging study of amygdala and medial prefrontal cortex responses to overtly presented fearful faces in posttraumatic stress disorder. *Archives of General Psychiatry, 62*, 273–281.

Siebert, M., Markowitsch, H. J., & Bartel, P. (2003). Amygdala, affect, and cognition: Evidence from ten patients with Urbach-Wiethe disease. *Brain, 126*, 2627–2637.

Sonntag, P., Gokalsing, E., Olivier, C., Robert, P., Burglen, F., Kauffmann-Muller, F., et al. (2003). Impaired strategic regulation of contents of conscious awareness in schizophrenia. *Consciousness and Cognition, 12*, 190–200.

Speckens, A. E., Ehlers, A., Hackmann, A., Ruths, F. A., & Clark, D. M. (2007). Intrusive memories and rumination in patients with post-traumatic stress disorder: A phenomenological comparison. *Memory, 15*, 249–257.

Staresina, B. P., & Davachi, L. (2006). Differential encoding mechanisms for subsequent associative recognition and free recall. *Journal of Neuroscience, 26*, 9162–9172.

Stein, M. B., Simmons, A. N., Feinstein, J. S., & Paulus, M. P. (2007). Increased amygdala and insula activation during emotion processing in anxiety-prone subjects. *American Journal of Psychiatry, 164*, 318–327.

Steinvorth, S., Levine, B., & Corkin, S. (2005). Medial temporal lobe structures are needed to re-experience remote autobiographical memories: Evidence from H.M. and W.R. *Neuropsychologia, 43*, 479–496.

Straube, T., Glauer, M., Dilger, S., Mentzel, H. J., & Miltner, W. H. (2006). Effects of cognitive-behavioral therapy on brain activation in specific phobia. *NeuroImage, 29*, 125–135.

Sullivan, E. V., & Marsh, L. (2003). Hippocampal volume deficits in alcoholic Korsakoff's syndrome. *Neurology, 61*, 1716–1719.

Summerfield, C., Greene, M., Wager, T., Egner, T., Hirsch, J., & Mangels, J. (2006). Neocortical connectivity during episodic memory formation. *PLoS Biology, 4*, e128.

Susman, E. J. (2006). Psychobiology of persistent antisocial behavior: Stress, early vulnerabilities and the attenuation hypothesis. *Neuroscience and Biobehavioral Reviews*, *30*, 376–389.

Sutherland, K., & Bryant, R. A. (2007). Autobiographical memory in posttraumatic stress disorder before and after treatment. *Behaviour Research and Therapy*, *45*, 2915–2923.

Sutherland, K., & Bryant, R. A. (2008). Social problem solving and autobiographical memory in posttraumatic stress disorder. *Behaviour Research and Therapy*, *46*, 154–161.

Svoboda, E., McKinnon, M. C., & Levine, B. (2006). The functional neuroanatomy of autobiographical memory: A meta-analysis. *Neuropsychologia*, *44*, 2189–2208.

Szeszko, P. R., Betensky, J. D., Mentschel, C., Gunduz-Bruce, H., Lencz, T., Ashtari, M., et al. (2006). Increased stress and smaller anterior hippocampal volume. *NeuroReport*, *17*, 1825–1828.

Tranel, D., & Hyman, B. T. (1990). Neuropsychological correlates of bilateral amygdala damage. *Archives of Neurology*, *47*, 349–355.

Tulving, E. (1972). Episodic and semantic memory. In E. Tulving & W. Donaldson (Eds.), *Organization of memory* (pp. 381–403). New York: Academic Press.

Tulving, E. (1987). Multiple memory systems and consciousness. *Human Neurobiology*, *6*, 67–80.

Tulving, E. (1995). Organization of memory: Quo vadis? In M. S. Gazzaniga (Ed.), *The cognitive neurosciences* (pp. 839–847). Cambridge, MA: MIT Press.

Tulving, E. (2002). Episodic memory: From mind to brain. *Annual Reviews of Psychology*, *53*, 1–25.

Tulving, E. (2005). Episodic memory and autonoesis: Uniquely human? In H. Terrace & J. Metcalfe (Eds.), *The missing link in cognition: Evolution of self-knowing consciousness* (pp. 3–56). New York: Oxford University Press.

Tulving, E., & Markowitsch, H. J. (1998). Episodic and declarative memory: Role of the hippocampus. *Hippocampus*, *8*, 198–204.

Uncapher, M. R., & Rugg, M. D. (2005a). Effects of divided attention on fMRI correlates of memory encoding. *Journal of Cognitive Neuroscience*, *17*, 1923–1935.

Uncapher, M. R., & Rugg, M. D. (2005b). Encoding and the durability of episodic memory: A functional magnetic resonance imaging study. *Journal of Neuroscience*, *25*, 7260–7267.

Vandekerckhove, M. M. P., Markowitsch, H. J., Mertens, M., & Woermann, F. G. (2005). Bi-hemispheric engagement in the retrieval of autobiographical episodes. *Behavioural Neurology*, *16*, 203–210.

Vargha-Khadem, F., Gadian, D. G., Watkins, K. E., Connely, A., Van Paeschen, W., & Mishkin, M. (1997). Differential effects of early hippocampal pathology on episodic and semantic memory. *Science*, *277*, 376–380.

Vargha-Khadem, F., Salmond, C. H., Watkins, K. E., Friston, K. J., Gadian, D. G., & Mishkin, M. (2003). Developmental amnesia: Effect of age at injury. *Proceedings of the National Academy of Sciences USA*, *100*, 10055–10060.

Velanova, K., Jacoby, L. L., Wheeler, M. E., McAvoy, M. P., Petersen, S. E., & Buckner, R. L. (2003). Functional-anatomic correlates of sustained and transient processing components engaged during controlled retrieval. *Journal of Neuroscience*, *23*, 8460–8470.

Vermetten, E., Schmahl, C., Lindner, S., Loewenstein, R. J., & Bremner, J. D. (2006).

Hippocampal and amygdalar volumes in dissociative identity disorder. *American Journal of Psychiatry*, *163*, 630–636.

Viard, A., Piolino, P., Desgranges, B., Chételat, G., Lebreton, K., Landeau, B., et al. (2007). Hippocampal activation for autobiographical memories over the entire lifetime in healthy aged subjects: An fMRI study. *Cerebral Cortex*, *17*, 2453–2467.

Wessa, M., Jatzko, A., & Flor, H. (2006). Retrieval and emotional processing of traumatic memories in posttraumatic stress disorder: Peripheral and central correlates. *Neuropsychologia*, *44*, 1683–1696.

Wheeler, M. A., & Stuss, D. T. (2003). Remembering and knowing in patients with frontal lobe injuries. *Cortex*, *39*, 827–846.

Wolf, O. T., Fujiwara, E., Luwinski, G., Kirschbaum, C., & Markowitsch, H. J. (2005). No morning cortisol response in patients with severe global amnesia. *Psychoneuroendocrinology*, *30*, 101–105.

Yasuno, F., Nishikawa, T., Nakagawa, Y., Ikejiri, Y., Tokunaga, H., Mizuta, I., et al. (2000). Functional anatomical study of psychogenic amnesia. *Psychiatry Research*, *99*, 43–57.

Yehuda, R., Harvey, P. D., Buchsbaum, M., Tischler, L., & Schmeidler, J. (2007). Enhanced effects of cortisol administration on episodic and working memory in aging veterans with PTSD. *Neuropsychopharmacology*, *32*, 2581–2591.

Zald, D. H. (2003). The human amygdala and the emotional evaluation of sensory stimuli. *Brain Research. Brain Research Reviews*, *41*, 88–123.

Zysset, S., Huber, O., Samson, A., Ferstl, E. C., & von Cramon, D. Y. (2003). Functional specialization within the anterior medial prefrontal cortex: A functional magnetic resonance imaging study with human subjects. *Neuroscience Letters*, *335*, 183–186.

14 The cognitive neuroscience of signed language

Applications to a working memory system for sign and speech

Jerker Rönnberg, Mary Rudner, and Catharina Foo

Introduction

The current chapter is about the scientific value of using sign language as a tool for understanding the interaction between language and cognition. Differences in sensory input channels between sign language and spoken language (visuospatial vs. auditory/audiovisual) and differences in the means of articulating the language (manual vs. oral) represent sensory and motor aspects of the languages that may contribute to disentangling neural substrates that are either shared or unique for several levels of comparative cognitive and communicative analysis. We will show that signed language may be profitably used to uncover behavioural and neural similarities and differences between the cognitive and neural bases of languages in different modalities. In particular, we focus on using sign language as a tool for testing critical assumptions about a working memory system for ease of language understanding. Since the linguistic status of sign language has been questioned – for example, in the debate about oral or manual methods of teaching the deaf (e.g., Smith & Campbell, 1997; Öhngren, 1992) – we commence our discussion by examining the evidence supporting this status and justifying the use of sign language as a tool for scrutinizing cognitive functions.

Sign language is a language

By now, many linguistic studies in different signed languages demonstrate that sign languages are languages like any spoken language, uniquely characterized by cultural, grammatical, and phonotactical constraints (Emmorey, 2002). Interestingly, differences and similarities among signed languages are not predictable from the particular constraints of the languages spoken in the same geographical region. For example, the differences between American Sign Language and British Sign Language are much greater than would be expected, considering the similarity between American English and British English (some standard references for the most commonly studied sign languages are American Sign Language (ASL): Stokoe, 1960; Stokoe,

Casterline, & Croneberg, 1965; British Sign Language (BSL): Sutton-Spence & Woll, 1998; Woll, 1990; French Sign Language (FSL): Courtin & Melot, 2005; German Sign Language (Deutsche Gebärdenspräche, DGS): Meyer et al., 2007; Swedish Sign Language (SSL): Bergman, 1982, 1983, 1990; Wallin, 1996).

Sign languages, like spoken languages, can be analysed at phonological, morphological, grammatical, and discourse levels (e.g., Lillo-Martin, 1997; Milkovic, Bradaric-Joncic, & Wilbur, 2007; Siple, 1997). It seems counterintuitive, at a superficial level, that a silent language should have a phonology, considering that the etymology of the word implicates sound. However, phonology can also be defined as the sublexical structure of language, and it is in this sense that sign language has a phonology. The phonological parameters of sign language are characterized by four sublexical aspects of lexical signs: shape, location relative to the body, movement, and orientation of the hands (Siple, 1997). Because signed and spoken languages share formal levels of analysis, they may be justifiably compared at these levels to investigate whether or not they share cognitive and neural systems. This provides a fruitful basis for investigating the extent to which the neural and cognitive base of language processing is dependent on the particular language modality.

Apart from linguistic data, behavioural and neuropsychological data attest that sign language is not just a gestural system tapping into visuospatial and/or motor networks of the brain but that it also has uniquely linguistic properties in common with spoken language. The Bellugi group was the first to systematically address similarities between signed and spoken languages. By studying aphasia, they discovered that sign language aphasias, just like spoken language aphasias, are caused by left hemisphere lesions (e.g., Bellugi, Poizner, & Klima, 1983; Poizner, Klima, & Bellugi, 1990). At a more analytical level, it was even more striking to observe that sign language aphasias are manifest in fluent and non-fluent forms, paralleling the classical Wernicke's and Broca's aphasias in terms of both expression and site of brain lesion (Hickok, Kritchevsky, Bellugi, & Klima, 1996b; Poizner, Klima, & Bellugi, 1987; Poizner et al., 1990).

Neuropsychological evidence not only demonstrates that sign language is dependent on the same neural systems as spoken language, it also shows that sign language performance is dissociated from performance on general visual and spatial tests. This is, of course, a crucial demonstration, adding to the parallelism of sign and speech observed for aphasias (Rönnberg, Söderfeldt, & Risberg, 2000). In particular, for right hemisphere lesion patients, visuospatial functions assessed by standard neuropsychological assessments may be selectively impaired, whereas language proficiency in both signers and speakers may be relatively unimpaired (Corina, Kritchevsky, & Bellugi, 1996; Poizner et al., 1987), and vice versa for left hemisphere patients (Hickok, Bellugi, & Klima, 1998; Hickok, Klima, & Bellugi, 1996a; Hickok, Say, Bellugi, & Klima, 1996c). Although sign language may be relatively spared in signers with right hemisphere lesions, it has been found that some specific language functions that depend on visuospatial processing may be compromised. These include processing of locative sentences and classifiers (Atkinson, Marshall, Woll, & Thacker, 2005) and facial negation (Atkinson, Campbell, Marshall, Thacker, & Woll, 2004). Furthermore, linguistic motor functions, relating to both sign and speech, can be spared while non-linguistic motor functions are impaired. For example, even though deaf native signers with Parkinson's disease and severely impaired general motor functions may show reduced sign language articulation in terms of amplitude of movement and facial expression, they may still produce qualitatively correct and comprehensible signs (Kegl, Cohen, & Poizner, 1999). Similarly, Hickok et al. (1996c) found no relationship between performance on apraxia tests and sign language performance in deaf native signers with brain lesions, and Marshall, Atkinson, Smulovitch, Thacker, and Woll (2004) found intact production of non-linguistic gesture in an aphasic signer. Thus, the general pattern is that even when the visuospatial and motor systems that support the production and comprehension of sign language are impaired, sign communication abilities may be relatively well preserved, suggesting that linguistic and non-linguistic visuospatial and motor components are driven by different and dissociable brain networks.

Furthermore, several brain imaging studies have shown that classical left hemisphere perisylvian language areas participate in perceiving signed languages at different levels of linguistic analysis (e.g., for the lexical level in JSL [Japanese Sign Language]: Nishimura et al., 1999; for sentence perception in ASL: Bavelier et al., 1998; Neville et al., 1997, 1998; for SSL discourse: Söderfeldt, Rönnberg, & Risberg, 1994a, 1994b; Söderfeldt et al., 1997). In addition, production of signs seems to activate Broca's area – as also would be expected on the basis of the lesion data (for BSL: McGuire et al., 1997). Thus, the imaging studies generally corroborate the lesion studies in supporting the thesis that sign language is a language, while at the same time unveiling new avenues for exciting research.

Common denominators for sign and speech in working memory

This chapter focuses the discussion of cognitive similarities between signed and spoken language to a working memory system conceptualized on the basis of common cognitive and neurofunctional denominators (Rönnberg, 2003a, 2003b). There are two categories of behavioural evidence that generally support the notion of similarities in *cognitive architecture*:

1 The classical effects of phonological similarity, articulatory suppression, and word length typically present in working memory for spoken items can also be observed with sign language (Wilson & Emmorey, 1997a, 1997b, 1998). By defining similarity in terms of (a) hand shape, (b) articulatory suppression as non-linguistic, irrelevant movements, and (c) word length as distance traversed by hand movement, Wilson and Emmorey

were able to elegantly demonstrate parallel empirical phenomena for ASL. Although short-term memory span is shorter for lexical signs than for words (Boutla, Supalla, Newport, & Bavelier, 2004; Rönnberg, Rudner, & Ingvar, 2004), ASL signing span is similar to English speaking span in tests designed to tap working memory resources in language production, in tasks that are not dependent on maintenance of serial order (Boutla et al., 2004).

2 Case studies of exceptionally skilled deaf communicators (Lyxell, 1994; Rönnberg, 1993; Rönnberg et al., 1999) have shown that expertise in speech understanding may be associated with superior complex working memory capacity. The important aspect in this context is that superior working memory capacity is the key factor irrespective of the hearing status, linguistic background, and habitual mode of communication of the individual. MM (Rönnberg et al., 1999) is moderately hearing impaired and a native bilingual in SSL and Swedish. SJ (Lyxell, 1994) is profoundly deaf since the age of 13 and communicates by speech and speechreading. GS (Rönnberg, 1993) is profoundly deaf since the age of 8 and communicates by speech, using his sense of touch to pick up vibrations from the larynx via the collarbone to supplement visual information about speech from lip movements. All three cases show working memory performance that far exceeds that of matched controls.

In addition to behavioural evidence, there are three categories of *neurofunctional* observation that suggest interesting and surprising convergences in neural networks underlying some potential pillars of a general working memory system; these relate to phonological, semantic, and syntactic levels of language processing. At the phonological level, syllabic judgments activate the planum temporale for both sign and speech, suggesting that at least some more global aspect of phonological processing is centred in the same neural sites (e.g., Pettito et al., 2000). At the semantic level, it has been demonstrated that retrieval of lexical items from distinct semantic categories is supported by distinct sites of the inferior temporal lobe, irrespective of whether the lexical items are signs or words (Emmorey et al., 2003). And, at the syntactic level, it has been shown that sentence processing is typically left-lateralized, irrespective of language, with crucial areas – such as the ventral part of the inferior frontal gyrus – showing no effect of language modality (i.e., comparing JSL with spoken Japanese: Sakai, Tatsuno, Suzuki, Kimura, & Ichida, 2005; for similar conclusions on BSL, see MacSweeney et al., 2006). In a working memory context, tasks based on serial recall or semantic retrieval produce similar inferior frontal and inferior temporal cortex activity for lexical signs and words (Rönnberg et al., 2004; Rudner, Fransson, Ingvar, Nyberg, & Rönnberg, 2007). Thus, both the cognitive and the neurofunctional evidence support a working memory system for language understanding that is independent of language modality.

Working memory system for ease of language understanding: Background and development

The cognitive and neurofunctional common denominators of sign and speech support a working memory model that is independent of language modality (Rönnberg, 2003a). In its general form, this model incorporates a system for interaction between multimodal language input (cf. Rönnberg et al., 1998a), long-term memory, and working memory. With the neurofunctional and cognitive similarities as a general frame, the more detailed similarities between sign and speech are modelled on the cognitive predictors that have been found to be crucial for ease of *speech* understanding (ESU) (Rönnberg et al., 1998a). The general model is about ease of *language* understanding (ELU) (Rönnberg, 2003a) and hence represents an extension of ESU. In this context, *understanding* refers to the extraction of lexical and semantic meaning from linguistic and paralinguistic signals (Lidestam, 2003) and *ease* refers to low processing costs and to absence of delays or misunderstandings (e.g., in a dialogue). Thus, in cognitive terms, ease implies implicit, automatic processing (Rönnberg, 2003a).

On modelling ESU

The details of the ESU model are based on the results of cognitive correlation studies that reveal direct cognitive predictors of sentence-based speechreading. These predictors include verbal inference-making (sentence completion: Lyxell & Rönnberg, 1989), word decoding (Lyxell & Rönnberg, 1991), and certain aspects of speed of information processing (lexical and semantic access speed: Rönnberg, 1990; rhyme decision speed: Lyxell, Rönnberg, & Samuelsson, 1994; Rönnberg, Andersson, Lyxell, & Spens, 1998b). Indirect predictors of sentence-based speechreading include the VN 130/P200 peak-to-peak amplitude measure in the visual evoked potential (Rönnberg, Arlinger, Lyxell, & Kinnefors, 1989); complex information processing and storage tasks, measured by the reading span task (Lyxell & Rönnberg, 1989); and verbal ability (Lyxell & Rönnberg, 1992). These indirect predictors are related to sentence-based speechreading *via* their relationships with the direct predictors.

The predictive strength of verbal inference-making in relation to sentence-based speechreading must be interpreted in the light of correlations between verbal inference-making and (a) complex processing and storage capacity, and verbal ability, and (b) word decoding, which relies on speed indices, in particular relating to rhyme and lexical access (for reviews of the evidence, see Rönnberg, 2003a, 2003b; Rönnberg et al., 1998a, 1998b). In short, phonologically mediated word-decoding speed, verbal ability, and working memory capacity are required to support intelligent guesswork needed for visual speech understanding (Rönnberg, 1995; Rönnberg et al., 1998a).

Before formulating an ESU model (Rönnberg, 2003a), we evaluated predictors of speech understanding under different *sensory* conditions. We were able to observe functional similarities that give grounds for cross-modal generalization. For example, the fact that GS performs at a normal level on phonological tasks (Rönnberg, 1993) suggests that speech mediated by visual-tactile means can be coded in non-auditory phonological representations. The quality of this kind of representation, which can be assessed by text-based rhyme tests, has also been shown to be an important predictor of visual–tactile speech-tracking skill (Andersson, Lyxell, Rönnberg, & Spens, 2001a, 2001b; Rönnberg, Andersson, Lyxell, & Spens, 1998b). This predictor has a function analogous to that of visual speech tracking (Andersson et al., 2001a, 2001b). In the same vein, data from profoundly deaf persons with cochlear implants collected by Lyxell et al. (1996, 1998) showed that audiovisual speech understanding, like visual speech understanding, is predicted by *phonological* ability and individual capacity for *simultaneous processing and storage of information* in working memory.

Thus, cognitive similarities relevant for a formulation of a general working memory system are apparent across sensory modes of transmitting speech information. In terms of general brain mechanisms supporting this claim, it is encouraging to note that both lipreading (Calvert et al., 1997; Lee et al., 2007; MacSweeney et al., 2004) and tactilely transmitted information about speech sounds (Levänen, 1998) are associated with activation of auditory and phonological cortical regions.

ESU: Threshold hypothesis

The set of case studies of exceptionally skilled deaf communicators and the studies of cognitive predictors of ESU prompted a theoretical formulation called the *threshold hypothesis* (Rönnberg, Samuelsson, & Lyxell, 1998c). This hypothesis generally states that low-level, bottom-up processing abilities are important up to a certain threshold only. The low-level abilities that are relevant in an ESU context are phonology and the speed of phonologically mediated lexical access, which support the machinery of implicit language perception (cf. Rönnberg, 1990, 2003a). Once the threshold is reached, the efficiency of visual, phonetic, and lexically supported perception is constrained by visual-neural, auditory-neural, and lexical access speed, as well as by the quality and speed with which phonological representations are accessed (Andersson, 2002; Pichora-Fuller, 2003). This means that, above the threshold, no communicative advantage can be gained from exceptional low-level abilities only.

Although low-level functions are not above threshold in our exceptionally skilled deaf communicators (SJ: Lyxell, 1994; GS: Rönnberg, 1993; MM: Rönnberg et al., 1999), top-down, high-level information-processing skills are remarkably superior (Rönnberg et al., 1998a, 1998c). It is these high-level skills that allow the individuals concerned to surpass the hypothetical threshold of low-level perceptual information extraction and hence attain extreme speech-understanding skills. Thus, speech understanding under difficult circumstances seems to depend on more compound and explicit cognitive processing skills.

ELU model

To build a general model that applies to both experts and non-experts, we need to take into account findings with respect to the factors that generally predict understanding of poorly specified linguistic input in the general population. This provides a more general and dynamic view of the interplay between implicit (i.e., phonologically mediated lexical access) and explicit (i.e., complex storage and processing) functions that contribute to ELU (Rönnberg, 2003a).

Four major, interacting parameters are proposed: the quality of extracted phonological representations in long-term memory (parameter P), phonologically mediated lexical access speed (parameter S), explicit storage and processing capacity (parameter C), and the degree of demand on explicit processing (parameter E). As long as the phonological information, which is perceived and extracted from the speech signal, can be *matched to* the phonological representations in long-term memory, with sufficient speed, then the process of unlocking the lexicon is assumed to be smooth and implicit, indicating a high degree of ESU.

Two assumptions should be noted here: (1) the input to the working memory system is typically multimodal or multisensory (Rönnberg et al., 1998a) and (2) the phonological parameter is based on the syllable. The latter assumption is founded on the fact that syllable processing is less effortful than phoneme processing (Andersson et al., 2001a, 2001b; Höien, Lundberg, Stanovitch, & Bjaalid, 1995; Rönnberg, 2003a) and is a better predictor of speech understanding (Andersson, 2002). In addition, it may be surmised that syllabic processing may involve abstract non-sound communalities, as syllabic judgments in sign and speech both activate similar neural sites (Petitto et al., 2000), and non-sound syllabic phonological information about speech may also be extracted from visual and visual-tactile signals (Andersson et al., 2001a, 2001b; Leybaert & Charlier, 1996; Rönnberg, 1993).

According to the model, when *mismatches* occur, due to phonological or contextual problems, demands on explicit processing (parameter E) are signalled by the system. Explicit processing involves retrospective and prospective comparisons between cues, hints, single words, and linguistic fragments that have been decoded from the discourse. It allows inferences to be made about what has been said at different points in time, as well as predictions and guesses concerning what is to come in the dialogue. To be able to make retrospective and prospective inferences, the individual needs to have the capacity to *store* information while *processing* and evaluating the information in the light of new input, as well as *accessing* long-term memory knowledge about objects, people, and situations, and finally *integrating* these different types of information (cf. Hannon & Daneman, 2001). These processes typically proceed implicitly and automatically when phonology and semantics work in tandem, but when the call for explicit processing is made by the system, the individual capacity to think about and elaborate on available information gains a key role. Explicit storage and processing capacity is crucial for compensatory purposes in the mismatch situation – for example, elderly people with sensory and speed losses need to be high on parameter C to compensate for these losses and retain functional language understanding (cf. Pichora-Fuller, 2003).

Although not explicitly stated in the Rönnberg (2003a) model, phonological extraction and mismatch problems may generally arise because of a poorly specified signal, a hearing impairment, or less precise phonological representations in long-term memory. A language signal may be poorly specified due to degradation of the remote signal or masking effects from background noise (e.g., Hygge, Rönnberg, Larsby, & Arlinger, 1992). Hearing may be impaired to varying degrees at different frequencies, and the effect of hearing impairment is modulated by type of signal-processing algorithm in the hearing aid and the degree to which residual hearing and signal amplification jointly produce a good-quality phonological percept. Lack of phonological precision (phonological degradation) in long-term memory may be caused by hearing impairment from an early age (Andersson, 2002), combined with a general lack of early phonological stimulation (Leybaert, 1998).

Generally, then, the need for explicit cognitive processing (parameter C) depends on the overall ratio between demands on explicit (E) and implicit (I) processes, that fluctuates naturally in a dialogue (for mathematical detail, see Rönnberg, 2003a). When the E/I ratio is larger than 1, the probability of explicit activation of processing and storage functions in working memory increases. Fluctuations in the ratio may be determined by a number of factors, such as rate and clarity of dialogue, as well as by topical and semantic coherence in the dialogue.

Recent work has empirically addressed some of the crucial assumptions of the ELU model. Here, we consider the mismatch and the similarity assumptions of the ELU model and how an episodic buffer for sign–speech interactions can be incorporated in the ELU system.

Mismatch assumption

The mismatch assumption (Rönnberg, 2003a) has recently been tested by manipulating signal-processing algorithms in hearing aids during speech recognition in noise (Foo, Rudner, Rönnberg, & Lunner, 2007; Rudner, Foo, Rönnberg, & Lunner, in press). In the test, 32 bilaterally fitted hearing-aid users with moderate hearing impairment of the sensorineural type were randomly assigned to either a non-linear (i.e., FAST, 40-ms, compression release settings) or a quasi-linear (i.e., SLOW, 640-ms, compression release settings) signal-processing algorithm during a 9-week training period. Before and after training, all participants were tested with two types of standardized Swedish speech recognition tests (Hagerman's sentence test: Hagerman, 1982; Hagerman & Kinnefors, 1995; the Swedish version of the Hearing In Noise Test (HINT): Hällgren, Larsby, & Arlinger, 2006; Nilsson, Soli, & Sullivan, 1994) in noise (modulated or unmodulated), with both the trained setting and the orthogonal non-trained settings. Quasi-linear amplification preserves syllable characteristics to a high degree, whereas nonlinear amplification results in syllabic compression, and thus a somewhat distorted sound at the syllable level (see, e.g., Dillon, 2001).

In the Foo et al. (2007) study, the mismatch test was between the pre-test compression release settings, which were the same for all participants (Digifocus II standard), and the *new* SLOW or *new* FAST settings, both of which were different from the original settings. Data revealed that speech recognition in noise was very well predicted by the reading span test (which measures explicit storage and processing capacity; Daneman & Merikle, 1996), indicating – as predicted by the ELU framework – that reliance would be high on explicit capacity under conditions of difficult signal processing (*r*s = .41 to .67, across noise conditions). That is to say, when a habitual mode of phonological processing is disrupted – as would be the case for a switch from pre-settings to FAST or to SLOW signal processing in noise – there is a higher probability of failure to match speech input to phonological representations in long-term memory. The patterns of correlation held true across type of speechreading test and type of noise and for both types of mismatch conditions. Even when dB loss was partialled out, correlations were still significant for all but one of the eight conditions, and when both dB loss and chronological age were partialled out, all but two of the conditions were still significant. This demonstrates a robust cognitive mismatch effect and shows that it has communicative and ecological validity.

The fact that the reading span test correlates with speech recognition in noise under mismatch conditions irrespective of speech recognition test and type of noise shows that it measures something important and general. In particular, the fact that correlations generalized from the Hagerman test based on predictable, constrained, and stereotyped materials (5-word sentences from a defined word pool) to HINT, which contains unpredictable, more naturalistic sentences varying in length and content, indicates a potential transfer to ecological speech understanding tests, with properties important for speech understanding in general.

In the Rudner et al. study (in press), we tested the mismatch assumption more analytically by evaluating how performance in the Hagerman and HINT sentences depended on the interaction between trained setting (FAST or SLOW) and the setting at post-training assessments (FAST or SLOW). That is, the matching conditions (i.e., FAST–FAST and SLOW–SLOW) were compared with the mismatching conditions (i.e., FAST–SLOW and SLOW–FAST). Using the matching conditions as baseline, we could observe systematic correlations of reading span performance with speech recognition in noise performance with the Hagerman sentences for mismatching conditions but not for the matching conditions. With HINT, the match–mismatch pattern was not apparent. Thus, the match–mismatch assumption receives repeated support from the experimental manipulations made for the Hagerman sentences, but not when it comes to HINT. The HINT sentences are more contextually rich and less constrained than the Hagerman sentences. It is possible that these contextual factors modulate the effect of phonological mismatch for HINT. This hypothesis is currently under investigation.

The original studies of mismatch negativity, which show a change-specific component of the auditory event-related potential elicited by changes in auditory stimulation, and many other applications by Näätänen and Kreegipuu (see chapter 15, this volume), as well as the recent observations of cognitive effects made for speech samples at our laboratory, seem to suggest a very general applicability of the mismatch principle. We conjecture that this effect may also be present for match–mismatch studies of sign language in the ELU context. Thus, sign language has yet to be evaluated to determine whether this assumption holds for both language modalities.

Similarity assumption

Based on the background data and the notion of common cognitive and neurofunctional denominators for sign and speech processing, Rönnberg (2003a) suggested that the C parameter, concerning explicit storage and processing capacity (i.e., estimated by the reading span test) could be generalized across language modality. One way of addressing the similarity assumption is by comparing estimates of parameter C for spoken and signed languages at the neurofunctional level.

In a PET study, Rönnberg et al. (2004) addressed this issue and found that explicit working memory (i.e., serial recall of 6-item lists) for unrelated signed words engaged bilateral parietal (dorsal stream), occipito-temporal (ventral stream) and left premotor cortical areas, whereas working memory for spoken words specifically engaged superior temporal areas. The similarity/difference test was carried out with participants who were bilingual in SSL and Swedish, some of whom were native signers and some of whom were early, non-native yet fluent users of sign language. In a recent fMRI study on native bilingual participants (Rudner et al., 2007), we replicated the sign-specific neural network in a 2-back task, as well as the speech-specific results (cf. Smith & Jonides, 1997). Thus, the specificity is stable across imaging method and type of working memory task. In this sense, the Rönnberg (2003a) model is falsified: *Explicit* working memory processing seems to recruit language-specific processing networks.

Although not manipulated in the two studies, *implicit* phonological processing seemed to be based on similar activity in left inferior frontal and inferior temporal areas (Rudner & Rönnberg, 2006), and this hypothesis is currently under investigation. The results are not due to task difficulty, differences in recoding operations, or production differences; thus, the results seem to reflect genuine, language-modality-specific explicit storage and processing differences but are suggestive of a lack of implicit language-specific differences (Rönnberg et al., 2004; Rudner & Rönnberg, 2006).

One current hypothesis is that native and non-native language skills may be reflected in distinct cortical networks for working memory. It has already been shown that native and non-native language skills may have different neural representations in both sign (Newman, Bavelier, Corina, Jezzard, & Neville, 2002) and speech (Kim et al, 2002). To investigate this possibility in the Rönnberg et al. (2004) study, we undertook a re-analysis of the data for the five native signers, excluding the three non-native users. Supporting the hypothesis of a different cortical network for native signers, it could be observed that the bilateral parietal activation shifted over to a more focal, left-sided, parietal activation for the native SSL users. This suggests that although all eight participants were fluent in sign language, native signing may be specifically associated with left-lateralized parietal engagement in working memory.

The data in Rönnberg et al. (2004) and Rudner et al. (2007) suggest that the specific parietal activity could be conceptualized in terms of a visuospatial array to support working memory processing for signed items (i.e., parameter C in the ELU system). In an earlier study on sign language perception and episodic encoding of discourse (i.e., a story that was to be later recalled), we also observed sign language specificity, although the effect was located in the ventral rather than the dorsal processing stream bilaterally (Söderfeldt et al., 1997). Thus, the evidence suggests that parameter C in the ELU system has a sign-specific component that is neurofunctionally associated with parietal regions.

Although the Söderfeldt et al. (1997) study was not designed to tap working memory, we were, in a subsequent study (Rönnberg, Söderfeldt, & Risberg, 1998d), able to tease apart an interaction between type of memory task (*episodic* recognition of words or *semantic* classification of words) and use of language modality (deaf participants perceiving *signed* SSL items and hearing participants listening to audiovisual *spoken* Swedish). We achieved this by measuring regional cerebral blood flow with a two-dimensional high-resolution system called Cortexplorer (Rönnberg et al., 1998d). The interaction revealed that semantic processing of both signs and words activated left-hemisphere perisylvian cortical areas, whereas episodic processing of words activated left-hemisphere areas and episodic processing of signs activated posterior right-hemisphere areas.

Thus, in the four studies (Rudner et al., 2007; Rönnberg et al., 1998d, 2004; Söderfeldt et al., 1997) the tasks represent different kinds of encoding-retrieval demands in explicit, working, and episodic memory. However, all tasks are associated with language-modality-specific neural representations for signed versus spoken episodes. In particular, they suggest that *parameter*

C in the ELU model is associated with posterior and parietal regions for sign language and the superior temporal lobes for speech.

Episodic buffer

A relatively recent addition to the concept of working memory is the episodic buffer. The role of the episodic buffer is to integrate information from different sensory sources and other cognitive systems, such as long-term memory, to form and bind together multidimensional representations (Baddeley, 2000; Repovs & Baddeley, 2006). Early work found that memory retrieval under bound conditions (e.g., when visual letters are bound to spatial locations) produces right prefrontal activity (Prabhakaran, Narayanan, Zhao, & Gabrielli, 2000). This finding fits with the notion that episodic buffer processing involves extensive executive and explicit processing resources to create the multidimensional representations. Similar right prefrontal activity has been reported for recall of bound auditory digits with spatial location (Zhang et al., 2004).

In more general terms, Repovs and Baddeley (2006) have distinguished between the *formation* and *maintenance* of bound information in the episodic buffer, where the conditions producing prefrontal activity (Prabhakaran et al., 2000; Zhang et al., 2004) primarily represent the maintenance of bound information. In the study by Rudner et al. (2007), we investigated both the formation and maintenance of lexical items, presented in either signed or spoken language versions. The task was a 2-back working memory task where – in the binding condition – participants had to match the meaning of a spoken lexical token with the meaning of a signed lexical token (or vice versa) to determine whether they were the same or not. Control conditions were unimodal signed or spoken lists where binding was not required to solve the task. The unique neural signature in the binding condition is located more posteriorly than in the Prabhakaran and Zhang studies – more precisely, in the right middle temporal lobe.

Two aspects are interesting to discuss in the present context. First, the data suggest that the initial assumption of the episodic buffer being a subsystem fractionated from the central executive – but still some part of frontal lobe function (Baddeley, 2000) – may not be supported by the non-frontal and right middle temporal activation observed in the Rudner et al. study (2007). In fact, this de-emphasis of the frontal lobes in episodic buffer processing was also demonstrated for a recent case of audiovisual integration across verbal items, where left temporal activity was shown (Suchan, Linnewerth, Köster, Daum, & Schmid, 2006). Recent behavioural data also agree with the neural findings such that there is no selective interference of attention-demanding distracter tasks on recall of bound vs. non-bound information, suggesting that executive functions are not a cardinal feature of episodic buffer processing (Allen, Baddeley, & Hitch, 2006). For a more extensive discussion on this matter, see Rudner and Rönnberg (2008).

Second, in terms of the ELU system proposed by Rönnberg (2003a), it seems that the confluence of sensory and semantic information described in terms of the episodic buffer may represent an important conceptual addition to the type of processing that occurs in the implicit mode. The assumption of a multimodal input system was introduced in the working memory model by Rönnberg et al. (1998a). It was recognized that under many ecological and disability-related linguistic conditions, there is a need to integrate phonological information in the auditory and visual channels (Rudner & Rönnberg, 2004; Summerfield, 1987), or visual and tactile channels (Andersson et al., 2001a, 2001b), in line with the general integrative functions of the episodic buffer. Generally, then, it is argued here that an episodic buffer function may be important for binding of all kinds of sensory *and* linguistic stimuli with a bearing on phonologically mediated lexical access in both signed and spoken discourse (Rönnberg, 1990).

Episodic buffer, implicit and explicit storage and processing

At this stage, the time is ripe to consider the similarities and differences between the episodic buffer (Repovs & Baddeley, 2006) and the ELU concept (Rönnberg, 2003a). Both concepts imply interaction between working memory and long-term memory, activation of long-term memory-based knowledge, multisensory contributions to episodic formation of stimuli, and maintenance of complex representations in a conscious, explicit state of mind for inference-making purposes. One of the major differences is that even in the implicit mode of information processing, the ELU system, unlike the episodic buffer, typically relies on integration and binding rather than separation and division of linguistic information. Moreover, the importance of information integration in the ELU model overshadows the loop specific effects that are prominent in Baddeley's model (Rudner et al., 2007). For, as we have seen, integration of modality specific information is fundamental to the compensatory communicative functioning of hearing impaired and deaf persons (Rönnberg et al., 1998a).

According to the ELU system, *buffer type function becomes apparent even at the perceptual streaming and implicit level of processing*. This way there is no conflict with the results that suggest separate, explicit storage sites for signed and spoken tokens (Rönnberg et al., 2004) and thus modality-specific fractionation of parameter C. Moreover, as long as episodic buffer function is implicit, the buffer notion is de-emphasized in the ELU system, because *r*apid, *a*utomatic *m*ultimodality *b*inding of *pho*nology (RAMBPHO) does not imply temporary storage or buffering of information. In the ELU system, such buffering is reserved, we argue, for conditions of mismatch and explicit storage and processing functions.

Multiple fractionations: Or many cortical sites to the same coin?

In behavioural correlation and regression studies addressing the explicit storage *and* processing component (i.e., parameter C) of the ELU system, we have typically employed complex and dual working memory span tasks such as the reading span test (e.g., Rönnberg, 1995). However, for methodological reasons we have based neurofunctional estimates of parameter C on relatively simple working memory tasks (Rönnberg et al., 2004; Rudner et al., 2007) that, relative to reading span, focus on storage and maintenance processing of items, without introducing simultaneous semantic processing of the items to be recalled. This means that our behavioural and neuroimaging studies have not addressed precisely the same cognitive functions. However, one recent study has addressed the neural correlates of the reading span test. In an fMRI study by Osaka et al. (2004), individuals with high storage and processing capacity according to the reading span test were compared with individuals with low capacity. The main task in the scanner was the reading span task. This task involves reading sentences, judging their semantic validity, and committing them to memory for subsequent recall. This task was contrasted with reading sentences and judging their semantic validity, but no recall. The findings were that individuals who were more successful at solving the reading span task, and thus had greater storage and processing capacity, showed net activation of the anterior cingulum, the inferior frontal gyrus, and the superior parietal lobes for this task compared to the reading baseline. This indicates that parameter C, defined in terms of complex working memory, is supported by a neural network including these specific regions. It is interesting to note that although this network includes the anterior cingulum, which is known to be sensitive to level of difficulty in working memory tasks (Barch et al., 1997), it does not include the dorsolateral prefrontal cortex, which is associated with working memory load (Braver et al., 1997). Furthermore, it does not include regions previously associated with episodic buffer processing, including the right prefrontal (Prabhakaran et al., 2000; Zhang et al., 2004) and middle temporal regions (Rudner et al., 2007). Although this fronto-parietal network is a good candidate for the neural substrate of parameter C, its modality specificity must be properly evaluated – for example, by comparing listening span with reading span, or by comparing signed working memory span tasks with reading or listening span tasks.

For the time being, we can only hypothesize that the parietal lobes represent a common visuospatial storage site for signed and written episodes, as well as non-linguistic visuospatial working memory representations (e.g., Zago & Tzourio-Mazoyer, 2002), and thus a key component of parameter C. Furthermore, assuming that frontal regions are less language-modality-specific in their operation, we could at least venture the idea that the frontal areas implicated in the Osaka et al. (2004) study would be replicated in another language modality (Cabeza & Nyberg, 2000). Thus, the data collected so far allows us to tentatively conclude that the neural network underpinning parameter C for sign and speech is distinct from the networks underpinning working memory load and the notion of the episodic buffer, irrespective of whether the comparison focuses on the right prefrontal activity found for maintenance of bound episodes (e.g., Prabhakaran et al., 2000) or on the right middle temporal activity found for formation and maintenance of bound sign–speech tokens (Rudner et al., 2007).

Episodic buffer and communication

We have argued in favour of a RAMBPHO function in the ELU context. This function serves to integrate multisensory, multilingual, and long-term memory-based information, and typically this type of information is perceptually bound in an implicit stream of information processing (cf. Lee et al., 2007), dissociated from parameter C functions (see Figure 14.1). Thus, it seems that, from a communicative point of view, the RAMBPHO functions play important roles. Online communicative demands typically do not allow for explicit reflection on combinations of different sensory and linguistic sources of information with long-term memory information. The key role played by the RAMBPHO function in the ELU system is assumed here to contribute to automatic integration of information, optimizing and facilitating rapid unlocking of the meaning of a message via bound multimodal information about phonology, in particular at the syllable level.

However, when phonological problems arise – that is, due to mismatching conditions – binding may be less successful, especially for the formation aspect of the process. Here, it seems likely that future work may show that the networks subserved by frontal regions, with respect both to the explicit

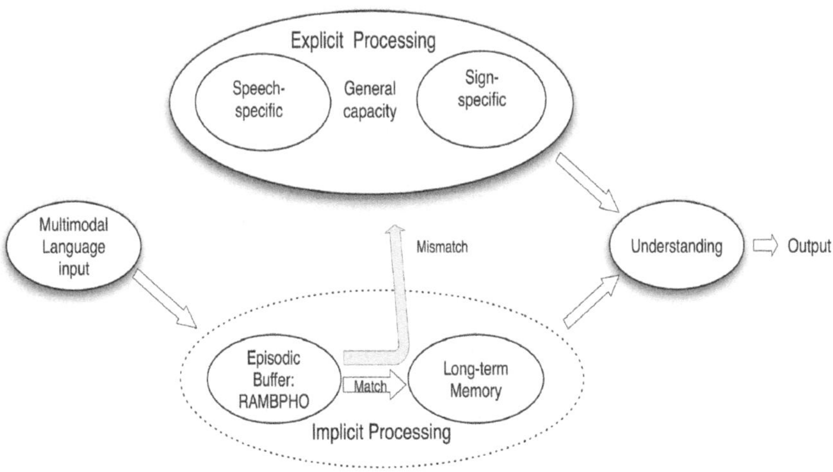

Figure 14.1 Working memory system for ELU.

maintenance aspect of binding in the episodic buffer and to the explicit processing part of parameter C, converge in their demands on executive functions. Thus, before we can reach firmer conclusions, further research is needed to disentangle exactly how explicit functions – estimated by dual tasks like reading span – compared to those involved in tasks demanding maintenance of bound information could work in tandem. Further work is also needed that uncover language-modality specificity for dual working memory span estimates of parameter C.

General conclusions

1. An abstract working memory system with implicit and explicit cognitive components and a specific neural representation serves well as a general model for ease of language understanding (ELU). It summarizes data from studies of cognitive predictors of speech understanding under various sensory conditions, as well as independent behavioural and neuroimaging data on working memory for sign and speech.
2. As long as phonological information extracted from the language signal can be rapidly matched with phonological representations in long-term memory, processing proceeds smoothly and implicitly. However, when mismatch occurs, greater reliance on explicit processing and storage capacity is suggested.
3. The mismatch assumption is supported by studies of aided speech recognition in noise, where performance under matching vs. non-matching conditions was compared. Performance in mismatch conditions produced systematically higher correlations with reading span performance than did matching conditions.
4. The assumption of similar *explicit* resources across the language modalities of sign and speech is not supported, as explicit working memory tasks engage modality-specific neural substrates. However, the similarity assumption seems to hold true for *implicit* processing of sign and speech.
5. The episodic buffer is assumed to serve important, communicatively relevant integrative functions. It represents formation and maintenance of multimodal representations in a new version of the ELU model, and this function *seems* to be neurally dissociated from explicit, complex, and simple working memory capacity estimates (parameter C), and from other executive functions.
6. In the ELU context, we have concluded that the *r*apid, *a*utomatic *m*ultimodality *b*inding of *pho*nology (RAMBPHO) is one aspect of the episodic buffer function that can be incorporated in the ELU model. Further research will have to delineate the extent to which buffering under mismatch conditions shares neural and cognitive resources with the explicit storage and processing functions of parameter C.

References

Allen, R. J., Baddeley, A. D., & Hitch, G. J. (2006). Is the binding of visual features in working memory resource-demanding? *Journal of Experimental Psychology: General*, *135*, 298–313.

Andersson, U. (2002). Deterioration of the phonological processing skills in adults with an acquired severe hearing loss. *European Journal of Cognitive Psychology*, *14*, 335–352.

Andersson, U., Lyxell, B., Rönnberg, J., & Spens, K.-E. (2001a). Cognitive predictors of visual speech understanding. *Journal of Deaf Studies and Deaf Education*, *6*, 103–115.

Andersson, U., Lyxell, B., Rönnberg, J., & Spens, K.-E. (2001b). A follow-up study on the effects of speech tracking training on visual speechreading of sentences and words: Cognitive prerequisites and chronological age. *Journal of Deaf Studies and Deaf Education*, *6*, 116–129.

Atkinson, J., Campbell, R., Marshall, J., Thacker, A., & Woll, B. (2004). Understanding "not": neuropsychological dissociations between hand and head markers of negation in BSL. *Neuropsychologia*, *42*, 214–229.

Atkinson, J., Marshall, J., Woll, B., & Thacker, A. (2005). Testing comprehension abilities in users of BSL following CVA. *Brain & Language*, *94*, 233–248.

Baddeley, A. D. (2000). The episodic buffer: A new component of working memory? *Trends in Cognitive Science*, *4*, 417–423.

Barch, D. M., Braver, T. S., Nystrom, L. E., Forman, S. D., Noll, D. C., & Cohen, J. D. (1997). Dissociating working memory from task difficulty in human prefrontal cortex. *Neuropsychologia*, *35*, 1373–1380.

Bavelier, D., Corina, D., Jezzard, P., Clark, V., Karni, A., Lalwani, A., et al. (1998). Hemispheric specialization for English and ASL: Left invariance–right variability. *NeuroReport*, *9*, 1537–1542.

Bellugi, U., Poizner, H., & Klima, E. S. (1983). Brain organization for language: Clues from sign aphasia. *Human Neurobiology*, *2*, 155–170.

Bergman, B. (1982). *Studies in Swedish sign language*. Doctoral dissertation, Institute of Linguistics, University of Stockholm, Sweden.

Bergman, B. (1983). Verbs and adjectives: Morphological processes in Swedish sign language. In: J. Kyle & B. Woll (Eds.), *Language in sign: An international perspective on sign language*. London: Croom Helm.

Bergman, B. (1990). Grammaticalisation of location. In: W. H. Edmondson & F. Karlsson (Eds.), SLR'87. *Papers from The Fourth International Symposium on Sign Language Research* (Lapeenranta, Finland). Hamburg: Signum-Press.

Boutla, M., Supalla, T., Newport, E. L., & Bavelier, D. (2004). Short-term memory span: Insights from sign language. *Nature Neuroscience*, *7*(9), 997–1002.

Braver, T. S., Cohen, J. D., Nystrom, L. E., Jonides, J., Smith, E. E., & Noll, D. C. (1997). A parametric study of prefrontal cortex involvement in human working memory. *NeuroImage*, *5*, 49–62.

Cabeza, R., & Nyberg, L. (2000). Imaging cognition II: An empirical review of 275 PET and fMRI studies. *Journal of Cognitive Neuroscience*, *12*(1), 1–47.

Calvert, G. A., Bullmore, E. T., Brammer, M. J., Campbell, R., Williams, S. C. R., McGuire, P. K., et al. (1997). Activation of auditory cortex during silent lipreading. *Science*, *276*, (5312), 593–596.

Corina, D., Kritchevsky, M., & Bellugi, U. (1996). Visual language processing and unilateral neglect: Evidence from American sign language. *Cognitive Neuropsychology*, *3*, 321–356.

Courtin, M., & Melot, A. M. (2005). Metacognitive development of deaf children: Lessons from the appearance-reality and false belief tasks. *Developmental Science*, *8*(1), 16–25.

Daneman, M., & Merikle, P M. (1996). Working memory and language comprehension: A meta-analysis. *Psychonomic Bulletin & Review*, *3*(4), 422–433.

Dillon, H. (2001). *Hearing aids*. Stuttgart: Thieme.

Emmorey, K. (2002). *Language, cognition and the brain: Insights from sign language research*. Mahwah, NJ: Lawrence Erlbaum Associates, Inc.

Emmorey, K., Grabowski, T., McCullough, S., Damasio, H., Ponto, L. B., Hichwa, D., et al. (2003). Neural systems underlying lexical retrieval for sign language. *Neuropsychologia*, *41*, 85–95.

Foo, C., Rudner, M., Rönnberg, J., & Lunner, T. (2007). Recognition of speech in noise with new hearing instrument compression release settings requires explicit cognitive storage and processing capacity. *Journal of American Academy of Audiology*, *18*, 553–566.

Hagerman, B. (1982). Sentences for testing speech-intelligibility in noise. *Scandinavian Audiology*, *11*, 79.

Hagerman, B., & Kinnefors, C. (1995). Efficient adaptive methods for measuring speech reception threshold in quiet and in noise. *Scandinavian Audiology*, *24*(1), 71–77.

Hällgren, M., Larsby, B., & Arlinger, S. (2006). A Swedish version of the Hearing In Noise Test (HINT) for measurement of speech recognition. *International Journal of Audiology*, *45*(4), 227–237.

Hannon, B., & Daneman, M. (2001). A new tool for measuring and understanding individual differences in the component processes of reading comprehension. *Journal of Educational Psychology*, *93*(1): 103–128.

Hickok, G., Bellugi, U., & Klima, E. S. (1998). What's right about the neural organization of sign language? A perspective on recent neuroimaging results. *Trends in Cognitive Sciences*, *2*, 465–467.

Hickok, G., Klima, E. S., & Bellugi, U. (1996a). The neurobiology of sign language and its implications for the neural basis of language. *Nature*, *381*, 699–702.

Hickok, G., Kritchevsky, M., Bellugi, U., & Klima, E. S. (1996b). The role of the frontal operculum in sign language aphasia. *Neurocase*, *5*, 373–380.

Hickok, G., Say, K., Bellugi, U., & Klima, E. S. (1996c). The basis for hemispheric asymmetries for language and spatial cognition: Clues from focal brain damage in two deaf signers. *Aphasiology*, *10*, 577–591.

Höien, T., Lundberg, I., Stanovitch, K., & Bjaalid, I.-K. (1995). Components of phonological awareness. *Reading and Writing*, *7*, 171–188.

Hygge, S., Rönnberg, J., Larsby, B., & Arlinger, S. (1992). Normal and hearing-impaired subjects' ability to just follow conversation in competing speech, reversed speech, and noise backgrounds. *Journal of Speech and Hearing Research*, *35*, 208–215.

Kegl. J., Cohen, H., & Poizner, H. (1999). Articulatory consequences of Parkinson's disease: Perspectives from two modalities. *Brain and Cognition*, *40*, 355–386.

Kim, J. J., Kim, M. S., Lee, J. S., Lee, D. S., Lee, M. C., & Kwon, J. S. (2002). Dissociation of working memory processing associated with native and second languages: PET investigation. *NeuroImage*, *15*, 879–891.

Lee, H.-J., Truy, E., Mamou, G., Sappey-Marinier, D., & Giraud, A-L. (2007). Visual speech circuits in profound acquired deafness: A possible role for latent multimodal connectivity. *Brain, 130*, 2929–2941.

Levänen, S. (1998). Neuromagnetic studies of human auditory cortex function and reorganization. *Scandinavian Audiology, Supplement 27*(49), 16.

Leybaert, J. (1998). Phonological representations in deaf children: The importance of early linguistic experience. *Scandinavian Journal of Psychology, 39*, 169–173.

Leybaert, J., & Charlier, B. L. (1996). Visual speech in the head: The effect of cued speech on rhyming, remembering, and spelling. *Journal of Deaf Studies and Deaf Education, 1*, 234–248.

Lidestam, B. (2003). Semantic framing of speech: Emotional and topical cues in perception of poorly specified speech [Doctoral dissertation, Linköping University, Sweden]. *Linköping Studies in Education and Psychology, 94*.

Lillo-Martin, D. (1997). The modular effects of sign language acquisition. In M. Marschark & V. S. Everhart (Eds.), *Relations of language and thought: The view from sign language and deaf children* (pp. 62–109). Oxford, UK: Oxford University Press.

Lyxell, B. (1994). Skilled speechreading: A single case study. *Scandinavian Journal of Psychology, 35*, 212–219.

Lyxell, B., Arlinger, S., Andersson, J., Bredberg, G., Harder, H., & Rönnberg, J. (1998). Phonological representation and speech understanding with cochlear implants in deafened adults. *Scandinavian Journal of Psychology, 39*, 175–179.

Lyxell, B., Arlinger, S., Andersson, J., Harder, H., Näsström, E., Svensson, H., et al. (1996). Information-processing capabilities and cochlear implants: Pre-operative predictors for speech understanding. *Journal of Deaf Studies and Deaf Education, 1*, 190–201.

Lyxell, B., & Rönnberg, J. (1989). Information-processing skills and speechreading. *British Journal of Audiology, 23*, 339–347.

Lyxell, B., & Rönnberg, J. (1991). Visual speech processing: Word decoding and word discrimination related to sentence-based speechreading and hearing-impairment. *Scandinavian Journal of Psychology, 32*, 9–17.

Lyxell, B., & Rönnberg, J. (1992). The relationship between verbal ability and sentence-based speechreading. *Scandinavian Audiology, 21*, 67–72.

Lyxell, B., Rönnberg, J., & Samuelsson, S. (1994). Internal speech functioning and speechreading in deafened and normal hearing adults. *Scandinavian Audiology, 23*, 179–185.

MacSweeney, M., Campbell, R., Woll, B., Brammer, M. J., Giampietro, V., David, A. S., et al. (2006). Lexical and sentential processing in British Sign Language. *Human Brain Mapping*, 27(1), 63–76.

MacSweeney, M., Campbell, R., Woll, B., Giampietro, V., David, A. S., McGuire, P. K., et al. (2004). Dissociating linguistic and nonlinguistic gestural communication in the brain. *NeuroImage, 22*(4), 1605–1618.

Marshall, J., Atkinson, J., Smulovitch, E., Thacker, A., & Woll., B. (2004). Aphasia in a user of British Sign Language: Dissociation between sign and gesture. *Cognitive Neuropsychology, 21*(5), 537–554.

McGuire, P. K., Robertson, D., Thacker, A., David, A. S., Kitson, N., Frackowiak, R. S. J., et al. (1997). Neural correlates of thinking in sign language. *NeuroReport, 8*, 695–698.

Meyer, M., Toepel, U., Keller, J., Nussbaumer, D., Zysset, S., & Friedrici, A. D. (2007).

Neuroplasticity of sign language: Implications from structural and functional brain imaging. *Restorative Neurology and Neuroscience, 25*, 335–351.

Milkovic, M., Bradaric-Joncic, S., & Wilbur, R. B. (2007). Information status and word order in Croatian Sign Language. *Clinical Linguistics & Phonetics, 21*(11), 1007–1017.

Newman, A. J., Bavelier, D., Corina, D., Jezzard, P., & Neville, H. J. (2002). A critical period for right hemisphere recruitment in American Sign Language processing. *Nature Neuroscience, 5*(1), 76–80.

Neville, H. J., Bavelier, D., Corina, D., Rauschecker, J., Karni, A., Lawani, A., et al. (1998). Cerebral organization for language in deaf and hearing subjects: Biological constraints and effects of experience. *Proceedings of the National Academy of Sciences USA, 95*, 922–929.

Neville, H. J., Coffey, S. A., Lawson, D. S., Fischer, A., Emmorey, K., & Bellugi, U. (1997). Neural systems mediating American Sign Language: Effects of sensory experience and age of acquisition. *Brain and Language, 57*, 285–308.

Nilsson, M. Soli, S. D., & Sullivan, J. A. (1994). Development of the Hearing In Noise Test for the measurement of speech reception thresholds in quiet and in noise. *Journal of the Acoustical Society of America, 95*, 1085–1099.

Nishimura, H., Hashikawa, K., Doi, K., Iwaki, T., Watanabe, Y., Kusuoka, H., et al. (1999). Sign language "heard" in the auditory cortex. *Nature, 397*, 116.

Öhngren, G. (1992). *Components of tactually mediated speechreading*. Unpublished doctoral thesis, Uppsala University, Sweden.

Osaka, N., Osaka, M., Kondo, H., Morishita, M., Fukuyama, H., & Shibasaki, H. (2004). The neural basis of executive function in working memory: An fMRI study based on individual differences. *NeuroImage, 21*, 623–631.

Petitto, L. A., Zatorre, R. J., Gauna, K., Nikelski, E. J., Dostie, D., Evans, A. C. (2000). Speech-like cerebral activity in profoundly deaf people processing signed languages: Implications for the neural basis of human language. *Proceedings of the National Academy of Sciences USA, 97*(25), 13961–13966.

Pichora-Fuller, K. (2003). Processing speed: Psychoacoustics, speech perception, and comprehension. *International Journal of Audiology, 42*, S59–S67.

Poizner, H., Klima, E. S., & Bellugi, U. (1987). *What the hands reveal about the brain*. Cambridge, MA: MIT Press.

Poizner, H., Klima, E. S., & Bellugi, U. (1990). Biological foundation of language: Clues from sign language. *Annual Review of Neuroscience, 13*, 283–307.

Prabhakaran, V., Narayanan, K., Zhao, Z., & Gabrielli, J. D. E. (2000). Integration of diverse information in working memory in the frontal lobe. *Nature Neuroscience, 3*, 85–90.

Repovs, G., & Baddeley, A. (2006). The multi-component model of working memory: Explorations in experimental cognitive psychology. *Neuroscience, 139*(1), 5–21.

Rönnberg, J. (1990). Cognitive and communicative function: The effects of chronological age and "handicap age". *European Journal of Cognitive Psychology, 2*, 253–273.

Rönnberg, J. (1993). Cognitive characteristics of skilled tactiling: The case of GS. *European Journal of Cognitive Psychology, 5*, 19–33.

Rönnberg, J. (1995). What makes a skilled speechreader? In G. Plant & K. Spens (Eds.), *Profound deafness and speech communication* (pp. 393–416). London: Whurr.

Rönnberg, J. (2003a). Cognition in the hearing impaired and deaf as a bridge between signal and dialogue: A framework and a model. *International Journal of Audiology, 42*: S68–S76.

Rönnberg, J. (2003b). Working memory, neuroscience, and language. In M. Marschark & P. E. Spencer (Eds.), *Oxford handbook of deaf studies, language, and education* (pp. 478–489). Oxford, UK: Oxford University Press.

Rönnberg, J., Andersson, J., Andersson, U., Johansson, K., Lyxell, B., & Samuelsson, S. (1998a). Cognition as a bridge between signal and dialogue: Communication in the hearing impaired and deaf. *Scandinavian Audiology, 27*(suppl. 49), 101–108.

Rönnberg, J., Andersson, J., Samuelsson, S., Söderfeldt, B., Lyxell, B., & Risberg, J. (1999). A speechreading expert: The case of MM. *Journal of Speech, Language, and Hearing Research, 42*, 5–20.

Rönnberg, J., Andersson, U., Lyxell, B., & Spens, K. (1998b). Vibrotactile speechreading support: Cognitive prerequisites for training. *Journal of Deaf Studies & Deaf Education, 3*, 143–156.

Rönnberg, J., Arlinger, S., Lyxell, B., & Kinnefors, C. (1989). Visual evoked potentials: Relation to adult speechreading and cognitive function. *Journal of Speech and Hearing Research, 32*, 725–735.

Rönnberg, J., Rudner, M., & Ingvar, M. (2004). Neural correlates of working memory for sign language. *Cognitive Brain Research, 20*, 165–182.

Rönnberg, J., Samuelsson, S., & Lyxell, B. (1998c). Conceptual constraints in sentence-based lipreading in the hearing impaired. In R. Campbell, B. Dodd, & D. Burnham (Eds.), *Hearing by eye: Part II. Advances in the psychology of speechreading and audiovisual speech* (pp. 143–153). London: Lawrence Erlbaum Associates.

Rönnberg, J., Söderfeldt, B., & Risberg, J. (1998d). Regional cerebral blood flow during signed and heard episodic and semantic tasks. *Applied Neuropsychology, 5*, 132–138.

Rönnberg, J., Söderfeldt, B., & Risberg, J. (2000). The cognitive neuroscience of signed language. *Acta Psychologica, 105*, 237–254.

Rudner, M., Foo, C., Rönnberg, J., & Lunner, T. (in press). Cognition and aided speech recognition in noise: Specific role for cognitive factors following nine-week experience with adjusted compression settings on hearing aids. *Scandinavian Journal of Psychology*.

Rudner, M., Fransson, P., Ingvar, M., Nyberg, L., & Rönnberg, J. (2007). Neural representation of binding lexical signs and words in the episodic buffer of working memory. *Neuropsychologia, 45*(10), 2258–2276.

Rudner, M., & Rönnberg, J. (2004). Perceptual saliency in the visual channel enhances explicit language processing. *Iranian Audiology, 3*(1), 16–26.

Rudner, M., & Rönnberg, J. (2006). Towards a functional ontology for working memory for sign and speech. *Cognitive Processing, 7*, S183–S186.

Rudner, M., & Rönnberg, J. (2008). The role of the episodic buffer in working memory for language processing. *Cognitive Processing, 9*, 19–28.

Sakai, K. L., Tatsuno, Y., Suzuki, K., Kimura, H., & Ichida, Y. (2005). Sign and speech: Amodal commonality in left hemisphere dominance for comprehension of sentences. *Brain, 128*, 1407–1417.

Siple, P. (1997). Universals, generalizability, and the acquisition of sign language. In M. Marschark & V. S. Everhart (Eds.), *Relations of language and thought: The view from sign language and deaf children* (pp. 24–61). Oxford, UK: Oxford University.

Smith, E. E., & Jonides, J. (1997). Working memory: A view from neuroimaging. *Cognitive Psychology*, *33*, 5–42.

Smith, M. E. G., & Campbell, P. (1997). Discourses on deafness: Social policy and the communicative habilitation of the deaf. *Canadian Journal of Sociology*, *22*, 437–456.

Söderfeldt, B., Ingvar, M., Rönnberg, J., Eriksson, L., Serrander, M., & Stone-Elander, S. (1997). Signed and spoken language perception studied by positron emission tomography. *Neurology*, *49*, 82–87.

Söderfeldt, B., Rönnberg, J., & Risberg, J. (1994a). Regional cerebral blood flow in sign-language users. *Brain and Language*, *46*, 59–68.

Söderfeldt, B., Rönnberg, J., & Risberg, J. (1994b). Regional cerebral blood flow during sign language perception: A comparison between deaf and hearing subjects with deaf parents. *Sign Language Studies*, *84*, 199–208.

Stokoe, W. C. (1960). Sign language structure: An outline of the visual communication systems of the American deaf. In *Studies in Linguistics: Occasional papers* (Vol. 8). Buffalo, NY: University of Buffalo.

Stokoe, W. C., Casterline, D., & Croneberg, C. (1965). *Dictionary of American Sign Language*. Washington, DC: Gallaudet College Press.

Suchan, B., Linnewerth, B. Köster, O., Daum, I., & Schmid, G. (2006). Cross-modal processing in auditory and visual working memory. *NeuroImage*, *29*, 853–858.

Summerfield, Q. (1987). Some preliminaries to a comprehensive account of audio-visual speech perception. In B. Dodd & R. Campbell (Eds.), *Hearing by eye: The psychology of lipreading* (pp. 3–51). Hillsdale, NJ: Lawrence Erlbaum Associates.

Sutton-Spence, R., & Woll, B. (1998). Fingerspelling as a resource for lexical innovation in British sign language. In M. K. Verma (Ed.), *Sociolinguistics, language and society: Language and development* (Vol. 5, pp. 10–143). New Delhi: Sage.

Wallin, L. (1996). *Polysynthetic signs in Swedish sign language*. Doctoral dissertation, Stockholm University, Sweden.

Wilson, K., & Emmorey, K. (1997a). A visuospatial "phonological" loop in working memory: Evidence from American Sign Language. *Memory & Cognition*, *25*, 313–320.

Wilson, K., & Emmorey, K. (1997b). Working memory for sign language: A window into the architecture of the working memory system. *Journal of Deaf Studies and Deaf Education*, *2*, 121–130.

Wilson, K., & Emmorey, K. (1998). A "word length" for sign language: Further evidence for the role of language in structuring working memory. *Memory & Cognition*, *26*, 584–591.

Woll, B. (1990). Sign language. In N. E. Collinge (Ed.), *An encyclopedia of language* (pp. 740–783). London: Routledge.

Zago, L., & Tzourio-Mazoyer, N. (2002). Distinguishing visuospatial working memory and complex mental calculation areas within the parietal lobes. *Neuroscience Letters*, *331*, 45–49.

Zhang, D., Zhang, X., Sun, X., Li, Z., Wang, Z., He, S., et al. (2004). Cross-modal temporal order memory for auditory digits and visual locations: An fMRI study. *Human Brain Mapping*, *22*(4), 280–289.

15 The mismatch negativity as an index of different forms of memory in audition

Risto Näätänen and Kairi Kreegipuu

The mismatch negativity (MMN) (illustrated in Figure 15.1) is an electromagnetic response to a discriminable change ("deviant") in any repetitive aspect ("standard") of auditory stimulation (Näätänen, Gaillard, & Mäntysalo, 1978; for reviews, see Näätänen, 2001; Näätänen & Winkler, 1999; Näätänen, Paavilainen, Rinne, & Alho, 2007). The MMN is initiated by an auditory change-detection process in which a difference is found between the deviant auditory event and the sensory-memory representation of the repetitive aspects of the preceding auditory stimulation. The MMN therefore provides an objective index of sound-discrimination accuracy (Lang et al., 1990; for a review, see Näätänen & Alho, 1997), and it is the only such index. This change-detection process occurs pre-perceptually in the auditory cortices, generating the auditory-cortex subcomponent of the MMN and triggering frontal-cortex processes that, in turn, generate the frontal subcomponent of the MMN and initiate an involuntary attention switch to auditory change (Giard, Perrin, Pernier, & Bouchet, 1990; Näätänen, 1990; Rinne, Alho, Ilmoniemi, Virtanen, & Näätänen, 2000). Consequently, the MMN generation does not result from the afferent processes elicited by the deviant stimuli or events – that is, separate, memory-related neuronal activity is involved rather than just the activation of new (or fresh) afferent elements, those activated by the deviants but not by the standards (for a review, see Näätänen, Jacobsen, & Winkler, 2005).

In the present article, we will review the different forms of auditory sensory memory as reflected by the MMN. Most MMN studies report MMNs originating from a discrepancy between the eliciting stimulus and that represented by a short-term, echoic, memory trace formed by the preceding stimuli in the same stimulus block and lasting for a few seconds. However, depending on the condition and stimuli, the MMN may also reflect long-term, or permanent, memory traces in audition, for both speech and non-speech stimuli. Finally, the MMN may also index the earliest and shortest form of memory – the sensory register, which is involved in the formation of sound perception – and even such auditory memory traces, that reflect automatic "intelligent" processes.

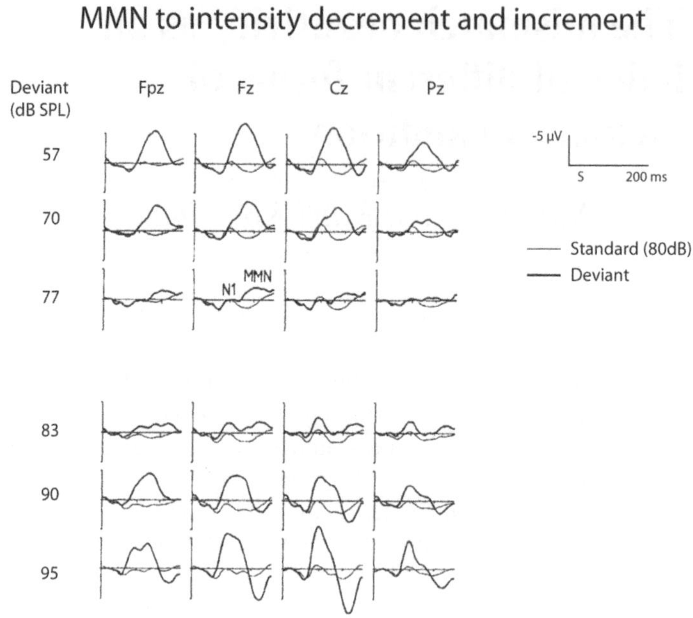

Figure 15.1 Grand average frontal-pole (Fpz), frontal (Fz), central (Cz), and parietal (Pz) event-related potentials to the 80-dB standard tone (thin line) and to the deviant tones of 6 different intensity levels presented in separate blocks. The N1 is marked to point out that whereas the N1 amplitude increases with increasing deviant-tone intensity (independent of the standard-tone intensity), the mismatch-negativity (MMN) amplitude increases and the MMN peak latency decreases with increasing distance from the standard (i.e., for deviants being both louder and softer than the standard). (From *Attention and Brain Function* (p. 140) by R. Näätänen, 1992. Copyright © 1992 Lawrence Erlbaum Associates, Inc. Reprinted with permission.)

The MMN as an index of short-term memory traces in audition

The MMN can only be elicited as long as there is a short-term memory trace of preceding auditory stimuli (Näätänen, Paavilainen, Alho, Reinikainen, & Sams, 1987). This duration is usually determined by prolonging the within-block constant inter-stimulus interval (ISI) until deviants no longer elicit an MMN. In young subjects, this duration may even be 10 sec (Böttscher-Gandor & Ullsperger, 1992; Sams, Hari, Rif, & Knuuttila, 1993), but in elderly ones, it is considerably shortened (Pekkonen et al., 1996). Furthermore, this age-related memory-trace duration decrease is expedited in chronic alcoholism (Polo, Escera, Gual, & Grau, 1999) and, in particular, in neurodegenerative brain diseases such as Alzheimer's disease (Pekkonen, Jousimäki,

Könönen, Reinikainen, & Partanen, 1994). These sensory-memory trace durations might therefore provide a (long searched for) general index of brain plasticity, whereas the sensitivity of the MMN response, as already mentioned, appears to serve as an objective index of sound-discrimination accuracy.

The MMN as an index of long-term memory traces in audition

When phoneme stimuli are used, then MMN data may also index the presence of mother-tongue, language-specific long-term memory traces. This occurs when mother-tongue speech sounds such as vowels of the language are used as deviant stimuli. Such stimuli elicit, in addition to the usual acoustic-change MMN component, one that indexes the presence of permanent language-specific memory traces. Such memory traces in the human brain were first reported by Näätänen et al. (1997) and Dehaene-Lambertz (1997). Näätänen et al. (1997) found that an infrequent vowel deviant presented in a sequence of native-language vowel standards elicited a larger-amplitude MMN when it was a typical exemplar of a vowel category in the subject's native language (Finnish) than when it was not a typical vowel in this language (/õ/ of the Estonian language, which does not exist in Finnish). Furthermore, the subsequent magnetoencephalography (MEG) recordings showed that the vowel-related MMN enhancement originated from the left posterior auditory cortex, a probable locus of the language-specific vowel traces. In contrast, the concomitant acoustic change necessarily accompanying the vowel change elicited a bilateral auditory-cortex MMN subcomponent. The authors proposed that these long-term or permanent traces serve as recognition patterns that are activated by the corresponding speech sounds, enabling one to correctly perceive them, and, in addition, that these traces provide reference information for pronunciation.

Furthermore, using a similar Finnish–Estonian cross-linguistic design, Cheour et al. (1998) obtained evidence suggesting that language-specific speech-sound memory traces develop between 6 and 12 months of age. The language-specific memory traces also tolerate wide acoustic variation, enabling one to correctly perceive the phonemes uttered, irrespective of the wide acoustic variation between different voices (see Shestakova et al., 2002). Hence, the phoneme-identity code must be identical in any sound perceived as, for instance, /e/, irrespective of whether it is uttered by a male, a female, or a child voice. The core property of this phoneme-identity code therefore must be its invariance in the midst of wide acoustical variation, suggesting that there must exist neuronal populations that detect such an invariance (Näätänen, 2001). Consistent with this, the existence of such types of neuronal populations in the human brain was shown by Paavilainen, Jaramillo, Näätänen, and Winkler's (1999) MMN data.

The MMN as an index of the very short form of auditory short-term memory (sensory register)

The MMN can also reflect the cumulation of sensory information underlying sound perception. Näätänen and Winkler (1999) proposed that the auditory sensory-memory trace is formed when the outcomes of the different parallel feature-specific processes cumulate on the neural mechanisms of auditory sensory memory. The neural sensory-memory trace then emerging (with this phase underlying perception) contains the highly stimulus-specific, feature-integrated sensory information present in perception and sensory memory. The authors further proposed that this integration process uses a sliding temporal window of some 150–200 ms in duration, called the temporal window of integration (TWI) (Näätänen, 1990). During the TWI, acoustic stimulation from the same source or channel (i.e., of similar acoustic parameters and approximately the same spatial origin) is integrated into a unitary auditory percept (Shinozaki et al., 2003). The emerging central sound representation usually enters conscious perception but may also remain subjectively silent, depending on the direction of attention and the strength of the parallel call-for-attention signals (Näätänen, 1992).

The TWI duration can be estimated on the basis of both behavioural and MMN data. Behavioural studies showed that loudness summation for brief sounds continues up to durations of about 200 ms (e.g., Scharf & Houtsma, 1986). Furthermore, in backward recognition-masking studies (Cowan, 1984; Hawkins & Presson, 1977, 1986; Massaro, 1970), when the mask followed the onset of a brief test stimulus (to be identified by the subject) with an interval shorter than 150–200 ms, then the test stimulus features were incompletely perceived. Hence, about 150–200 ms from stimulus onset appear to be needed for the completion of the trace development, and thus for a fully elaborated percept to emerge. (For supporting MMN data from the backward-masking paradigm, see Winkler & Näätänen, 1992, 1994; Winkler, Reinikainen, & Näätänen, 1993.)

Furthermore, an infrequent stimulus omission elicits an MMN only when the constant stimulus onset asynchrony (SOA) is shorter than 150 ms (Yabe, Tervaniemi, Reinikainen, & Näätänen, 1997; Yabe et al., 1998). Yabe et al. (1997) suggested that auditory input is processed in approximately 150–170-ms temporal segments (TWI); therefore, stimulus omission from this time window initiated by the onset of the preceding stimulus elicited an MMN, whereas stimulus omission occurring thereafter did not (i.e., with SOAs > 150 ms).

The TWI may also be crucial for speech perception and musical experience. Both depend on the simultaneous psychological presence of auditory stimulation from a time window of some short duration rather than from any given instant. Thus, auditory perception does not correspond to the immediately present acoustic reality but, rather, to the outcome of temporal integration over the immediate past of some 150–200 ms (TWI). Näätänen (1990) proposed that the continuously sliding temporal window of integration actually provides this temporally stretched psychological presence. The TWI may considerably expand in time "the 'psychological presence' in audition relative to the timeless 'cutting edge' of the physical presence that continuously turns the future into the past" (Näätänen, 1990, p. 275).

The MMN as an index of extrapolatory and other "intelligent" traces

Finally, we will review MMN evidence for automatic "primitive sensory intelligence" at the level of the auditory cortex. In these "abstract-feature" MMN studies, there is no physically identical, repetitive standard stimulus but, rather, a class of several physically different "standard" stimuli that obey some common rule.

In the first of these studies, Saarinen, Paavilainen, and Schröger (1992) presented their subjects with tone pairs. The frequency level of the tone pairs varied randomly over a wide range, there being no physically identical, repetitive standard stimulus. Instead, the constant feature of the standard pairs was an "abstract" or "second-order" one – namely, the *direction* of the frequency change within a tone pair: all standard pairs were ascending pairs, whereas the deviants were descending pairs. Thus, the abstract attribute was based on a rule defining the *relationship* between the simple physical, first-order, attributes of the two tones forming a pair. Nevertheless, an MMN was elicited by the deviant pairs in an ignore condition. This result showed that the preattentively formed sensory representations were of an abstract nature, corresponding to simple concepts ("rise", "fall"). Hence, auditory cortex was capable of automatically deriving a common invariant feature from a set of individual varying physical events. (For similar results in children aged 8–14 years, see Gumenyuk et al., 2003.) Furthermore, Korzyukov, Winkler, Gumenyuk, and Alho (2003), using a similar paradigm, and MEG recordings, localized the source of the abstract-feature MMN at the auditory cortex. (For studies showing abstract-feature MMNs in newborns, see Ruusuvirta, Huotilainen, Fellman, & Näätänen, 2004; Carral et al., 2005.)

Similarly, in music, we recognize melodies irrespective of the key into which they are transposed or the instrument on which they are played. Tervaniemi, Rytkönen, Schröger, Ilmoniemi, and Näätänen's (2001) posed standard stimuli consisted of a melodic pattern that was randomly presented at different frequency levels (simulating a melody randomly played in different keys). It was found that occasional slight contour changes in the patterns widely varying in the frequency level elicited an MMN in subjects ignoring sound stimuli (but only after some training and only in musicians who perform music primarily without a score).

Furthermore, the MMN mechanism also forms extrapolatory traces representing the forthcoming stimuli on the basis of the regularities or trends automatically detected in the auditory past. Tervaniemi, Maury, and

Näätänen (1994) presented a long sequence of steadily descending tones. It was found that an occasional ascending tone or a tone repetition elicited an MMN (Figure 15.2).

Very recently, Paavilainen, Arajärvi, and Takegata (2007) used sound stimuli that varied in two features, duration and frequency, being either short (50 ms) or long (150 ms), and low (1,000 Hz) or high (1,500 Hz). All four possible combinations (short–low, short–high, long–low, long–high) were equiprobably presented with a short constant ISI. Furthermore, the duration of each stimulus predicted the frequency of the *next* stimulus as follows: (1) if the present stimulus is short in duration, then the next stimulus will be low in frequency; and (2) if the present stimulus is long in duration, then the next stimulus will be high in frequency. Occasional deviant events breaking these rules (e.g., a high-pitched stimulus following a short stimulus) elicited an MMN, in an ignore condition.

In the subsequent attend conditions, subjects were asked to press a button to any stimuli they found somehow "strange" or "deviant". (The rules were not explained to them.) An MMN was again elicited, although subjects could detect only 15% of the deviant events, and none of them could verbally express the rules in the later interviews. The results suggest that the neural mechanism modelling the auditory environment may automatically learn the co-variation between the features of the successive events and make predictions regarding the forthcoming stimuli. Furthermore, if the predictions are not fulfilled, then the MMN is generated.

Hence, the information extracted by the sensory-memory mechanisms often seems to be in an implicit form, not directly available to conscious processes and difficult to express verbally (see also Winkler, Cowan, Csépe, Czigler, & Näätänen, 1996a). Such reports of rich dynamic encoding of stimulus pattern can even be viewed in terms of (potentially) available and (actually) accessible information in memory (Tulving & Pearlstone, 1966) or perception (Allik, 1999). It means that in the case of multiple stimuli varying in one or more dimensions, the amount of potentially available information (i.e., number of different representations, "higher-order categories", or "grouping rules") can in principle be infinite. Technically, it is achieved by "presenting variable standards" (e.g., Paavilainen, Simola, Jaramillo, Näätänen, & Winkler, 2001; van Zuijen, Simoens, Paavilainen, Näätänen, & Tervaniemi, 2007) or using the multi-deviant condition recently introduced as the "Optimum I paradigm" (Näätänen, Pakarinen, Rinne, & Takegata, 2004). Thus, a particular internal representation can well be approached by means of a deviant stimulus serving as a retrieval cue for encoded information. The information is both available and accessible when the MMN response – usually a sensitive index of discrimination ability (cf. the direct comparison of MMN and behavioural discrimination in Kujala, Kallio, Tervaniemi, & Näätänen, 2001; Paavilainen et al., 2007; van Zuijen et al., 2007) – is elicited.

In conclusion, the MMN studies reviewed above suggest that the central

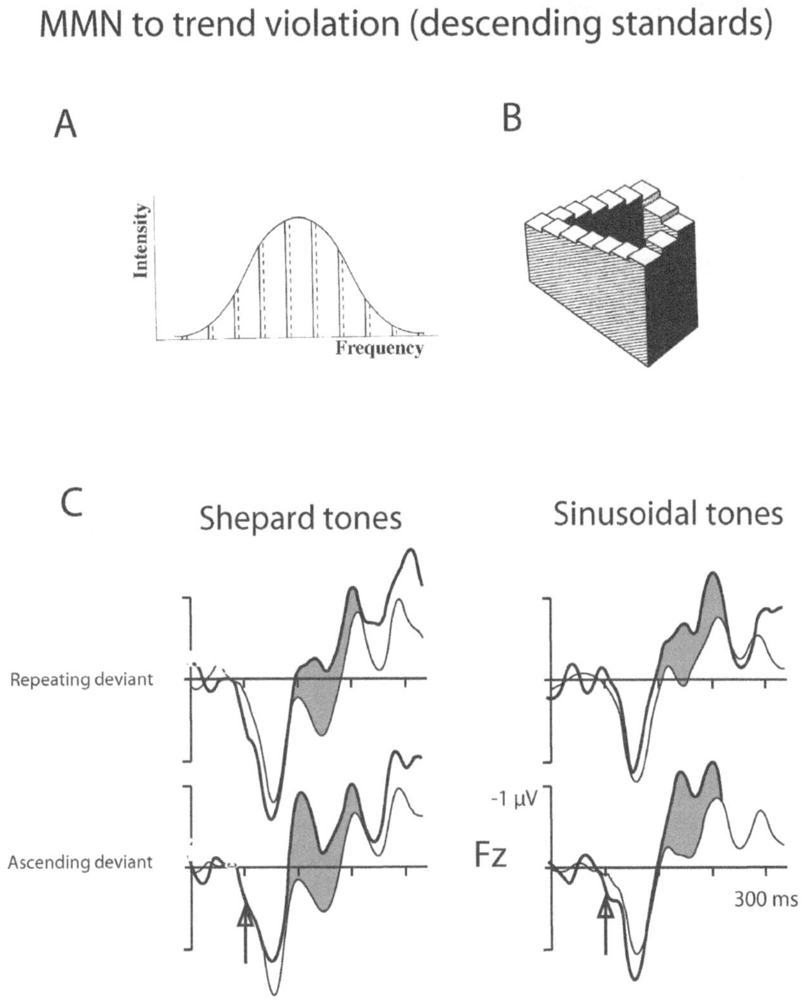

Figure 15.2 (a) Spectrum of an individual Shepard sound that, when presented in ascending or descending sequences of 12 sounds in 1-semitone steps, causes a pitch to ascend or descend in an endless manner. One Shepard sound consists of 10 frequency components, of 1 octave apart, with a bell-shaped spectrum. While a 12-tone series of Shepard sounds is delivered, the tone-height perception (which is equivalent to the sense of octave) is made to disappear by manipulating the sound spectrum. (b) A visual analogy of the Shepard illusion – the endlessly ascending or descending stairs. (c) The event-related potentials (ERPs) recorded at the frontal (Fz) electrode from reading subjects to Shepard (left) and sinusoidal (right) tones (thin line: standard stimulus; thick line: deviant stimulus). The left column shows a regularly descending Shepard sound sequence randomly replaced by a repeating (top) or an ascending (bottom) tone (deviant). The right column shows a regularly descending sinusoidal tone sequence with occasional repetitive (top) or ascending (bottom) deviants. The arrow indicates the deviant-stimulus onset and the shadowed area the statistically significant part of the mismatch negativity. Adapted with permission from Tervaniemi, M., Maury, S., & Näätänen, R. (1994). Neural representations of abstract stimulus features in the human brain as reflected by the mismatch negativity, *NeuroReport*, *5*, 844–846.

auditory system performs surprising cognitive operations, such as generalization leading to simple concept formation, rule extraction, and the anticipation of the next stimulus even at the pre-attentive level, demonstrating a kind of "primitive sensory intelligence" in the auditory cortex (for a review, see Näätänen, Tervaniemi, Sussman, Paavilainen, & Winkler, 2001).

Concluding overview and summary

As we have discussed in this chapter, the MMN can reflect several different hierarchically organized forms of auditory sensory memory starting from the earliest, most primitive one, which reflects the cumulation of sensory data extracted by different feature-detection activity – that is, Cowan's (1984, 1988) short form of auditory sensory memory. Consequently, the MMN seems to reflect online the emergence of a sound percept by illustrating the formation of the memory trace carrying the central sound representation. Moreover, MMN data also describe the route of this sensory information, from stimulus change to conscious perception, by shedding light on the prerequisites and mechanisms of the involuntary attention switch to auditory change (for a review, see Näätänen & Winkler, 1999). This sequence of cerebral events is initiated by predominantly right frontal-cortex activation (Giard et al., 1990) that appears to express a call for attention (Öhman, 1979) triggered with a very brief temporal delay (Rinne et al., 2000) by the preperceptual auditory-cortex change-detection signal. The occurrence of the subsequent attention switch is in turn reflected by the elicitation of a P3a component peaking at about 250 ms from stimulus onset (Squires, Squires, & Hillyard, 1975). This attention switch is indexed by a transient deterioration of primary-task performance accompanying MMN elicitation (Escera, Alho, Winkler, & Näätänen, 1998; Schröger, 1996).

Furthermore, MMN data also illustrate the relation between perception and memory in audition by showing that the rapid build-up of the sensory-memory trace corresponds to the perception of a sound and the gradual decay of this trace to sensory memory of this sound.

This sensory-memory development and decay can be observed, although indirectly, online with the MMN for stimuli presented in a stimulus block or session, but, as already mentioned, the MMN also enables one to probe long-term or permanent memory traces such as those of the phonemes or words of the mother tongue or even those learned later in the life (Winkler et al., 1999). Moreover, quite surprisingly, the MMN can also reflect higher-order linguistic phenomena such as grammar and semantic meaning, therefore being, in fact, capable of reflecting the hierarchical structure of the system of the language representations in the brain, from the smallest linguistic units – the phonemes – to semantic meaning (Pulvermüller, Härle, & Hummel, 2001a; Pulvermüller & Shtyrov, 2003; Pulvermüller, Shtyrov, Kujala, & Näätänen, 2004; Pulvermüller et al., 2001b; Shtyrov, Hauk, & Pulvermüller, 2004; for a review, see Pulvermüller, 2002). Does this correspond to the idea of levels of processing (Craik & Lockhart, 1972) – the well-known rule indicating that the deeper the processing of material has been (e.g., phonological, rhyme, semantic), the better the memory trace will be? On a very large scale, this is true. The TWI is long enough for registering stimuli but not for the fine elaboration of stimulus information, and it was recently demonstrated that subjects who were able to develop explicit knowledge (meaning, presumably, deeper processing) of the standard stimuli also expressed a larger-amplitude MMN (van Zuijen et al., 2007). At the same time, the optimal ISIs for the MMN in multiple-deviant conditions seem to be shorter than those in classical single-deviant conditions, most likely due to the higher working memory load (e.g., cf. Grau, Escera, Yago, & Polo, 1998; Paavilainen et al., 2001; van Zuijen et al., 2007).

Moreover, the MMN can also, at least in part, account for the predominantly left-hemispheric language processing in the brain by indicating the presence of the speech-sound traces mainly in the left hemisphere. In addition, the MMN data can also illustrate the special property of the speech-sound traces – that is, their ability to represent and recognize the invariant phoneme code in the midst of acoustic variation, accounting for the correct phoneme perception irrespective of the speaker-voice characteristics and sentence context. Furthermore, with regard to music perception, the MMN enables one to understand the perception and recognition of a familiar melody irrespective of the key in which the melody is played (for a review, see Tervaniemi & Brattico, 2004).

Finally, the MMN has also revealed a novel category of memory traces, those expressing the operation of automatic intelligent sensory processes such as the extrapolatory ones, anticipatory traces developing on the basis of the regularities encoded by the memory traces of the past (Winkler, Cowan, Csépe, Czigler, & Näätänen, 1996a; Winkler, Karmos, & Näätänen, 1996b; for a review, see Näätänen et al., 2001).

References

Allik, J. (1999). Available and accessible information in memory and vision. In E. Tulving (Ed.), *Memory, consciousness and the brain: The Tallinn conference* (pp. 7–17). Philadelphia, PA: Psychology Press.

Böttscher-Gandor, C., & Ullsperger, P. (1992). Mismatch negativity in event-related potentials to auditory stimuli as a function of varying interstimulus interval. *Psychophysiology*, *29*, 546–550.

Carral, V., Huotilainen, M., Ruusuvirta, T., Fellman, V., Näätänen, R., & Escera, C. (2005). A kind of auditory "primitive intelligence" already present at birth. *European Journal of Neuroscience*, *21*, 3201–3204.

Cheour, M., Ceponiene, R., Lehtokoski, A., Luuk, A., Allik, J., Alho, K., et al. (1998). Development of language-specific phoneme representations in the infant brain. *Nature Neuroscience*, *1*, 351–353.

Cowan, N. (1984). On short and long auditory stores. *Psychological Bulletin*, *96*, 341–370.

Cowan, N. (1988). Evolving conceptions of memory storage, selective attention, and their mutual constraints within the human information-processing system. *Psychological Bulletin, 104*, 163–191.

Craik, F. I. M., & Lockhart, R. S. (1972). Levels of processing: A framework for memory research. *Journal of Verbal Learning and Verbal Behaviour, 11*, 671–684.

Dehaene-Lambertz, G. (1997). Electrophysiological correlates of categorical phoneme perception in adults. *NeuroReport, 8*, 919–924.

Escera, C., Alho, K., Winkler, I., & Näätänen, R. (1998). Neural mechanisms of involuntary attention switching to novelty and change in the acoustic environment. *Journal of Cognitive Neuroscience, 10*, 590–604.

Giard, M. H., Perrin, F., Pernier, J., & Bouchet, P. (1990). Brain generators implicated in processing of auditory stimulus deviance: A topographic event-related potential study. *Psychophysiology, 27*, 627–640.

Grau, C., Escera, C., Yago, E., & Polo, M. D. (1998). Mismatch negativity and sensory memory evaluation: A new faster paradigm. *NeuroReport, 9*, 2451–2456.

Gumenyuk, V., Korzyukov, O., Alho, K., Winkler, I., Paavilainen, P., & Näätänen, R. (2003). Electric brain responses indicate preattentive processing of abstract acoustic regularities in children. *NeuroReport, 14*, 1411–1415.

Hawkins, H. L., & Presson, J. C. (1977). Masking and perceptual selectivity in auditory recognition. In S. Dornic (Ed.), *Attention and Performance VI* (pp. 195–211). Hillsdale, NJ: Lawrence Erlbaum Associates, Inc.

Hawkins, H. L., & Presson, J. C. (1986). Auditory information processing. In K. R. Boff, L. Kaufman, & J. P. Thomas (Eds.), *Handbook of perception and human performance* (Vol. 2, pp. 261–264). New York: Wiley.

Korzyukov, O., Winkler, I., Gumenyuk, V. I., & Alho, K. (2003). Processing abstract auditory features in the human auditory cortex. *NeuroImage, 20*, 2245–2258.

Kujala, T., Kallio, J., Tervaniemi, M., & Näätänen, R. (2001). Mismatch negativity as an index of temporal processing in audition. *Clinical Neurophysiology, 112*, 1712–1719.

Lang, H. A., Nyrke, T., Ek, M., Aaltonen, O., Raimo, I., & Näätänen, R. (1990). Pitch discrimination performance and auditory event-related potentials. In C. H. M. Brunia, A. W. K. Gaillard, A. Kok, G. Mulder, & M. N. Verbaten (Eds.), *Psychophysiological brain research* (Vol. 1, pp. 294–298). Tilburg, The Netherlands: Tilburg University Press.

Massaro, D. W. (1970). Retroactive interference in short-term recognition memory for pitch. *Journal of Experimental Psychology, 83*, 32–39.

Näätänen, R. (1990). The role of attention in auditory information processing as revealed by event-related potentials and other brain measures of cognitive function. *Behavioral and Brain Sciences, 13*, 201–288.

Näätänen, R. (1992). *Attention and brain function*. Hillsdale, NJ: Lawrence Erlbaum Associates, Inc.

Näätänen, R. (2001). The perception of speech sounds by the human brain as reflected by the mismatch negativity (MMN) and its magnetic equivalent MMNm [Presidential Address]. *Psychophysiology, 38*, 1–21.

Näätänen, R., & Alho, K. (1997). Mismatch negativity: The measure for central sound representation accuracy. *Audiology & Neuro-Otology, 2*, 341–353.

Näätänen, R., Gaillard, A. W. K., & Mäntysalo, S. (1978). Early selective-attention effect on evoked potential reinterpreted. *Acta Psychologica, 42*, 313–329.

Näätänen, R., Jacobsen, T., & Winkler, I. (2005). Memory based or afferent processes in mismatch negativity (MMN): A review of the evidence. *Psychophysiology*, *42*, 25–32.

Näätänen, R., Lehtokoski, A., Lennes, M., Cheour, M., Huotilainen, M., Iivonen, A., et al. (1997). Language-specific phoneme representations revealed by electric and magnetic brain responses. *Nature*, *385*, 432–434.

Näätänen, R., Paavilainen, P., Alho, K., Reinikainen, K., & Sams, M. (1987). Inter-stimulus interval and the mismatch negativity. In L. Barber & T. Blum, (Eds.), *Evoked potentials III* (pp. 392–397). London: Butterworths.

Näätänen, R., Paavilainen, P., Rinne, T., & Alho, K. (2007). The mismatch negativity (MMN) in basic research of central auditory processing: A review. *Clinical Neurophysiology*, *118*, 2544–2590.

Näätänen, R., Pakarinen, S., Rinne, T., & Takegata, R. (2004). The mismatch negativity (MMN): Towards the optimal paradigm. *Clinical Neurophysiology*, *115*, 140–144.

Näätänen, R., Tervaniemi, M., Sussman, E., Paavilainen, P., & Winkler, I. (2001). "Primitive intelligence" in the auditory cortex. *Trends in Neurosciences*, *24*, 283–288.

Näätänen, R., & Winkler, I. (1999). The concept of auditory stimulus representation in neuroscience. *Psychological Bulletin*, *125*, 826–859.

Öhman, A. (1979). The orienting response, attention and learning: An information-processing perspective. In H. D. Kimmel, E. H. van Olst, & J. F. Orlebeke (Eds.), *The orienting reflex in humans* (pp. 443–471). Hillsdale, NJ: Lawrence Erlbaum Associates, Inc.

Paavilainen, P., Arajärvi, P., & Takegata, R. (2007). Preattentive detection of nonsalient contingencies between auditory features. *NeuroReport*, *18*, 159–163.

Paavilainen, P., Jaramillo, M., Näätänen, R., & Winkler, I. (1999). Neuronal populations in the human brain extracting invariant relationships from acoustic variance. *Neuroscience Letters*, *265*, 179–182.

Paavilainen, P., Simola, J., Jaramillo, M., Näätänen, R., & Winkler, I. (2001). Preattentive extraction of abstract feature conjunctions from auditory stimulation as reflected by the mismatch negativity (MMN). *Psychophysiology*, *38*, 359–365.

Pekkonen, E., Jousimäki, V., Könönen, M., Reinikainen, K., & Partanen, J. (1994). Auditory sensory memory impairment in Alzheimer's disease: An event-related potential study. *NeuroReport*, *5*, 2537–2540.

Pekkonen, E., Rinne, T., Reinikainen, K., Kujala, T., Alho, K., & Näätänen, R. (1996). Aging effects on auditory processing: An event-related potential study. *Experimental Aging Research*, *22*, 171–184.

Polo, M. D., Escera, C., Gual, A., & Grau, C. (1999). Mismatch negativity and auditory sensory memory in chronic alcoholics. *Alcoholism: Clinical and Experimental Research*, *23*, 1744–1750.

Pulvermüller, F. (2002). A brain perspective on language mechanisms: From discrete neuronal ensembles to serial order. *Progress in Neurobiology*, *67*, 85–111.

Pulvermüller, F., Härle, M., & Hummel, F. (2001a). Walking or talking? Behavioral and neurophysiological correlates of action verb processing. *Brain and Language*, *78*, 143–168.

Pulvermüller, F., Kujala, T., Shtyrov, Y., Simola, J., Tiitinen, H., Alku, P., et al. (2001b). Memory traces for words as revealed by the mismatch negativity. *NeuroImage*, *14*, 607–616.

Pulvermüller, F., & Shtyrov, Y. (2003). Automatic processing of grammar in the human brain as revealed by the mismatch negativity. *NeuroImage, 20*, 159–172.

Pulvermüller, F., Shtyrov, Y., Kujala, T., & Näätänen, R. (2004). Word-specific cortical activity as revealed by the mismatch negativity (MMN). *Psychophysiology, 41*, 106–112.

Rinne, T., Alho, K., Ilmoniemi, R. J., Virtanen, J., & Näätänen, R. (2000). Separate time behaviors of the temporal and frontal mismatch negativity sources. *NeuroImage, 12*, 14–19.

Ruusuvirta, T., Huotilainen, M., Fellman, V., & Näätänen, R. (2004). Newborn human brain identifies repeated auditory feature conjunctions of low sequential probability. *European Journal of Neuroscience, 20*, 2819–2821.

Saarinen, J., Paavilainen, P., & Schröger, E. (1992). Representation of abstract attributes of auditory stimuli in the human brain. *NeuroReport, 3*, 1149–1151.

Sams, M., Hari, R., Rif, J., & Knuuttila, J. (1993). The human auditory sensory memory trace persists about 10 s: Neuromagnetic evidence. *Journal of Cognitive Neuroscience, 5*, 363–370.

Scharf, B., & Houtsma, A. J. (1986). Audition II: Loudness, pitch, localization, aural distortion, pathology. In K. R. Boff, L. Kaufman, & J. P. Thomas (Eds.), *Handbook of perception and human performance: Vol. 1. Sensory processes and perception* (pp. 15.1–15.60). New York: Wiley.

Schröger, E. (1996). A neural mechanism for involuntary attention shifts to changes in auditory stimulation. *Journal of Cognitive Neuroscience, 8*, 527–539.

Shestakova, A., Brattico, E., Huotilainen, M., Galunov, V., Soloviev, A., Sams, M., et al. (2002). Abstract phoneme representations in the left temporal cortex: Magnetic mismatch negativity study. *NeuroReport, 13*, 1813–1816.

Shinozaki, N., Yabe, H., Sato, Y., Hiruma, T., Sutoh, T., Matsuoka, T., et al. (2003). Spectrotemporal window of integration of auditory information in the human brain, *Cognitive Brain Research, 17*, 563–571.

Shtyrov, Y., Hauk, O., & Pulvermüller, F. (2004). Distributed neuronal networks for encoding category-specific semantic information: The mismatch negativity to action words. *European Journal of Neuroscience, 19*, 1083–1092.

Squires, N. K., Squires, K. C., & Hillyard, S. A. (1975). Two varieties of long-lasting positive waves evoked by unpredictable auditory stimuli. *Electroencephalography and Clinical Neurophysiology, 38*, 387–401.

Tervaniemi, M., & Brattico, E. (2004). From sounds to music: Towards understanding the neurocognition of musical sound perception. *Journal of Consciousness Studies, 11*, 9–27.

Tervaniemi, M., Maury, S., & Näätänen, R. (1994). Neural representations of abstract stimulus features in the human brain as reflected by the mismatch negativity. *NeuroReport, 5*, 844–846.

Tervaniemi, M., Rytkönen, M., Schröger, E., Ilmoniemi, R. J., & Näätänen, R. (2001). Superior formation of cortical memory traces for melodic patterns in musicians. *Learning & Memory, 8*, 295–300.

Tulving, E., & Pearlstone, Z. (1966). Availability and accessibility of information in memory for words. *Journal of Verbal Learning and Verbal Behaviour, 5*, 381–391.

van Zuijen, T. L., Simoens, V. L., Paavilainen, P., Näätänen, R., & Tervaniemi, M. (2007). Implicit, intuitive and explicit knowledge of abstract regularities in sound sequence: An event-related potential study. *Journal of Cognitive Neuroscience, 18*, 1292–1303.

Winkler, I., Cowan, N., Csépe, V., Czigler, I., & Näätänen, R. (1996a). Interactions between transient and long-term auditory memory as reflected by the mismatch negativity. *Journal of Cognitive Neuroscience*, *8*, 403–415.

Winkler, I., Karmos, G., & Näätänen, R. (1996b). Adaptive modeling of the unattended acoustic environment reflected in the mismatch negativity event-related potential. *Brain Research*, *742*, 239–252.

Winkler, I., Kujala, T., Tiitinen, H., Sivonen, P., Alku, P., Lehtokoski, A., et al. (1999). Brain responses reveal the learning of foreign language phonemes. *Psychophysiology*, *36*, 638–642.

Winkler, I., & Näätänen, R. (1992). Event-related potentials in auditory backward recognition masking: A new way to study the neurophysiological basis of sensory memory in humans. *Neuroscience Letters*, *140*, 239–242.

Winkler, I., & Näätänen, R. (1994). The effects of auditory backward masking on event-related brain potentials. *Electroencephalography and Clinical Neurophysiology*, *44*, 185–189.

Winkler, I., Reinikainen, K., & Näätänen, R. (1993). Event-related brain potentials reflect echoic memory in humans. *Perception & Psychophysics*, *53*, 443–449.

Yabe, H., Tervaniemi, M., Reinikainen, K., & Näätänen, R. (1997). Temporal window of integration revealed by MMN to sound omission. *NeuroReport*, *8*, 1971–1974.

Yabe, H., Tervaniemi, M., Sinkkonen, J., Huotilainen, M., Ilmoniemi, R. J., & Näätänen, R. (1998). Temporal window of integration of auditory information in the human brain. *Psychophysiology*, *35*, 615–619.

16 Imaging genomics

Brain alterations associated with the *APOE* genotype

Johanna Lind and Lars Nyberg

Introduction

Traditionally, most neuroscience research has focused on universal features. Neuroimaging is no exception. The majority of studies until now have aimed at mapping common brain characteristics that are shared by a large population. However, as evidenced by a growing trend in the research literature, more recent neuroimaging studies have shifted focus to also pay attention to individual variability and dynamic variation. For instance, recent results have revealed substantial inter-individual variance in how the brain processes various cognitive tasks (Grabner et al., 2007; Hariri et al., 2003) or emotions (Hamann & Canli, 2004), as well as individual differences in brain development (Bengtsson et al., 2005) and aging (Cabeza, Anderson, Locantore, & McIntosh, 2002; Persson et al., 2006b; Raz et al., 2005). This shift in attention – from more general characteristics towards individual variance – can probably be seen as a natural next step after the successful mapping project, but it should also be ascribed to rapid advances in non-invasive brain imaging techniques, as well as to recent insights into the human genome and genetic variation (International Human Genome Sequencing Consortium, 2001; Venter et al., 2001).

Although environmental factors (e.g., intensive learning and physical training) have also been acknowledged (Bengtsson et al., 2005; Colcombe et al., 2006), most studies focusing on individual variance have emphasized genetic variation as the central determinant (Plomin, Owen, & McGuffin, 1994; Thompson et al., 2001; Winterer & Goldman, 2003). In contrast to traditional neuroscience research, inter-individual variance has always been a central topic of genetics, with particular focus on so-called single nucleotide polymorphisms (SNPs). Genes, or DNA, are composed of nucleotide sequences (A-C-T-G) of various lengths. SNPs occur when a single nucleotide in the genome differs between members of a species (or between paired chromosomes in an individual). For example, a certain proportion of the population may have a C in the same position as others have a T (Figure 16.1). About 10 million SNPs (representing less than 1% of the total human DNA sequence) are believed to characterize the genetic diversity in

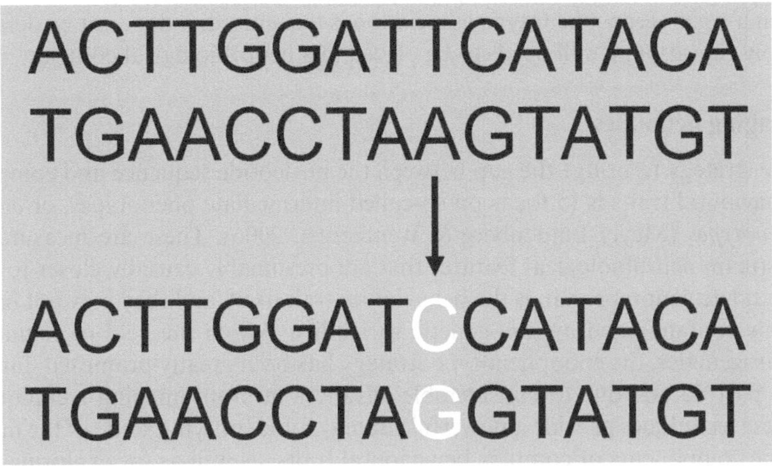

Figure 16.1 A single nucleotide polymorphism. Small changes in the DNA sequence such as these can have significant phenotypic effects, including, for example, on cognitive abilities and disease susceptibility. (This figure is published in colour at http://www.cognitiveneurosciencearena.com/brain-scans/.)

the worldwide population. A majority of these have no functional consequences – that is, the SNP is silent or is in a non-coding area of the gene. Functional SNPs, on the other hand, might induce changes in the expression or behaviour of corresponding protein products, ultimately resulting in significant overt variability in cognition, behaviour, anatomy, physiology, and so forth, as well as vulnerability to various diseases.

One of the main challenges of genetic research today is to understand the relationship between genome sequence variation within human populations and phenotypic diversity. A central part of this comprehensive quest concerns genetic impact on brain and behaviour – a research area lately referred to as *cognitive neurogenetics* (Goldberg & Weinberger, 2004). Quantitative genetic research has consistently validated the importance of inheritance for many complex dimensions of human behaviour, including cognitive abilities, temperament, personality, and intelligence (Plomin et al., 1994). Extensive evidence for genetic influence has also been presented for nearly all behavioural disorders; representative examples include schizophrenia, major affective disorder, and Alzheimer's disease (Sawa & Snyder, 2002; Serretti, Olgiati, & De Ronchi, 2007). Nevertheless, previous efforts to link specific genetic polymorphisms to behavioural phenotypes or clinical diagnosis have commonly failed (Menzel, 2002; Petrill et al., 1997; Plomin et al., 1995; Riley & McGuffin, 2000). This is probably because the effect of any single gene on complex traits is likely to be small, and because valid relationships may easily be obscured by substantial non-genetic variability of traditional behavioural measures. For example, neuropsychological test results or clinical evaluations might be influenced by test-taking strategy, motivation, or test monitoring. In addition, even if a genotype–phenotype association is recognized, it does not by default imply causation; it still needs to be placed in a neurobiological context.

Imaging genomics

One strategy to bridge the gap between the nucleotide sequence and complex behavioural traits is to focus on so-called intermediate phenotypes, or *endophenotypes* (Meyer-Lindenberg & Weinberger, 2006). These are measurable upstream neurobiological features that are presumably causally closer to the candidate genotype than is the behavioural trait itself, and they may not be as easily contaminated by non-genetic variability. Within the field of cognitive neurogenetics, the endophenotype strategy has been greatly promoted during the past decade due to considerable advances in brain imaging techniques. These techniques provide a powerful strategy for identifying some of the more basic components of complex behavioural traits, as well as for exploring the bottom-up consequences of gene actions. Also, by allowing rapid acquisition of hundreds of repeated measures of brain function at the level of information processing within a single subject, brain imaging increases statistical power and hence sensitivity to small effects. As a consequence, imaging studies might require considerably fewer subjects to detect significant genetic influences on brain function as compared to behavioural studies (tens versus hundreds).

Structural imaging

Brain imaging techniques can broadly be divided into two categories: structural imaging and functional imaging. Structural imaging is used to measure brain volume or the volume of subregions, or to look at diffuse changes in grey or white matter, or to assess localized lesions. The most common technique for experimental structural imaging is magnetic resonance imaging – (MRI, including diffusion tensor imaging, DTI). For example, Thompson et al. (2001) used structural MRI to study inter-individual differences in cortical grey matter between twins. They found that genetic factors significantly influenced several cortical structures, including frontal regions, and that frontal grey matter differences predicted individual differences in cognitive performance (Spearman's *g*). These findings also suggest that genes involved in cortical determination could contribute to familial liability for diseases that affect cortical integrity.

Functional imaging: Electrophysiological techniques

Functional imaging includes several techniques; usually, the choice is based on whether high temporal or high spatial resolution is of main interest. Electrophysiological methods can provide near real-time temporal resolution accuracy (10–100 ms) for the recorded neuronal activity by measuring either the electric field change (electroencephalography: EEG), or magnetic field change (magnetoencephalography: MEG) associated with the neuronal depolarization. However, because the measurement is performed outside the skull, the signal is distorted and "smoothed" by the bone, with loss of spatial resolution as a result. A successful example of using EEG for studying gene–behaviour relationships was provided by Leonard et al. (2002): Previous genetic linkage and biochemical studies have suggested that the nicotinic acetylcholine receptor subunit gene *CHRNA7* is a susceptibility gene for schizophrenia, as well as for an auditory attentional processing (gating or inhibition) deficit (Freedman et al., 1997). The attentional process is hypothesized to play a role in schizophrenic symptoms such as hallucinations and disorganization, and it can be indexed by the so-called P50 EEG response. Leonard et al. were able to demonstrate that a functional polymorphism in the *CHRNA7* gene was associated with inter-individual variability in the ability to inhibit the P50 response to repeated auditory stimuli. This effect was demonstrated both in normal controls and in schizophrenic patients and showed stronger association to the genotype than did a clinical diagnosis of schizophrenia. This study illustrates nicely that genetic associations that are weak on the level of the clinical phenotype can be more penetrant on the neurobiological level.

Functional imaging: Hemodynamic techniques

In contrast to the electrophysiological methods, hemodynamic techniques – functional magnetic resonance imaging (fMRI), positron emission tomography (PET), single photon emission computerized tomography (SPECT) – measure neuronal activity indirectly through the associated changes in metabolism and blood flow. This provides relatively high spatial resolution (1–10 mm), but rather low temporal resolution (hundreds of milliseconds for fMRI, several seconds for PET and SPECT), being limited by the rate of the much slower hemodynamic changes that accompany neuronal activation.

Functional MRI is commonly used to index brain activity that corresponds to various mental operations. For example, fMRI has been used to explore individual differences in episodic memory processing (Egan et al., 2003; Hariri et al., 2003). Previous studies *in vitro* and in experimental animals have shown that the brain-derived neurotrophic factor (*BDNF*) gene plays a crucial role in hippocampal long-term potentiation associated with learning and memory (Poo, 2001). Egan et al. (2003) found that a G-to-A polymorphism in the human *BDNF* gene induced differences in intracellular processing and secretion of the corresponding protein, which in turn was associated with inter-individual differences in episodic memory performance. The same group of researchers then used fMRI ($n = 28$) to explore the impact of *BDNF* genotype on memory-related hippocampal processing and found that an interaction of *BDNF* alleles and hippocampal response during memory encoding was a strong predictor of behavioural accuracy (Hariri et al., 2003). These findings highlight the power of functional neuroimaging for exploring the impact of genetic variation at the level of information processing in specific brain regions or circuits in relatively small samples of subjects.

Functional MRI has also been successfully employed to elucidate the relationship between the dopamine-regulating gene catechol-O-methyltransferase (*COMT*) and risk for schizophrenia (Egan et al., 2001; Heinz & Smolka, 2006; see also Bäckman & Nyberg, chapter 11, this volume). Several previous studies have suggested that the *COMT* gene is crucial for working memory and prefrontal information processing through its impact on dopamine activity (Braver, Barch, & Cohen, 1999; Gasparini, Fabrizio, Bonifati, & Meco, 1997; Gogos et al., 1998). A functional polymorphism in the human *COMT* gene causes a substitution of the amino acid valine (val) to methionin (met) in the peptide sequence, which in turn affects the thermolability of the protein so that at body temperature the val-variant *COMT* catabolizes dopamine much faster than its met counterpart (Lachman et al., 1996). Despite the long hypothesized role of dopamine in schizophrenia and findings of abnormal prefrontal executive functions in schizophrenic patients, the evidence for an association between *COMT* genotype and schizophrenia per se have been weak and inconsistent (for a review, see Riley & McGuffin, 2000). Egan and colleagues (2003) hypothesized that the high-activity val allele would result in faster degradation of dopamine at the synapse and thereby impair prefrontal functioning. They studied a large sample of schizophrenic patients, their healthy siblings, and controls ($n = 458$) and found that *COMT* genotype predicated task performance in an allele dosage fashion: met/met > met/val > val/val, across the sample. In addition, by using fMRI ($n = 11–16$), the authors were also able to demonstrate that val allele carriers consistently displayed a less efficient physiological response in the prefrontal cortex (PFC) (i.e., greater PFC activity) for a fixed level of task performance than did subjects with the met allele. The pattern of abnormal prefrontal brain function in the val allele carriers was analogous to that which had been identified earlier in patients with schizophrenia and in their healthy siblings (Callicott et al., 2000; Cannon et al., 2000; Weinberger, Berman, & Zec, 1986), suggesting that it was a biological reflection of genetic risk for schizophrenia. The authors concluded that the *COMT* val allele impairs prefrontal cognition and physiology by increasing prefrontal dopamine catabolism, which thereby in turn increases risk for schizophrenia.

In contrast to fMRI, which is completely non-invasive, PET requires an injection of a radioactive tracer isotope. The PET technique is commonly used to measure the expression and function of specific proteins and metabolites, during both activated (Zubieta et al., 2003) and resting-state (Drzezga et al., 2005) conditions. For instance, the *COMT* val/met polymorphism has been associated with, in addition to schizophrenia (Egan et al., 2001), inter-individual differences in adaptation and response to pain. This relationship was clarified by Zubieta et al. (2003), using PET and C^{11} carfentanil (a μ-opioid receptor-selective radiotracer). Pain responses are mediated through the dopamine-dependent μ-opioid system. Zubieta et al. (2003) were able to demonstrate that varying levels of dopamine metabolism, conferred by the *COMT* polymorphism, are associated with downstream alterations in the functional responses of the μ-opioid neurotransmitter system and that these effects ultimately induced differences in sensory and affective ratings of pain. In another PET study, Drzezga et al. (2005) used PET and [^{18}F]luorodeoxyglucose (a tracer that indexes glucose conversion) to study characteristic abnormalities of resting-state cerebral glucose metabolism in patients with Alzheimer's disease (AD), in relation to the polymorphic gene *Apolipoprotein E* (*APOE*). The authors found that the metabolic abnormalities were more pronounced in carriers of the AD-risk allele *APOE*ε4, compared to non-carriers, which in turn may be related to individual differences in clinical disease expression (although this assumption remains to be clarified).

Apolipoprotein E and the brain

Clearly, genes can influence human behaviour and increase the risk for various brain disorders through a number of pathways, including receptor modulation, neurotransmitter modulation, or synaptic plasticity. While, for example, receptor subunit genes are likely to exert rather specific or discrete effects on the brain, genes controlling the degradation of a family of neurotransmitters may have a more general impact, as may those genes that modulate the efficiency of neuronal repair or plasticity. The most studied gene in the latter category is the *APOE* gene, coding for a lipid-carrying protein involved in cell maintenance and repair (for reviews, see Mahley, 1988; Mahley & Rall, 2000). Two well-known SNPs in the *APOE* gene give rise to three common *APOE* alleles (ε2, ε3, and ε4), with three corresponding protein isoforms (E2, E3, and E4) (Figure 16.2). E3 is by far the most common and seems to be the normal isoform in every known function of the protein, whereas E4 and E2 are less common and can each be dysfunctional. APOE-E4, in particular, seems to have a global detrimental effect on the CNS and has been associated with a number of clinical conditions, with AD being the most acknowledged. Although several potential effects of the *APOE* gene have been suggested to contribute to the increased risk for AD (for reviews, see Huang, Qiu, von Strauss, Winblad, & Fratiglioni, 2004; Huang, 2006), the precise underlying mechanisms are as yet largely unknown.

The focus of the remaining parts of this chapter will be to discuss new findings from our own lab regarding relationships between the *APOE* genotype and brain structure and function. The risk allele *APOE*ε4 has been associated with cognitive decline, especially in episodic memory (Nilsson et al., 2006; Small, Rosnick, Fratiglioni, & Bäckman, 2004), and a number of neuroimaging studies have reported structural and functional brain alterations in non-demented carriers of *APOE*ε4 (Bookheimer et al., 2000; Reiman et al., 2004; Smith et al., 1999; Tohgi et al., 1997) – findings that have tentatively been interpreted as early signs of impending AD. However, the results have been inconsistent, and the impact of *APOE* remains unclear. For instance,

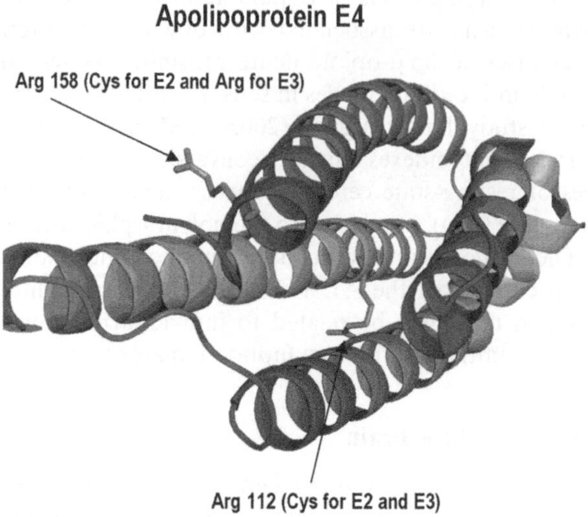

Figure 16.2 A 3d-rendering of the APOE-E4 isoform. The two SNPs (at amino acid positions 112 and 158) are indicated by arrows. APOE-E4 has arginine in both positions, whereas APOE-E3 has cysteine and arginine, respectively, and APOE-E2 has cysteine in both positions. (This figure is published in colour at http://www.cognitiveneurosciencearena.com/brain-scans/.)

there is inconsistency regarding the direction of activity alterations (decreased vs. increased), and it is still unclear how the observed changes correspond to changes in cognition and ultimately dementia. We will here address the issue of whether response alterations associated with *APOE*ε4 represent preclinical markers of AD or, rather, reflect detrimental consequences of the risk allele per se.

All of the presented studies are based on the same study sample, including 60 healthy individuals (age range = 49–79 years), collected from the ongoing longitudinal Betula prospective cohort study (Nilsson, Adolfsson, Bäckman, de Frias, Molander, & Nyberg, 2004; Nilsson et al., 1997). The data include structural and functional brain imaging, as well as longitudinal neuropsychological testing. All subjects had gone through extensive cognitive testing and medical examination (including *APOE* genotyping). Of the subjects, 30 were carriers of at least one copy of *APOE*ε4: 10 were homozygous (ε44), and 20 were heterozygous (ε34). The remaining 30 subjects carried two copies of *APOE*ε3 and served as controls. In addition, to examine possible dose effects of *APOE*ε4 (Lind et al., 2006c), three subgroups consisting of 10 subjects each were composed: *APOE*ε44, *APOE*ε34, and *APOE*ε33. All groups were closely matched according to sex, age, and length of education. Critically, all accessible data imply that all participants were cognitively intact at time of data collection (Table 16.1; for details, see Lind et al., 2006c).

Table 16.1 Sample characteristics

	APOEε4[a] (*N* = 30)	*APOEε33* (*N* = 30)	*APOEε44* (*N* = 10)	*APOEε34* (*N* = 10)	*APOEε33* (*N* = 10)
Female/male	19/11	18/12	9/1	7/3	8/2
Age	65.3 (7.9)	66.6 (8.3)	61.2 (9.4)	65.0 (8.5)	64 (11.1)
Range	49–74	49–79	49–74	49–74	50–79
Education (yrs)	10.6 (3.5)	10.2 (3.3)	11.7 (3.1)	10.7 (4.0)	11.8 (3.1)
Range	6–17	6–16	8–16	6–17	9–16
MMSE	28.2 (1.5)	27.9 (1.7)	28.5 (1.4)	28.4 (1.4)	28.1 (2.1)
Range	24–30	24–30	26–30	26–30	24–30
SRB	25.0 (2.4)	22.6 (4.8)	23.7 (2.8)	25.3 (2.4)	23.2 (3.8)
Range	16–29	11–29	16–26	22–29	17–28
AD in family (*N*)	2	0	0	1	0

Note: Means and standard deviations (in parentheses). MMSE = Mini Mental State Examination (maximum = 30). SRB = word comprehension (maximum = 30). AD in family = first-degree family history of AD. The three right-most columns represent the matched subgroups.
[a] Carriers of at least one copy of the *APOEε*4 allele: 10 with *APOEε*4/4; 20 with *APOEε*3/4.

APOE and grey matter

Clinical AD is associated with severe brain atrophy. The most prominent effects are seen in medial temporal lobe structures (Braak, Braak, & Bohl, 1993), including the entorhinal cortex and the hippocampus, which are well-known to be crucial for episodic memory functioning (Nyberg et al., 1996; Squire & Zola-Morgan, 1991). Several studies of AD patients have indicated that morphological loss is more severe in carriers of *APOEε*4 compared to non-carriers (Geroldi et al., 1999; Juottonen, Lehtovirta, Helisalmi, Reikkinen, & Soininen, 1998; Lehtovirta et al., 1995), whereas similar studies of non-demented subjects have yielded mixed results. Jack et al. (1998), for instance, studied hippocampal volumes in 62 demented and 125 cognitively normal subjects (mean age = 79 years) and found no differences on the basis of *APOE* genotype. Neither did a study by Killiany et al. (2002), which investigated entorhinal and hippocampal volumes among subjects with normal cognition, memory difficulties, and mild dementia (see also Han et al., 2007; Jernigan et al., 2001; Schmidt et al., 1996; Small et al., 1995). In contrast to these negative findings, Plassman et al. (1997) reported that non-demented *APOEε*4-carriers (mean age = 63 years) had smaller left and right hippocampal volumes as compared to non-carriers, despite the fact that the two groups did not differ in performance on neuropsychological tests. Tohgi et al. (1997) extended this finding by observing significantly reduced right hippocampal size and a trend towards smaller left hippocampal volume in cognitively intact *APOEε*4-carriers as young as in their forties (age range = 39–80 years).

There are also studies of non-demented subjects that failed to detect differences in absolute sizes between *APOE* genotype groups but instead observed other alterations associated with the *APOE*ε4 allele (Cohen, Small, Lalonde, Friz, & Sunderland, 2001; Moffat, Szekely, Zonderman, Kabani, & Resnick, 2000; Soininen et al., 1995). For instance, Soininen et al. (1995) found no differences in normalized measurements of right or left hippocampal volume in elderly (mean age = 69 years) *APOE*ε4-carriers, but they reported that normal hippocampal right > left asymmetry was diminished. In a longitudinal study, Moffat et al. (2000) found no *APOE*-related difference in absolute size at the start of the study, whereas *APOE*ε4-carriers (mean age = 69 years) in comparison to non-carriers displayed a significantly steeper rate of hippocampal atrophy over a 3-year follow-up period. Similar results were reported by Cohen et al. (2001).

Hippocampal volume and recognition memory performance

In our study (Lind et al., 2006b), we collected structural MRI data for 30 carriers and 30 non-carriers of *APOE*ε4 with equal cognitive status. We also had the subjects perform a word categorization task that promoted incidental encoding of a word list and measured recognition memory performance – that is, previously displayed words were randomly intermixed with completely new words and the subjects responded yes or no to whether or not they recognized the word from before. Manual outlining of the hippocampus revealed a right-sided volume reduction in carriers of *APOE*ε4 as compared to non-carriers (Figure 16.3a). We also found that the difference was most pronounced before the age of 65, possibly as a function of normal age-related hippocampal atrophy among non-carriers in older ages (Figure 16.3b). These findings are well in line with the results reported by Tohgi et al. (1997), who observed right-sided atrophy in non-demented carriers of *APOE*ε4 as early as age 40.

We also noted that the *APOE*ε4-carriers made more false alarms in the recognition memory test, and that the number of false alarms correlated significantly with right hippocampus volume. The increased tendency to say that non-studied items are familiar may relate to difficulties assessing relative novelty/familiarity, as there is ample evidence that hippocampus – in particular, the right hippocampus – is crucial for novelty detection (Martin, 1999; Strange, Fletcher, Henson, Friston, & Dolan, 1999; Tulving, Markowitsch, Kapur, Habib, & Houle, 1994). Related to this, Weiss et al. (2004) reported that right hippocampal atrophy in schizophrenic patients correlated with false-alarm rate, and studies of AD patients have demonstrated that intact hippocampal function is important for correctly rejecting previously non-studied words in tests of recognition memory (Lekeu et al., 2003). The observation of structural changes in the right hippocampus is also convergent with functional imaging findings showing diminished right-sided hippocampal novelty response in carriers of *APOE*ε4 (see below) (Han et al., 2007; Lind et al., 2006c; Trivedi et al., 2006).

Collectively, studies of *APOE*ε4-related atrophy, including our own study

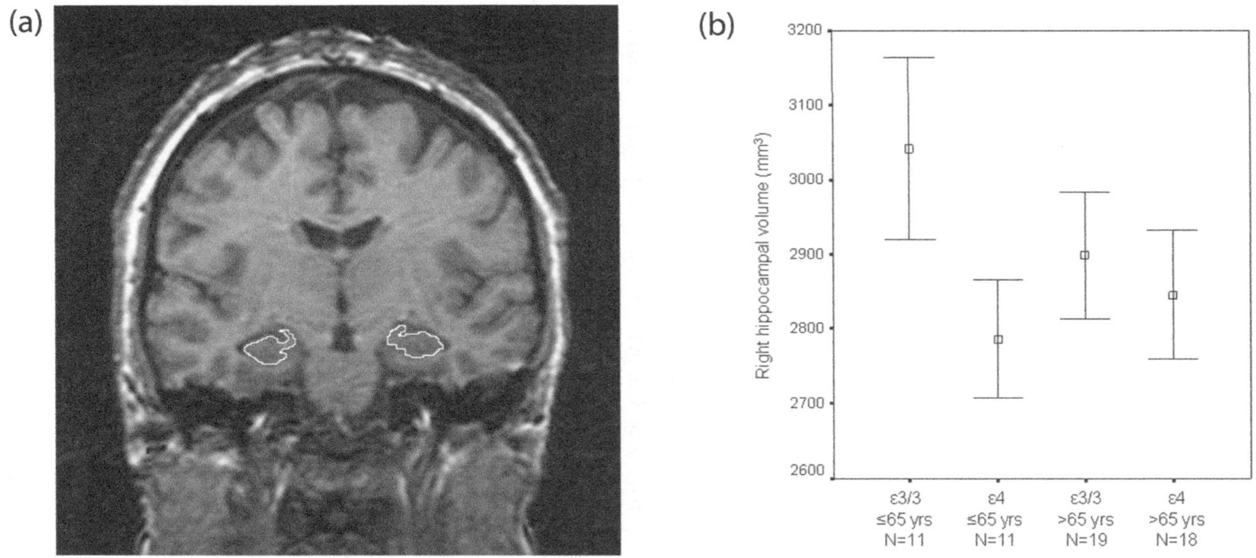

Figure 16.3 (a) Manually outlined hippocampus on coronal MRI slices. (b) Group differences in hippocampal volume as a function of *APOE* genotype and chronological age (≤65 years vs. >65 years). Bars show mean standard error of the mean (*$p < .05$; Student's *t* test, one-tailed). (Lind et al., 2006b.) (This figure is published in colour at http://www.cognitiveneurosciencearena.com/brain-scans/.)

(Lind et al., 2006b), indicate that the hippocampal region is most affected, particularly on the right side (Lehtovirta et al., 1995; Soininen et al., 1995; Tohgi et al., 1997). In contrast, total cerebral volume seems not to differ by genotype (e.g., Cohen et al., 2001; Lehtovirta et al., 1995; Moffat et al., 2000; but see Yasuda et al., 1998, who reported larger global brain volume for *APOE*ε4-carriers). The finding of *APOE*ε4-related atrophy in relatively young subjects (Lind et al., 2006b; Tohgi et al., 1997) raises the question whether smaller hippocampal volume in *APOE*ε4-carriers represents early-onset atrophy or an inherent trait. Support for the former was presented by Rose and colleagues (referred to by Scarmeas & Stern, 2006), who studied 50 healthy paediatric subjects on two occasions, at ages 10 and 12, and found no evidence for a relationship between *APOE* status and hippocampal volume.

APOE and white matter

Although AD has traditionally been considered a disease of the grey matter, there are several reports of abnormal white matter integrity in AD patients (Bozzali et al., 2002; Bronge, Bogdanovic, & Wahlund, 2002; Englund, Brun, & Alling, 1988; Hanyu et al., 1998; Meyer, Kawamura, & Terayama, 1992; Yoshiura et al., 2002). In contrast to normal aging, which is commonly associated with white matter atrophy in frontal regions of the brain (Head et al., 2004; Janowsky, Kaye, & Carper, 1996), AD patients display greatest changes in posterior regions, preferentially in callosal fibre systems (Biegon et al., 1994; Teipel et al., 1999, 2003).

In a study by Skoog et al. (1998), it was found that the combination of white matter lesions and the presence of an *APOE*ε4 allele increased the risk for AD in an elderly population at the age of 85. This finding led Bronge et al. (1999) to further evaluate the relation between white matter lesions and the *APOE* genotype. Bronge et al. (1999) studied T2-weighted magnetic resonance images of AD patients and found that homozygous *APOE*ε44-carriers had more extensive white matter lesions than did heterozygous carriers and non-carriers. The authors also noticed the absence of an age correlation for white matter lesions in *APOE*ε4-carriers (in contrast to non-carriers), and they concluded that white matter lesions in *APOE*ε4-carriers may represent a pathological process related to the aetiology of AD. De Leeuw et al. (2004) investigated a possible interaction effect of *APOE* genotype and hypertension on white matter lesions and found that carriers of ε4 had significantly increased subcortical white matter lesion volume as compared to non-carriers, irrespective of hypertension. In a recent study, Nierenberg et al. (2005) used diffusion tensor imaging (DTI) to compare healthy *APOE*ε4-carriers (mean age = 68 years) and non-carriers (mean age = 67 years). It was found that ε4-carriers had disrupted white matter microstructure in the parahippocampal gyrus, in the absence of regional or global atrophy.

Microstructural alterations in the posterior corpus callosum and the hippocampus

Taken together, not many studies have examined the integrity of white matter in healthy *APOE*ε4-carriers. We therefore decided to use DTI for this purpose. DTI measures the amount of non-randomness (so-called fractional anisotropy: FA) of water diffusion within tissues, which makes DTI a powerful tool for assessing microstructural changes in white matter integrity and connectivity. Based on previous findings (Biegon et al., 1994; Teipel et al., 1999, 2003), we expected to see alterations in posterior parts of the brain. Three regions of interest (ROIs) were examined: the genu, body, and splenium of the corpus callosum. As hypothesized, in comparison to non-carriers, carriers of *APOE*ε4 showed a significant decline in FA values in the posterior part of the corpus callosum (splenium). This difference was significant for both young (<65 years) and old (>65 years) individuals. In addition, exploratory whole-brain analyses revealed reduced FA values for *APOE*ε4-carriers in the occipitofrontal fasciculus and in the body/posterior corpus callosum, as well as in the left hippocampus. Our findings, together with those of Nierenberg et al. (2005), suggest that the presence of *APOE*ε4 may influence microstructural white matter integrity well before onset of AD.

APOE and brain activation: Resting-state findings

Resting-state PET studies of AD patients show a highly consistent pattern of reduced blood flow and glucose utilization in parietal, temporal, and posterior cingulate regions, with later spreading to prefrontal cortices (Alexander, Chen, Pietrini, Rapoport, & Reiman, 2002; Frackowiak et al., 1981; Lehtovirta et al., 1996, 1998; Mielke et al., 1998; Smith et al., 1992). Similar reductions have been observed among non-demented *APOE*ε4-carriers (Reiman et al., 1996, 2001, 2004; Small et al., 1995, 2000). For instance, Small et al. (2000) studied subjects with normal memory performance (mean age = 66 years) and found that a single copy of the *APOE*ε4 allele was associated with lowered inferior parietal, temporal, and posterior cingulate cortical metabolism. Moreover, a longitudinal follow-up study revealed that lower baseline metabolism predicted cognitive decline among carriers of the *APOE*ε4 allele two years later and, also, that the greatest metabolic decline over time was observed in the parietal and temporal regions (see Figure 16.4). Reiman and colleagues (2004) extended these findings by observing similar metabolic reductions in cognitively intact *APOE*ε4-carriers even before the age of 40 (age range 20–39 years).

APOE and brain activation: Task-associated findings

In line with resting-state studies, it has been found that AD patients (Bäckman, Small, & Fratiglioni, 2001; Grossman et al., 2003; Kato, Knopman, & Liu,

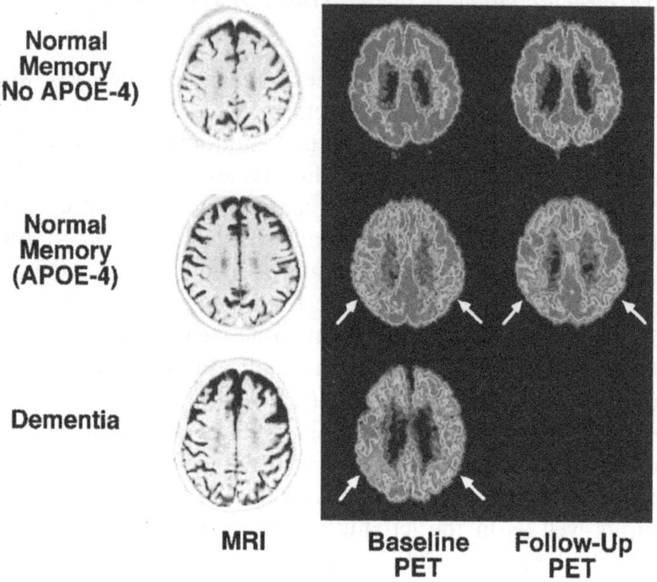

Figure 16.4 Examples of PET images (co-registered to each subject's baseline MRI scan) for a non-demented woman without the *APOE*ε4 allele, a non-demented woman with the *APOE*ε4 allele, and a demented woman with *APOE*ε4. Middle column: Compared with the non-demented subject without *APOE*ε4, the non-demented *APOE*ε4 carrier had 18% (*right*) and 12% (*left*) lower inferior parietal cortical metabolism, whereas the demented woman's parietal cortical metabolism was 20% (*right*) and 22% (*left*) lower, as well as there being a more widespread metabolic dysfunction due to disease progression. Final column: Two-year follow-up scans for the non-demented subjects showed minimal parietal cortical decline for the woman without *APOE*ε4, but bilateral parietal cortical decline for the non-demented woman with *APOE*ε4, who also met clinical criteria for mild AD at follow-up. (Small et al., 2000.) (This figure is published in colour at http://www.cognitiveneurosciencearena.com/brain-scans/.)

2001; Machulda et al., 2003; Rombouts et al., 2000), as well as non-demented *APOE*ε4-carriers (Mondadori et al., 2007; Smith et al., 1999, 2005; Trivedi et al., 2006) display reduced neuronal activation in medial temporal lobe (MTL) and temporo-parietal regions during performance of various cognitive tasks. For instance, Smith et al. (1999) compared fMRI activation between *APOE*ε4-carriers with a family history of AD versus non-carriers with no family history of AD (mean age = 52 years) during an object-naming task. Carriers of the ε4 allele showed diminished task-related activity in the infero-temporal cortex, and a follow-up four years later revealed a greater longitudinal decline in fMRI response in the same region among the ε4-carriers (Smith et al., 2005). Mondadori et al. (2007) studied young (mean age = 22 years) healthy individuals and found that carriers of *APOE*ε4 had smaller learning-related brain activations compared with carriers of *APOE*ε2 and ε3.

Differences were seen during both encoding and retrieval and included several regions – for example, the hippocampus, the right frontal gyrus, and the right precuneus. Moreover, as may seem somewhat counterintuitive, it was also found that greater decreases in these regions among the *APOE*ε4-carriers correlated with better learning. The authors suggested that the relatively smaller activations in carriers of *APOE*ε4 reflected a more economic use of the neural resources.

However, observations of reduced task-associated brain activity among at-risk subjects have not been consistent; several studies have reported increased, rather than decreased, response (Bondi, Houston, Eyler, & Brown, 2005; Bookheimer et al., 2000; Dickerson et al., 2005; Fleisher et al., 2005; Han et al., 2007; Smith et al., 2002; Wishart et al., 2006). Bookheimer et al. (2000) performed fMRI while 14 *APOE*ε4-carriers and 16 matched non-carriers (age range = 47–82 years) with mild memory complaints but normal cognitive performance memorized and recalled unrelated pairs of words. When contrasted against resting periods, the magnitude and spatial extent of brain activation during memory performance was greater in several regions, including hippocampus, parietal, and prefrontal regions among *APOE*ε4-carriers, as compared to non-carriers. In addition, *APOE*ε4-carriers performed worse on a delayed-recall test, and longitudinal assessment indicated that greater baseline brain activation correlated with verbal memory decline two years later. The authors suggested a compensatory hypothesis, whereby subjects at increased risk for AD need to perform additional cognitive work in order to accomplish the task. Bondi et al. (2005) found that cognitively normal (mean age = 76 years) *APOE*ε4-carriers showed greater fMRI response in the fusiform gyrus, parietal cortex, and frontal gyrus compared to *APOE*ε33-carriers, when subjects had to discriminate novel pictures from a single repeating picture. This study also reported that *APOE*ε4-carriers displayed greater activation in the right MTL, but reduced activation in the left MTL, compared to ε33-carriers. In addition, there was a correlation between memory ability on a word list learning task and right and left hippocampal activation during picture encoding (positive in ε33-carriers and negative or zero in ε4-carriers). Han et al. (2007) assessed brain activity while subjects memorized novel and familiar word-pairs. They found that non-demented *APOE*ε4-carriers (mean age = 77 years) displayed greater activation than did non-carriers in multiple right hemisphere regions for previously encoded word-pairs relative to fixation. Moreover, in contrast to non-carriers, *APOE*ε4-carriers displayed greater response to familiar words than to novel words in the right hippocampus, which is the inverse of what is normally seen (i.e., novel > repeated).

Reduced brain activation during incidental episodic memory encoding

Clearly, there are conflicting data on the relationship between *APOE*ε4 and brain activity in non-demented subjects. To further elucidate this issue, we conducted a large-scale fMRI study of healthy carriers and non-carriers of

*APOE*ε4 (Lind et al., 2006c). Measurements were taken while participants performed a simple semantic categorization task that promoted incidental encoding of a word list. Critically, behavioural results – word classification accuracy, response time, and post-scan recognition memory (hits minus false alarms) – showed no differences between groups. In contrast, fMRI data analyses – categorization task versus resting-state baseline – revealed that *APOE*ε4-carriers had significantly lower task-associated brain activity in the left inferior parietal cortex, Brodmann area (BA) 39 (XYZ = −44, −56, 36), and bilaterally in the anterior cingulate region (22, 12, 26; and −18, 30, 24) as compared to non-carriers. In addition, for the first time with fMRI, a genetic dose effect was observed in the parietal region such that homozygous *APOE*ε4-carriers exhibited greater reduction than did heterozygous carriers – a finding that clearly strengthens the relationship between the gene and the observed effect (Figure 16.5).

Moreover, contrasts of processing novel versus familiar items revealed an abnormal response in the right hippocampus in the *APOE*ε4 group (30, −30, −8), mainly expressed as diminished sensitivity to the relative novelty of stimuli. This result corresponds well with our findings of reduced right hippocampal volume and the accompanying increase of false alarms in the recognition memory test for the *APOE*ε4-carriers (Lind et al., 2006b). It is also well in line with the findings by Trivedi et al. (2006), who used a comparable fMRI paradigm (i.e., contrasted processing of novel vs. familiar items) and observed a reduced novelty response in the right hippocampal region for

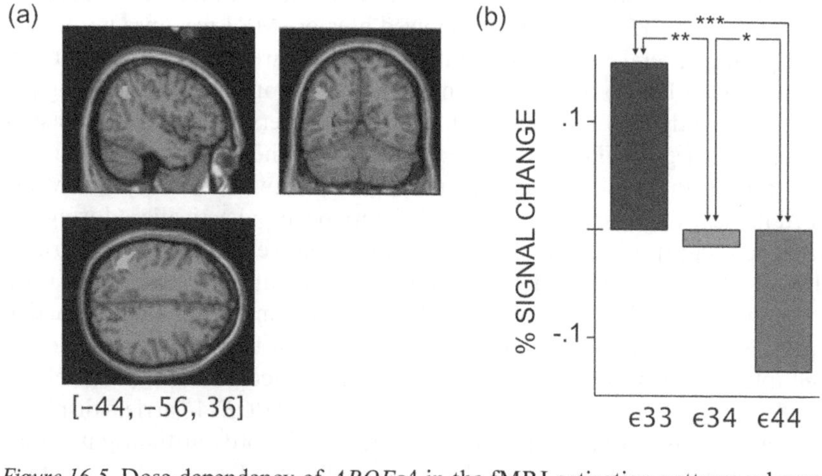

Figure 16.5 Dose-dependency of *APOE*ε4 in the fMRI activation pattern: subgroup comparisons of left parietal response. (a) The search was constrained by means of a functional ROI derived from the main group contrast (ε4 non-carriers vs. ε4 carriers; $n = 60$). (b) The dose of *APOE*ε4 predicted failure to recruit the left parietal region (XYZ = −44, −56, 36) (*$p < .1$; **$p < .05$; ***$p < .01$; one-tailed). (Lind et al., 2006c.) (This figure is published in colour at http://www.cognitiveneurosciencearena.com/brain-scans/.)

*APOE*ε4-carriers (mean age = 53 years) as compared to non-carriers (see also Han et al., 2007).

Our observation of reduced parietal activation in non-demented *APOE*ε4-carriers is consistent with previous fMRI studies (Elgh, Larsson, Eriksson, & Nyberg, 2003; Smith et al., 1999; Trivedi et al., 2006) and also with resting-state PET studies showing substantial hypometabolism in the parietal cortex, both in AD patients (Alexander et al., 2002; Frackowiak et al., 1981; Smith et al., 1992) and in healthy carriers of *APOE*ε4 (Reiman et al., 2004). It is possible that these two features – that is, reduced activity responses and diminished metabolism – are related, as previous research has demonstrated that regional metabolic rate is coupled to regional cerebral blood flow, and both of these features are coupled to neural response (Logothetis & Wandell, 2004; Mosconi, De Santi, Rusinek, Convit, & de Leon, 2004). An underlying mechanism to the observed alterations may be localized neuronal pathology (Boxer et al., 2003; Mega et al., 1999; Morishima-Kawashima et al., 2000). For instance, Boxer et al. (2003) reported that atrophy in AD patients was particularly prominent in the inferior parietal cortex, suggesting that this region is affected very early in the course of the disease. Another possibility is that the observed alterations reflect disruption of upstream regions of the functional network, resulting in decreased synaptic input. Support for this view was provided by Meguro et al. (2001) who demonstrated that damage to the densely connected hippocampal region induced hypometabolism in the parietal cortex. This notion can also be related to our findings of structural alterations in both grey (Lind et al., 2006b) and white (Persson et al., 2006a) matter in the hippocampal region among the *APOE*ε4-carriers. It could also be stressed that white matter tracts of the splenium originate from temporo-parietal regions of the brain (Conturo et al., 1999). Our DTI study (Persson et al., 2006a) provided evidence for microstructural changes of white matter integrity in the posterior corpus callosum in the studied *APOE*ε4-carriers. Thus, the observation of altered parietal activation in *APOE*ε4-carriers may, at least in part, be related to atrophy in the posterior corpus callosum. Taken together, it is possible that early structural and metabolic brain abnormalities coexist or interact to produce the observed activation pattern in carriers of the AD-risk allele *APOE*ε4.

Can reduced brain activation forecast memory decline?

The next critical question in this context is, of course, whether the observed alterations can be used to predict negative outcome. To gain further insight in this matter, we analysed longitudinal follow-up behavioural data for the *APOE*ε4-carriers in our study (Lind et al., 2006a). The specific aim was to examine whether a diminished fMRI response in the parietal region that differentiated between carriers and non-carriers of *APOE*ε4 predicted memory decline within the group of at-risk individuals. Behavioural data were collected at two test occasions, approximately five years apart (before and after the fMRI data collection; Lind et al., 2006c), and the participants ($n = 18$) were divided into two groups based on their longitudinal memory performance ("decline" vs. "non-decline"). Both groups showed equal behavioural performance at the initial examination as well as at the time for fMRI data collection. The post-hoc fMRI analyses revealed that those *APOE*ε4-carriers that later dropped in episodic memory performance displayed significantly lower activation in the parietal cortex than did those that remained stable; the analyses also revealed that the locus of this effect overlapped with the previously observed parietal region in BA39 (Lind et al., 2006c) (Figure 16.6a). Moreover, further analyses revealed that the parietal activation correlated significantly with the relative change in episodic memory performance over time (Figure 16.6b). In other words, the parietal diminution was most pronounced for those *APOE*ε4-carriers who later experienced memory decline.

In conclusion, our studies of the *APOE* genotype in relation to functional brain activation suggest that genetic risk for AD, in symptom-free individuals, translates into reduced brain activity in regions pertinent to the disease, including the hippocampus and the parietal cortex, and, moreover, that parietal cortex alterations can predict memory decline in non-demented *APOE*ε4-carriers and hence possibly progression to AD.

(a)

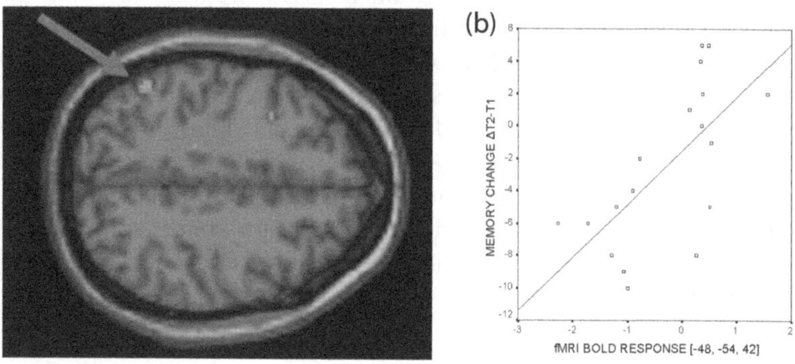

Figure 16.6 (a) A group-contrast (*APOE*ε4 decliners vs. *APOE*ε4 non-decliners) revealed diminished parietal activation for subjects who later experienced memory decline. The locus of this effect (XYZ = −48, −54, 42) overlapped with the previously observed region (Figure 16.5a). (Lind et al., 2006c.) (b) The parietal response correlated significantly with subsequent episodic memory change, such that lower parietal activation was related to poorer subsequent memory (Lind et al., 2006a). (This figure is published in colour at http://www.cognitiveneurosciencearena.com/brain-scans/.)

Discussion

Functional alterations in carriers of APOEε4: Decreases versus increases

Although there are several lines of evidence supporting our conclusion that genetic risk for AD translates into reduced brain activation (e.g., Reiman et al., 2004; Small et al., 2000; Smith et al., 1999; Trivedi et al., 2006), our findings are at odds with studies showing increased activation in non-demented carriers of *APOE*ε4 (e.g., Bondi et al., 2005; Bookheimer et al., 2000; Smith et al., 2002). The exact reasons for the contradictory findings are not known, although several demographic and methodological differences might account for the discrepancies. For instance, individual variance among the *APOE*ε4-carriers should be considered; as indicated by our follow-up study outlined above (Lind et al., 2006a), it may be that ε4-carriers that are predestined to develop AD differ from ε4-carriers that will remain healthy. Other important factors include sample sizes, age and cognitive status of subjects, as well as choice of cognitive task. For example, Bookheimer et al. (2000), who observed a relative increase in fMRI signal in *APOE*ε4-carriers, used a relatively demanding task (to memorize and recall unrelated pairs of words), whereas we used a fairly simple task (semantic categorization). In addition, the *APOE*ε4-carriers in the Bookheimer et al. study performed worse than controls on a delayed recall test and also showed a significant decline in memory performance two years later. In contrast, the *APOE*ε4-carriers in our study had cognitive test results that were equal to their non-carrier counterparts, both at time of scanning and two years later (see Lind et al., 2006c).

Strikingly, most studies that relate *APOE*ε4 to decreased brain activation (Mondadori et al., 2007; Smith et al., 1999, 2005; Trivedi et al., 2006) have used relatively simple tasks (e.g., picture naming or picture recognition) and also examined subjects at a relatively young age (mean age <57 years). In contrast, a majority of the studies that report increased brain activation for *APOE*ε4-carriers (Bondi et al., 2005; Bookheimer et al., 2000; Fleisher et al., 2005; Han et al., 2007; Wishart et al., 2006) have used relatively demanding tasks (e.g., intentional encoding), and examined either elderly *APOE*ε4-carriers (mean age > 75 years) (Bondi et al., 2005; Han et al., 2007) or *APOE*ε4-carriers that express lower memory performance than controls (Bookheimer et al., 2000; Wishart et al., 2006).

The role of APOE: An AD-susceptibility gene versus a neuronal repair gene

Based on the examples outlined above, the tentative conclusion emerges that genetic risk for AD in otherwise normal individuals initially translates into decreased brain activation, particularly in regions that are pertinent to AD (including the hippocampal and parietal regions). But eventually, with increasing age and – presumably – emerging AD pathology, compensatory effects and associated brain activation come into play, especially in response to more demanding cognitive tasks. A further distinction in this matter is that the former reflects consequences associated with the risk allele per se (albeit the magnitude of these alterations might still correspond to the degree of AD susceptibility: see Lind et al., 2006a; Small et al., 2000), whereas the latter is more closely related to actual AD pathology.

Several studies have demonstrated that the ε4 allele of the *APOE* gene is associated with inefficient neuronal repair processes (Mahley & Rall, 2000). For instance, APOE-E4 appears to be deficient in stimulating neurite outgrowth in response to cellular injury and degeneration and, moreover, appears to interfere with the normal protective effect of APOE-E3 (Buttini et al., 2000). It is likely that this fragility makes the brain more vulnerable to insults, including the effects of normal aging, independently of AD pathology. This view is consistent with findings of brain alterations in healthy *APOE*ε4-carriers in midlife or earlier, even decades before average age of AD onset (Reiman et al., 2004; Tohgi et al., 1997). It should also be mentioned that relatively smaller brain activation in young healthy carriers of *APOE*ε4, in comparison with carriers of *APOE*ε3 and *APOE*ε2, has been interpreted to reflect a more economic use of the neural resources (Mondadori et al., 2007). This is clearly an interesting notion, not the least from an evolutionary point of view since a possible advantageous effect of *APOE*ε4 in childhood and early adulthood could explain its existence and further persistence in humans (see also Gerdes, 2003).

However, over time, the (detrimental) effects of *APOE*ε4 could make the brain more susceptible to AD pathology and thereby hasten disease development – not only as a result of poor neuronal protection, but also through direct interactions between the APOE protein and the neuronal hallmarks of AD. For instance, it has been reported that the E4 isoform of APOE binds more strongly to the beta-amyloid peptide that may facilitate plaque formation (Strittmatter et al., 1993). It has also been demonstrated that E4 binds less efficiently to microtubule-associated protein tau, which renders tau vulnerable to phosphorylation and therefore neurofibrillary tangles formation (Polvikoski et al., 1995; Strittmatter et al., 1993).

As a result of the expanding pathology, it might eventually become necessary to perform additional cognitive work in order to bring behavioural performance to a normal level – as indicated by increased brain activations in at-risk individuals (e.g., Bookheimer et al., 2000). In particular, frontal and temporal areas that are important for executive functions and semantic memory might be increasingly engaged. However, there are limits to the functional compensation, and when a critical threshold of brain pathology is reached, the subject exhibits a period of rapid decline of cognitive abilities, accompanied by reduced functional brain activity. In support of this cascade model, fMRI studies commonly reveal significantly decreased brain activity in clinical AD patients (Bäckman et al., 1999; Grossman et al., 2003; Kato et al., 2001; see also Persson & Nyberg, 2006).

Hence, according to the compensatory interpretation, overactivity in *APOE*ε4-carriers can be viewed as a positive feature as it might prolong the preclinical, asymptomatic phase of AD. On the other hand, compensatory processes, especially in combination with episodic memory decline, are likely a preclinical marker of impending dementia. Thus, healthy *APOE*ε4-carriers with no functional alterations (or reduced activations) are probably better off than those showing overactivation. The worst case might be *APOE*ε4 in combination with memory impairment and no compensatory alterations at all.

In summary, several lines of evidence suggest that the effects of *APOE* genotype on brain function and structure are broad, early, but enduring and are possibly expressed unevenly over the lifespan and not limited to AD. To further clarify the life-long influence of *APOE* on the brain, more longitudinal follow-ups and careful sample selection are warranted.

Imaging genetics: Future outlook

In closing, this chapter has emphasized the value of combining independent streams of information, such as structural and functional neuroimaging, together with clinical and neuropsychological assessment for elucidating genotype–phenotype relations beyond simple statistical association. However, although the rapidly growing literature shows that single polymorphisms can be reliably linked to individual differences in brain structure and function, associations between single genes and any given phenotype are clearly simplifications; a more complete account of individual variance in gene–brain–behaviour relations must go beyond this point by also considering multiple interacting genetic polymorphisms within a gene (Bray et al., 2003), between separate genes (de Quervain & Papassotiropoulos, 2006; Espeseth et al., 2006), and between genes and the environment (Caspi et al., 2003). For instance, the frequency of the *APOE*ε4 allele appears to be higher in northern regions of Europe than in southern regions without significantly affecting the ultimate risk effects of the gene (Douglas, 2002; Gerdes, Klausen, Sihm, & Faergeman, 1992), and not all *APOE*ε4-carriers develop dementia (Henderson et al., 1995; Myers et al., 1996). This strongly indicates that the effects of *APOE* can be modified by other factors.

Genetic polymorphisms may also be expressed unevenly over the lifespan. Genes with a role in neuronal support and repair functions might be expressed more strongly in response to demand for neuronal repair – for example, following brain injury or in the presence of aging. This is consistent with studies showing that *APOE*ε4 is associated with detrimental effects on the brain, including cognitive decline, in middle-aged and older adults, whereas tests on children and young adults have revealed no effects (Deary et al., 2002; Scarmeas & Stern, 2006; Turic, Fisher, Plomin, & Owen, 2001) or possibly even advantageous effects (Mondadori et al., 2007). Certainly, more studies need to be done of younger subject samples. Also noteworthy, a meta-analysis (including 38 studies) by Small et al. (2004) showed that the effect size for *APOE*ε4 on psychometric functions such as global cognitive functioning and episodic memory was maximal for middle-aged groups and declined with age thereafter. This indicates that a simple model of progressive decline due to impaired neuronal repair mechanisms does not capture the whole complexity of how *APOE*ε4 affects brain function.

Nevertheless, although there are still achievements to be made in the fast-moving research field of imaging genomics, this translational approach already has the potential not only to reform our understanding of inter-individual variance in gene–behaviour relations, but also to point the way to better diagnostic strategies and to new treatment targets for various brain disorders.

References

Alexander, G. E., Chen, K., Pietrini, P., Rapoport, S. I., & Reiman, E. M. (2002). Longitudinal PET evaluation of cerebral metabolic decline in dementia: A potential outcome measure in Alzheimer's disease treatment studies. *American Journal of Psychiatry*, *159*, 738–745.

Bäckman, L., Andersson, J. L. R., Nyberg, L., Winblad, B., Nordberg, A., & Almkvist, O. (1999). Brain regions associated with episodic retrieval in normal aging and Alzheimer's disease. *Neurology*, *52*, 1861–1870.

Bäckman, L., Small, B. J., & Fratiglioni, L. (2001). Stability of the preclinical episodic memory deficit in Alzheimer's disease. *Brain*, *124*, 96–102.

Bengtsson, S. L., Nagy, Z., Skare, S., Forsman, L., Forssberg, H., & Ullen, F. (2005). Extensive piano practicing has regionally specific effects on white matter development. *Nature Neuroscience*, *8*, 1148–1150.

Biegon, A., Eberling, J. L., Richardson, B. C., Roos, M. S., Wong, S. T., Reed, B. R., et al. (1994). Human corpus callosum in aging and Alzheimer's disease: A magnetic resonance imaging study. *Neurobiology of Aging*, *15*, 393–397.

Bondi, M. W., Houston, W. S., Eyler, L. T., & Brown, G. G. (2005). fMRI evidence of compensatory mechanisms in older adults at genetic risk for Alzheimer disease. *Neurology*, *64*, 501–508.

Bookheimer, S. Y., Strojwas, M. H., Cohen, M. S., Saunders, A. M., Pericak-Vance, M. A., Mazziotta, J. C., et al. (2000). Patterns of brain activation in people at risk for Alzheimer's disease. *New England Journal of Medicine*, *343*, 450–456.

Boxer, A. L., Rankin, K. P., Miller, B. L., Schuff, N., Weiner, M., Gorno-Tempini, M. L., et al. (2003). Cinguloparietal atrophy distinguishes Alzheimer disease from semantic dementia. *Archives of Neurology*, *60*, 949–956.

Bozzali, M., Falini, A., Franceschi, M., Cercignani, M., Zuffi, M., Scotti, G., et al. (2002). White matter damage in Alzheimer's disease assessed in vivo using diffusion tensor magnetic resonance imaging. *Journal of Neurology, Neurosurgery, and Psychiatry*, *72*, 742–746.

Braak, H., Braak, E., & Bohl, J. (1993). Staging of Alzheimer-related cortical destruction. *European Neurology*, *33*, 403–408.

Braver, T. S., Barch, D. M., & Cohen, J. D. (1999). Cognition and control in schizophrenia: A computational model of dopamine and prefrontal function. *Biological Psychiatry*, *46*, 312–328.

Bray, N. J., Buckland, P. R., Williams, N. M., Williams, H. J., Norton, N., Owen, M. J., et al. (2003). A haplotype implicated in schizophrenia susceptibility is associated with reduced COMT expression in human brain. *American Journal of Human Genetics*, *73*, 152–161.

Bronge, L., Bogdanovic, N., & Wahlund, L. O. (2002). Postmortem MRI and histopathology of white matter changes in Alzheimer brains. *Dementia and Geriatric Cognitive Disorders*, *13*, 205–212.

Bronge, L., Fernaeus, S. E., Blomberg, M., Ingelson, M., Lannfelt, L., Isberg, B., et al. (1999). White matter lesions in Alzheimer patients are influenced by apolipoprotein E genotype. *Dementia and Geriatric Cognitive Disorders*, *10*, 89–96.

Buttini, M., Akeefe, H., Lin, C., Mahley, R. W., Pitas, R. E., Wyss-Coray, T., et al. (2000). Dominant negative effects of apolipoprotein E4 revealed in transgenic models of neurodegenerative disease. *Neuroscience*, *97*, 207–210.

Cabeza, R., Anderson, N. D., Locantore, J. K., & McIntosh, A. R. (2002). Aging gracefully: Compensatory brain activity in high-performing older adults. *NeuroImage*, *17*, 1394–1402.

Callicott, J. H., Bertolino, A., Mattay, V. S., Langheim, F. J. P., Duyn, J., Coppola, R., et al. (2000). Physiological dysfunction of the dorsolateral prefrontal cortex in schizophrenia revisited. *Cerebral Cortex*, *10*, 1078–1092.

Cannon, T. D., Huttunen, M. O., Lonnqvist, J., Tuulio-Henriksson, A., Pirkola, T., Glahn, D., et al. (2000). The inheritance of neuropsychological dysfunction in twins discordant for schizophrenia. *American Journal of Human Genetics*, *67*, 369–382.

Caspi, A., Sugden, K., Moffitt, T. E., Taylor, A., Craig, I. W., Harrington, H., et al. (2003). Influence of life stress on depression: Moderation by a polymorphism in the 5-HTT gene. *Science*, *301*, 386–389.

Cohen, R. M., Small, C., Lalonde, F., Friz, J., & Sunderland, T. (2001). Effect of apolipoprotein E genotype on hippocampal volume loss in aging healthy women. *Neurology*, *57*, 2223–2228.

Colcombe, S. J., Erickson, K. I., Scalf, P. E., Kim, J. S., Prakash, R., McAuley, E., et al. (2006). Aerobic exercise training increases brain volume in aging humans. *Journal of Gerontology. Series A, Biological Sciences and Medical Sciences*, *61*, 1166–1170.

Conturo, T. E., Lori, N. F., Cull, T. S., Akbudak, E., Snyder, A. Z., Shimony, J. S., et al. (1999). Tracking neuronal fiber pathways in the living human brain. *Proceedings of the American Academy of Sciences USA*, *96*, 10422–10427.

Deary, I. J., Whiteman, M. C., Pattie, A., Starr, J. M., Hayward, C., Wright, A. F., et al. (2002). Cognitive change and the APOE epsilon 4 allele. *Nature*, *418*, 932.

de Leeuw, F.-E., Richard, F., de Groot, J. C., van Duijn, C. M., Hofman, A., van Gijn, J., et al. (2004). Interaction between hypertension, APOE, and cerebral white matter lesions. *Stroke*, *35*, 1057–1060.

de Quervain, D. J.-F., & Papassotiropoulos, A. (2006). Identification of a genetic cluster influencing memory performance and hippocampal activity in humans. *Proceedings of the American Academy of Sciences USA*, *103*, 4270–4274.

Dickerson, B. C., Salat, D. H., Greve, D. N., Chua, E. F., Rand-Giovannetti, E., Rentz, D. M., et al. (2005). Increased hippocampal activation in mild cognitive impairment compared to normal aging and AD. *Neurology*, *65*, 404–411.

Douglas, C. E. (2002). Mortality differences by APOE genotype estimated from demographic synthesis. *Genetic Epidemiology*, *22*, 146–155.

Drzezga, A., Riemenschneider, M., Strassner, B., Grimmer, T., Peller, M., Knoll, A., et al. (2005). Cerebral glucose metabolism in patients with AD and different APOE genotypes. *Neurology*, *64*, 102–107.

Egan, M. F., Goldberg, T. E., Kolachana, B. S., Callicott, J. H., Mazzanti, C. M., Straub, R. E., et al. (2001). Effect of COMT Val108/158 Met genotype on frontal lobe function and risk for schizophrenia. *Proceedings of the American Academy of Sciences USA*, *98*, 6917–6922.

Egan, M. F., Kojima, M., Callicott, J. H., Goldberg, T. E., Kolachana, B. S., Bertolino, A., et al. (2003). The BDNF val66met polymorphism affects activity-dependent secretion of BDNF and human memory and hippocampal function. *Cell*, *112*, 257–269.

Elgh, E., Larsson, A., Eriksson, S., & Nyberg, L. (2003). Altered prefrontal brain activity in persons at risk for Alzheimer's disease: An fMRI study. *International Psychogeriatrics*, *15*, 121–133.

Englund, E., Brun, A., & Alling, C. (1988). White matter changes in dementia of Alzheimer's type: Biochemical and neuropathological correlates. *Brain*, *111*, 1425–1439.

Espeseth, T., Greenwood, P. M., Reinvang, I., Fjell, A. M., Walhovd, K. B., Westlye, L. T., et al. (2006). Interactive effects of APOE and CHRNA4 on attention and white matter volume in healthy middle-aged and older adults. *Cognitive, Affective, & Behavioral Neuroscience*, *6*, 31–43.

Fleisher, A. S., Houston, W. S., Eyler, L. T., Frye, S., Jenkins, C., Thal, L. J., et al. (2005). Identification of Alzheimer disease risk by functional magnetic resonance imaging. *Archives of Neurology*, *62*, 1881–1888.

Frackowiak, R. S., Pozzilli, C., Legg, N. J., Du, Boulay, G. H., Marshall, J., Lenzi, G. L., et al. (1981). Regional cerebral oxygen supply and utilization in dementia: A clinical and physiological study with oxygen-15 and positron tomography. *Brain*, *104*, 753–778.

Freedman, R., Coon, H., Myles-Worsley, M., Orr-Urtreger, A., Olincy, A., Davis, A., et al. (1997). Linkage of a neurophysiological deficit in schizophrenia to a chromosome 15 locus. *Proceedings of the American Academy of Sciences USA*, *94*, 587–592.

Gasparini, M., Fabrizio, E., Bonifati, V., & Meco, G. (1997). Cognitive improvement during tolcapone treatment in Parkinson's disease. *Journal of Neural Transmission*, *17*, 92–99.

Gerdes, L. U. (2003). The common polymorphism of apolipoprotein E: Geographical aspects and new pathophysiological relations. *Clinical Chemistry and Laboratory Medicine*, *41*, 628–631.

Gerdes, L. U., Klausen, I. C., Sihm, I., & Faergeman, O. (1992). Apolipoprotein E polymorphism in a Danish population compared to findings in 45 other study populations around the world. *Genetic Epidemiology*, *9*, 155–167.

Geroldi, C., Pihlajamaki, M., Laakso, M. P., DeCarli, C., Beltramello, A., Bianchetti, A., et al. (1999). APOE-ε4 is associated with less frontal and more medial temporal lobe atrophy in AD. *Neurology*, *53*, 1825–1832.

Gogos, J. A., Morgan, M., Luine, V., Santha, M., Ogawa, S., Pfaff, D., et al. (1998). Catechol-O-methyltransferase-deficient mice exhibit sexually dimorphic changes in catecholamine levels and behavior. *Proceedings of the American Academy of Sciences USA*, *95*, 9991–9996.

Goldberg, T. E., & Weinberger, D. R. (2004). Genes and the parsing of cognitive processes. *Trends in Cognitive Sciences*, *8*, 325–335.

Grabner, R. H., Ansari, D., Reishofer, G., Stern, E., Ebner, F., & Neuper, C. (2007). Individual differences in mathematical competence predict parietal brain activation during mental calculation. *NeuroImage*, *38*, 346–356.

Grossman, M., Koenig, P., Glosser, G., DeVita, C., Moore, P., Rhee, J., et al. (2003). Neural basis for semantic memory difficulty in Alzheimer's disease: An fMRI study. *Brain*, *126*, 292–311.

Hamann, S., & Canli, T. (2004). Individual differences in emotion processing. *Current Opinion in Neurobiology*, *14*, 233–238.

Han, S. D., Houston, W. S., Jak, A. J., Eyler, L. T., Nagel, B. J., Fleisher, A. S., et al. (2007). Verbal paired-associate learning by APOE genotype in non-demented older adults: fMRI evidence of a right hemispheric compensatory response. *Neurobiology of Aging*, *28*, 238–247.

Hanyu, H., Sakurai, H., Iwamoto, T., Takasaki, M., Shindo, H., & Abe, K. (1998). Diffusion-weighted MR imaging of the hippocampus and temporal white matter in Alzheimer's disease. *Journal of the Neurological Sciences*, *156*, 195–200.

Hariri, A. R., Goldberg, T. E., Mattay, V. S., Kolachana, B. S., Callicott, J. H., Egan, M. F., et al. (2003). Brain-derived neurotrophic factor val66met polymorphism affects human memory-related hippocampal activity and predicts memory performance. *Journal of Neuroscience*, *23*, 6690–6694.

Head, D., Buckner, R. L., Shimony, J. S., Williams, L. E., Akbudak, E., Conturo, T. E., et al. (2004). Differential vulnerability of anterior white matter in nondemented aging with minimal acceleration in dementia of the Alzheimer type: Evidence from diffusion tensor imaging. *Cerebral Cortex*, *14*, 410–423.

Heinz, A., & Smolka, M. N. (2006). The effects of catechol-O-methyltransferase genotype on brain activation elicited by affective stimuli and cognitive tasks. *Reviews in the Neurosciences*, *17*, 359–367.

Henderson, A. S., Easteal, S., Jorm, A. F., Mackinnon, A. J., Korten, A. E., Christensen, H., et al. (1995). Apolipoprotein E allele epsilon 4, dementia, and cognitive decline in a population sample. *Lancet*, *346*, 1387–1390.

Huang, W., Qiu, C., von Strauss, E., Winblad, B., & Fratiglioni, L. (2004). APOE Genotype, family history of dementia, and Alzheimer disease risk: A 6-year follow-up study. *Archives of Neurology*, *61*, 1930–1934.

Huang, Y. (2006). Apolipoprotein E and Alzheimer disease. *Neurology*, *66*, S79–85.

International Human Genome Sequencing Consortium. (2001). Initial sequencing and analysis of the human genome. *Nature*, *409*, 860–921.

Jack, C. J., Petersen, R. C., Xu, Y. C., O'Brien, P. C., Waring, S. C., Tangalos, E. G., et al. (1998). Hippocampal atrophy and apolipoprotein E genotype are independently associated with Alzheimer's disease. *Annals of Neurology*, *43*, 303–310.

Janowsky, J. S., Kaye, J. A., & Carper, R. A. (1996). Atrophy of the corpus callosum in Alzheimer's disease versus healthy aging. *Journal of the American Geriatric Society*, *44*, 798–803.

Jernigan, T. L., Archibald, S. L., Fennema-Notestine, C., Gamst, A. C., Stout, J. C., Bonner, J., et al. (2001). Effects of age on tissues and regions of the cerebrum and cerebellum. *Neurobiology of Aging*, *22*, 581–594.

Juottonen, K., Lehtovirta, M., Helisalmi, S., Reikkinen, P. J. Sr, & Soininen, H. (1998). Major decrease in the volume of the entorhinal cortex in patients with

Alzheimer's disease carrying the apolipoprotein E epsilon 4 allele. *Journal of Neurology, Neurosurgery, and Psychiatry*, *65*, 322–327.

Kato, T., Knopman, D., & Liu, H. (2001). Dissociation of regional activation in mild AD during visual encoding: A functional MRI study. *Neurology*, *57*, 812–816.

Killiany, R. J., Hyman, B. T., Gomez-Isla, T., Moss, M. B., Kikinis, R., Jolesz, F., et al. (2002). MRI measures of entorhinal cortex vs hippocampus in preclinical AD. *Neurology*, *58*, 1188–1196.

Lachman, H. M., Papolos, D. F., Saito, T., Yu, Y. M., Szumlanski, C. L., & Weinshilboum, R. M. (1996). Human catechol-O-methyltransferase pharmacogenetics: Description of a functional polymorphism and its potential application to neuropsychiatric disorders. *Pharmacogenetics*, *6*, 243–250.

Lehtovirta, M., Kuikka, J., Helisalmi, S., Hartikainen, P., Mannermaa, A., Ryynanen, M., et al. (1998). Longitudinal SPECT study in Alzheimer's disease: Relation to apolipoprotein E polymorphism. *Journal of Neurology, Neurosurgery, and Psychiatry*, *64*, 742–746.

Lehtovirta, M., Laakso, M. P., Soininen, H., Helisalmi, S., Mannermaa, A., Helkala, E. L., et al. (1995). Volumes of hippocampus, amygdala and frontal lobe in Alzheimer patients with different apolipoprotein E genotypes. *Neuroscience*, *67*, 65–72.

Lehtovirta, M., Soininen, H., Laakso, M. P., Partanen, K., Helisalmi, S., Mannermaa, A., et al. (1996). SPECT and MRI analysis in Alzheimer's disease: Relation to apolipoprotein E epsilon 4 allele. *Journal of Neurology, Neurosurgery, and Psychiatry*, *60*, 644–649.

Lekeu, F., Van der, Linden, M., Degueldre, C., Lemaire, C., Luxen, A., Franck, G., et al. (2003). Effects of Alzheimer's disease on the recognition of novel versus familiar words: Neuropsychological and clinico-metabolic data. *Neuropsychology*, *17*, 143–154.

Leonard, S., Gault, J., Hopkins, J., Logel, J., Vianzon, R., Short, M., et al. (2002). Association of promoter variants in the α7 nicotinic acetylcholine receptor subunit gene with an inhibitory deficit found in schizophrenia. *Archives of General Psychiatry*, *59*, 1085–1096.

Lind, J., Ingvar, M., Persson, J., Sleegers, K., Van Broeckhoven, C., Adolfsson, R., et al. (2006a). Parietal cortex activation predicts memory decline in apolipoprotein E-ε4 carriers. *NeuroReport*, *17*, 1683–1686.

Lind, J., Larsson, A., Persson, J., Ingvar, M., Nilsson, L.-G., Bäckman, L., et al. (2006b). Reduced hippocampal volume in non-demented carriers of the apolipoprotein E-ε4: Relation to chronological age and recognition memory. *Neuroscience Letters*, *396*, 23–27.

Lind, J., Persson, J., Ingvar, M., Larsson, A., Cruts, M., Van Broeckhoven, C., et al. (2006c). Reduced functional brain activity response in cognitively intact apolipoprotein E epsilon4 carriers. *Brain*, *129*, 1240–1248.

Logothetis, N. K., & Wandell, B. A. (2004). Interpreting the BOLD signal. *Annual Review of Physiology*, *66*, 735–769.

Machulda, M. M., Ward, H. A., Borowski, B., Gunter, J. L., Cha, R. H., O'Brien, P. C., et al. (2003). Comparison of memory fMRI response among normal, MCI, and Alzheimer's patients. *Neurology*, *61*, 500–506.

Mahley, R. W. (1988). Apolipoprotein E: Cholesterol transport protein with expanding role in cell biology. *Science*, *240*, 622–630.

Mahley, R. W., & Rall, S. C. (2000). Apolipoprotein E: Far more than a lipid transport protein. *Annual Review of Genomics and Human Genetics*, *1*, 507–537.

Martin, A. (1999). Automatic activation of the medial temporal lobe during encoding: Lateralized influences of meaning and novelty. *Hippocampus, 9*, 62–70.

Mega, M. S., Chu, T., Mazziotta, J. C., Trivedi, K. H., Thompson, P. M., Shah, A., et al. (1999). Mapping biochemistry to metabolism: FDG-PET and amyloid burden in Alzheimer's disease. *NeuroReport, 10*, 2911–2917.

Meguro, K., LeMestric, C., Landeau, B., Desgranges, B., Eustache, F., & Baron, J. C. (2001). Relations between hypometabolism in the posterior association neocortex and hippocampal atrophy in Alzheimer's disease: A PET/MRI correlative study. *Journal of Neurology, Neurosurgery, and Psychiatry, 71*, 315–321.

Menzel, S. (2002). Genetic and molecular analyses of complex metabolic disorders: Genetic linkage. *Annals of the New York Academy Sciences, 967*, 249–257.

Meyer, J. S., Kawamura, J., & Terayama, Y. (1992). White matter lesions in the elderly. *Journal of the Neurological Sciences, 110*, 1–7.

Meyer-Lindenberg, A., & Weinberger, D. R. (2006). Intermediate phenotypes and genetic mechanisms of psychiatric disorders. *Nature Reviews Neuroscience, 7*, 818–827.

Mielke, R., Kessler, J., Szelies, B., Herholz, K., Wienhard, K., & Heiss, W. D. (1998). Normal and pathological aging – findings of positron-emission-tomography. *Journal of Neural Transmission, 105*, 821–837.

Moffat, S. D., Szekely, C. A., Zonderman, A. B., Kabani, N. J., & Resnick, S. M. (2000). Longitudinal change in hippocampal volume as a function of apolipoprotein E genotype. *Neurology, 55*, 134–136.

Mondadori, C. R. A., de Quervain, D. J. F., Buchmann, A., Mustovic, H., Wollmer, M. A., Schmidt, C. F., et al. (2007). Better memory and neural efficiency in young apolipoprotein E ε4 carriers. *Cerebral Cortex, 17*, 1934–1947.

Morishima-Kawashima, M., Oshima, N., Ogata, H., Yamaguchi, H., Yoshimura, M., Sugihara, S., et al. (2000). Effect of apolipoprotein E allele ε4 on the initial phase of amyloid β-protein accumulation in the human brain. *American Journal of Pathology, 157*, 2093–2099.

Mosconi, L., De Santi, S., Rusinek, H., Convit, A., & de Leon, M. (2004). Magnetic resonance and PET studies in the early diagnosis of Alzheimer's disease. *Expert Review of Neurotherapeutics, 4*, 831–849.

Myers, R. H., Schaefer, E. J., Wilson, P. W., D'Agostino, R., Ordovas, J. M., Espino, A., et al. (1996). Apolipoprotein E epsilon4 association with dementia in a population-based study: The Framingham study. *Neurology, 46*, 673–677.

Nierenberg, J., Pomara, N., Hoptman, M. J., Sidtis, J. J., Ardekani, B. A., & Lim, K. O. (2005). Abnormal white matter integrity in healthy apolipoprotein E epsilon4 carriers. *NeuroReport, 22*, 1369–1372.

Nilsson, L.-G., Adolfsson, R., Bäckman, L., Cruts, M., Nyberg, L., Small, B. J., et al. (2006). The influence of APOE status on episodic and semantic memory: Data from a population-based study. *Neuropsychology, 20*, 645–657.

Nilsson, L.-G., Adolfsson, R., Bäckman, L., de Frias, C. M., Molander, B., & Nyberg, L. (2004). Betula: A prospective cohort study on memory, health and aging. *Aging, Neuropsychology, and Cognition, 11*, 134–148.

Nilsson, L.-G., Bäckman, L., Erngrund, K., Nyberg, L., Adolfsson, R., Bucht, G., et al. (1997). The Betula prospective cohort study: Memory, health, and aging. *Aging, Neuropsychology, and Cognition, 4*, 1–32.

Nyberg, L., McIntosh, A. R., Cabeza, R., Habib, R., Houle, S., & Tulving, E. (1996). General and specific brain regions involved in encoding and retrieval of events:

What, where, and when. *Proceedings of the American Academy of Sciences USA, 93*, 11280–11285.

Persson, J., Lind, J., Larsson, A., Ingvar, M., Cruts, M., Van, Broeckhoven, C., et al. (2006a). Altered brain white matter integrity in healthy carriers of the APOE ε4 allele: A risk for AD? *Neurology, 66*, 1029–1033.

Persson, J., & Nyberg, L. (2006). Altered brain activity in healthy seniors: What does it mean? *Progress in Brain Research, 157*, 45–56.

Persson, J., Nyberg, L., Lind, J., Larsson, A., Nilsson, L.-G., Ingvar, M., et al. (2006b). Structure-function correlates of cognitive decline in aging. *Cerebral Cortex, 16*, 907–915.

Petrill, S. A., Ball, D., Eley, T., Hill, L., Plomin, R., McClearn, G. E., et al. (1997). Failure to replicate a QTL association between a DNA marker identified by EST00083 and IQ. *Intelligence, 25*, 179–184.

Plassman, B. L., Welsh Bohmer, K. A., Bigler, E. D., Johnson, S. C., Anderson, C. V., Helms, M. J., et al. (1997). Apolipoprotein E epsilon 4 allele and hippocampal volume in twins with normal cognition. *Neurology, 48*, 985–989.

Plomin, R., McClearn, G. E., Smith, D. L., Skuder, P., Vignetti, S., Chorney, M. J., et al. (1995). Allelic associations between 100 DNA markers and high versus low IQ. *Intelligence, 21*, 31–48.

Plomin, R., Owen, M. J., & McGuffin, P. (1994). The genetic basis of complex human behaviors. *Science, 264*, 1733–1739.

Polvikoski, T., Sulkava, R., Haltia, M., Kainulainen, K., Vuorio, A., Verkkoniemi, A., et al. (1995). Apolipoprotein E, dementia, and cortical deposition of β-amyloid protein. *New England Journal of Medicine, 333*, 1242–1248.

Poo, M.-M. (2001). Neurotrophins as synaptic modulators. *Nature Reviews. Neuroscience, 2*, 24–32.

Raz, N., Lindenberger, U., Rodrigue, K. M., Kennedy, K. M., Head, D., Williamson, A., et al. (2005). Regional brain changes in aging healthy adults: General trends, individual differences and modifiers. *Cerebral Cortex, 15*, 1676–1689.

Reiman, E. M., Caselli, R. J., Chen, K., Alexander, G. E., Bandy, D., & Frost, J. (2001). Declining brain activity in cognitively normal apolipoprotein E epsilon 4 heterozygotes: A foundation for using positron emission tomography to efficiently test treatments to prevent Alzheimer's disease. *Proceedings of the American Academy of Sciences USA, 98*, 3334–3339.

Reiman, E. M., Caselli, R. J., Yun, L. S., Chen, K., Bandy, D., Minoshima, S., et al. (1996). Preclinical evidence of Alzheimer's disease in persons homozygous for the epsilon 4 allele for apolipoprotein E. *New England Journal of Medicine, 334*, 752–758.

Reiman, E. M., Chen, K., Alexander, G. E., Caselli, R. J., Bandy, D., Osborne, D., et al. (2004). Functional brain abnormalities in young adults at genetic risk for late-onset Alzheimer's dementia. *Proceedings of the American Academy of Sciences USA, 101*, 284–289.

Riley, B. P., & McGuffin, P. (2000). Linkage and associated studies of schizophrenia. *American Journal of Medical Genetics, 97*, 23–44.

Rombouts, S. A., Barkhof, F., Veltman, D. J., Machielsen, W. C. M., Witter, M. P., et al. (2000). Functional MR imaging in Alzheimer's disease during memory encoding. *American Journal of Neuroradiology, 21*, 1869–1875.

Sawa, A., & Snyder, S. H. (2002). Schizophrenia: Diverse approaches to a complex disease. *Science, 296*, 692–695.

Scarmeas, N., & Stern, Y. (2006). Imaging studies and APOE genotype in persons at risk for Alzheimer's disease. *Current Psychiatry Reports*, *8*, 11–17.

Schmidt, H., Schmidt, R., Fazekas, F., Semmler, J., Kapeller, P., Reinhart, B., et al. (1996). Apolipoprotein E e4 allele in the normal elderly: Neuropsychologic and brain MRI correlates. *Clinical Genetics*, *50*, 293–299.

Serretti, A., Olgiati, P., & De Ronchi, D. (2007). Genetics of Alzheimer's disease: A rapidly evolving field. *Journal of Alzheimer's Disease*, *12*, 73–92.

Skoog, I., Hesse, C., Aevarsson, O., Landahl, S., Wahlstrom, J., Fredman, P., et al. (1998). A population study of APOE genotype at the age of 85: Relation to dementia, cerebrovascular disease, and mortality. *Journal of Neurology, Neurosurgery, and Psychiatry*, *64*, 37–43.

Small, B. J., Rosnick, C. B., Fratiglioni, L., & Bäckman, L. (2004). Apolipoprotein E and cognitive performance: A meta-analysis. *Psychology and Aging*, *19*, 592–600.

Small, G. W., Ercoli, L. M., Silverman, D. H., Huang, S. C., Komo, S., Bookheimer, S. Y., et al. (2000). Cerebral metabolic and cognitive decline in persons at genetic risk for Alzheimer's disease. *Proceedings of the American Academy of Sciences USA*, *97*, 6037–6042.

Small, G. W., Mazziotta, J. C., Collins, M. T., Baxter, L. R., Phelps, M. E., Mandelkern, M. A., et al. (1995). Apolipoprotein E type 4 allele and cerebral glucose metabolism in relatives at risk for familial Alzheimer disease. *Journal of the American Medical Association*, *273*, 942–947.

Smith, C. D., Andersen, A. H., Kryscio, R. J., Schmitt, F. A., Kindy, M. S., Blonder, L. X., et al. (1999). Altered brain activation in cognitively intact individuals at high risk for Alzheimer's disease. *Neurology*, *53*, 1391–1396.

Smith, C. D., Andersen, A. H., Kryscio, R. J., Schmitt, F. A., Kindy, M. S., Blonder, L. X., et al. (2002). Women at risk for AD show increased parietal activation during a fluency task. *Neurology*, *58*, 1197–1202.

Smith, C. D., Kryscio, R. J., Schmitt, F. A., Lovell, M. A., Blonder, L. X., Rayens, W. S., et al. (2005). Longitudinal functional alterations in asymptomatic women at risk for Alzheimer's disease. *Journal of Neuroimaging*, *15*, 271–277.

Smith, G. S., de Leon, M. J., George, A. E., Kluger, A., Volkow, N. D., McRae, T., et al. (1992). Topography of cross-sectional and longitudinal glucose metabolic deficits in Alzheimer's disease: Pathophysiologic implications. *Archives of Neurology*, *49*, 1142–1150.

Soininen, H., Partanen, K., Pitkanen, A., Hallikainen, M., Hanninen, T., Helisalmi, S., et al. (1995). Decreased hippocampal volume asymmetry on MRIs in nondemented elderly subjects carrying the apolipoprotein E epsilon 4 allele. *Neurology*, *45*, 391–392.

Squire, L. R., & Zola-Morgan, S. (1991). The medial temporal lobe memory system. *Science*, *253*, 1380–1386.

Strange, B. A., Fletcher, P. C., Henson, R. N., Friston, K. J., & Dolan, R. J. (1999). Segregating the functions of human hippocampus. *Proceedings of the American Academy of Sciences USA*, *96*, 4034–4039.

Strittmatter, W. J., Saunders, A. M., Schmechel, D., Pericak-Vance, M., Enghild, J., Salvesen, G. S., et al. (1993). Apolipoprotein E: High-avidity binding to beta-amyloid and increased frequency of type 4 allele in late-onset familial Alzheimer disease. *Proceedings of the American Academy of Sciences USA*, *90*, 1977–1981.

Teipel, S. J., Bayer, W., Alexander, G. E., Bokde, A. L. W., Zebuhr, Y., Teichberg, D., et al. (2003). Regional pattern of hippocampus and corpus callosum atrophy in Alzheimer's disease in relation to dementia severity: Evidence for early neocortical degeneration. *Neurobiology of Aging, 24*, 85–94.

Teipel, S. J., Hampel, H., Pietrini, P., Alexander, G. E., Horwitz, B., Daley, E., et al. (1999). Region-specific corpus callosum atrophy correlates with the regional pattern of cortical glucose metabolism in Alzheimer disease. *Archives of Neurology, 56*, 467–473.

Thompson, P. M., Cannon, T. D., Narr, K. L., van Erp, T., Poutanen, V.-P., Huttunen, M., et al. (2001). Genetic influences on brain structure. *Nature Neuroscience, 4*, 1253–1258.

Tohgi, H., Takahashi, S., Kato, E., Homma, A., Niina, R., Sasaki, K., et al. (1997). Reduced size of right hippocampus in 39- to 80-year-old normal subjects carrying the apolipoprotein E epsilon4 allele. *Neuroscience Letters, 236*, 21–24.

Trivedi, M., Schmitz, T., Ries, M., Torgerson, B., Sager, M., Hermann, B., et al. (2006). Reduced hippocampal activation during episodic encoding in middle-aged individuals at genetic risk of Alzheimer's Disease: A cross-sectional study. *BMC Medicine, 4*, 1.

Tulving, E., Markowitsch, H. J., Kapur, S., Habib, R., & Houle, S. (1994). Novelty encoding networks in the human brain: Positron emission tomography data. *NeuroReport, 5*, 2525–2528.

Turic, D., Fisher, P. J., Plomin, R., & Owen, M. J. (2001). No association between apolipoprotein E polymorphisms and general cognitive ability in children. *Neuroscience Letters, 299*, 97–100.

Venter, J. C., Adams, M. D., Myers, E. W., Li, P. W., Mural, R. J., Sutton, G. G., et al. (2001). The sequence of the human genome. *Science, 291*, 1304–1351.

Weinberger, D. R., Berman, K. F., & Zec, R. (1986). Physiologic dysfunction of dorsolateral prefrontal cortex in schizophrenia. I. Regional cerebral blood flow evidence. *Archives of General Psychiatry, 43*, 114–124.

Weiss, A. P., Zalesak, M., DeWitt, I., Goff, D., Kunkel, L., & Heckers, S. (2004). Impaired hippocampal function during the detection of novel words in schizophrenia. *Biological Psychiatry, 55*, 668–675.

Winterer, G., & Goldman, D. (2003). Genetics of human prefrontal function. *Brain Research Reviews, 43*, 134–163.

Wishart, H. A., Saykin, A. J., Rabin, L. A., Santulli, R. B., Flashman, L. A., Guerin, S. J., et al. (2006). Increased brain activation during working memory in cognitively intact adults with the APOE ε4 allele. *American Journal of Psychiatry, 163*, 1603–1610.

Yasuda, M., Mori, E., Kitagaki, H., Yamashita, H., Hirono, N., Shimada, K., et al. (1998). Apolipoprotein E ε4 allele and whole brain atrophy in late-onset Alzheimer's disease. *American Journal of Psychiatry, 155*, 779–784.

Yoshiura, T., Mihara, F., Ogomori, K., Tanaka, A., Kaneko, K., & Masuda, K. (2002). Diffusion tensor in posterior cingulate gyrus: Correlation with cognitive decline in Alzheimer's disease. *NeuroReport, 13*, 2299–2302.

Zubieta, J.-K., Heitzeg, M. M., Smith, Y. R., Bueller, J. A., Xu, K., Xu, Y., et al. (2003). COMT val158met genotype affects μ-opioid neurotransmitter responses to a pain stressor. *Science, 299*, 1240–1243.

Author index

Subject index

Please note: Page entries in **bold** refer to tables and figures.